THE NONINVASIVE EVALUATION OF HEMODYNAMICS
IN CONGENITAL HEART DISEASE

Developments in Cardiovascular Medicine

VOLUME 114

The titles published in this series are listed at the end of this volume.

THE NONINVASIVE EVALUATION OF HEMODYNAMICS IN CONGENITAL HEART DISEASE

Doppler Ultrasound Applications in the Adult and Pediatric Patient with Congenital Heart Disease

Edited by

JAMES V. CHAPMAN

Scientific Research Coordinator in Clinical Ultrasound,
Department of Cardiology, University Medical Center, Gent, Belgium

and

GEORGE R. SUTHERLAND

Director of Echocardiography Laboratory,
Department of Cardiology, Thorax Center, Erasmus University, Rotterdam, The Netherlands

KLUWER ACADEMIC PUBLISHERS

DORDRECHT / BOSTON / LONDON

Library of Congress Cataloging-in-Publication Data

The Noninvasive evaluation of hemodynamics in congenital heart disease
  : Doppler ultrasound applications in the adult and pediatric patient
  with congenital heart disease / [edited by] James V. Chapman, George
  R. Sutherland.
      p.   cm. -- (Developments in cardiovascular medicine ; 114)
   Includes index.

   1. Congenital heart disease--Diagnosis--Congresses. 2. Doppler
echocardiography--Congresses. 3. Laser Doppler blood flowmetry-
-Congresses.   I. Chapman, J. V. II. Sutherland, George R., MB.
III. Series: Developments in cardiovascular medicine ; v. 114.
   [DNLM: 1. Echocardiography, Doppler. 2. Heart Defects,
Congenital--diagnosis. 3. Hemodynamics.   W1 DE997VME v. 114 / WG
220 N813]
   RC687.N66   1990
   616.1'2043--dc20
   DNLM/DLC
   for Library of Congress   90-5172

ISBN-13: 978-94-010-6776-8   e-ISBN-13: 978-94-009-0647-1
DOI: 10.1007/ 978-94-009-0647-1

Published by Kluwer Academic Publishers,
P.O. Box 17, 3300 AA Dordrecht, The Netherlands.

Kluwer Academic Publishers incorporates
the publishing programmes of
D. Reidel, Martinus Nijhoff, Dr W. Junk and MTP Press.

Sold and distributed in the U.S.A. and Canada
by Kluwer Academic Publishers,
101 Philip Drive, Norwell, MA 02061, U.S.A.

In all other countries, sold and distributed
by Kluwer Academic Publishers Group,
P.O. Box 322, 3300 AH Dordrecht, The Netherlands.

Printed on acid-free paper

Preface

The noninvasive evaluation of hemodynamics in congenital heart disease is an application for which Doppler ultrasound is ideally suited. The pediatric cardiac sonographer has used 2D and TM imaging for several years to study the structural abnormalities associated with various lesions. Pulsed Doppler, continuous wave Doppler, and more recently, color flow mapping techniques have been used to study the pathophysiology, and to make quantitative measurements thereof. To those already working in pediatric echocardiography, this book is intended to serve as a guide to the applications of the various Doppler modalities in specific abnormalities.

The other group for which this text is intended are the adult cardiac sonographers who see the occasional patient with congenital heart disease in their echocardiography laboratories. The incidence of congenital heart disease is not decreasing. As more patients survive to child bearing age, the adult cardiologist sees more and more referrals from the pediatric cardiologist to follow up the parent with corrected congenital heart disease, and in many smaller institutions, to examine their offspring as well. For this group, the book is intended to serve as a reference which gives a basic description of the pathology, the relevant parameters to observe, and a guide to the Doppler applications used to make these observations.

While there are a few books available on the subject of echocardiography in congenital heart disease, they do not usually go into much detail on noninvasive assessment of the pathophysiology. It is our hope that this text fills that gap.

The editors
May, 1990

Contributors

James V. Chapman BSc, RDCS
Scientific Research Coordinator
in Clinical Ultrasound
Department of Cardiology, University Medical Center Gent, Belgium

Alan G. Fraser MB, ChB, MRCP
Department of Cardiology, Thorax Center, Rotterdam, The Netherlands

Beat Friedli MD
Professor of Pediatric Cardiology
Department of Pediatric Cardiology, University Medical Center, University of Geneva, Switzerland

Howard M. McAlpine MB, ChB, MRCP
Department of Cardiology, Thorax Center, Rotterdam, The Netherlands

Ingrid Oberhaensli MD
Director of Echocardiography Laboratory
Department of Pediatric Cardiology, University Medical Center, University of Geneva, Switzerland

Naryswamy Sreeram MD
Department of Cardiology, Thorax Center, Rotterdam, The Netherlands

Oliver F.W. Stümper MD
Department of Cardiology, Thorax Center, Rotterdam, The Netherlands

George R. Sutherland MD, ChB, FRCP
Director of Echocardiography Laboratory,
Department of Cardiology, Thorax Center, Rotterdam, The Netherlands

Acknowledgments

I would like to thank several people who have helped me both directly and indirectly in the writing of this text. Throughout the technical chapters I have borrowed extensively from the explanations of Bjørn Angelsen Dr. Techn. and Kjell Kristoffersen Dr. Techn., and thank them for helping me understand difficult technical issues. I would like to acknowledge Alberto Meguira M.Sc. and Phillip Brun M.D. from CHU Creteil. Much of my chapter on blood flow measurements was based on their works in our earlier collaboration "Basic Concepts in Cardiac Doppler". I would like to extend my thanks to David J. Sahn M.D., UC San Diego, who introduced me to pediatric echocardiography and initiated my interest in this application, and to David T. Linker M.D., who as an engineer, adult, and pediatric cardiologist, offered an interesting perspective on the multidisciplinary field in which we work. My thanks to Lenny van Kooten for secretarial assistance, and finally , I would like to dedicate my work on this book to my wife Sandra and son Jamie for the hours of neglect imposed upon them during its writing and layout.

J. Chapman / Gent 4/90.

I should like to thank the following colleagues whose help and tution has been invaluable during the past ten years. I was fortunate to be introduced to both two-dimensional echocardiography and fluteplaying by Dr. Gert-Jan van Mil during my stay in Utrecht. Dr. Stewart Hunter in Newcastle convinced me that echocardiographers need not be bad golfers. During my stay in Trondheim, Prof. Liv Hatle not only taught me much about cardiac utrasound, but also tried to convince me that cross-country skiing was a viable substitute for downhill skiing. I would like to thank Professor Jos Roelandt, whose help and encouragement during the past three years in Thoraxcentrum has been greatly appreciated and who has taught me much about wines from Pomerol, second hand BMW's and the need to wax your skis before a race. I hope my advice to him on Speyside malts was as good.

G.R. Sutherland / Rotterdam 4/90.

Table of Contents

IV THE NORMAL EXAMINATION TECHNIQUE

J.V. CHAPMAN

V OBSTRUCTIVE LESIONS IN CONGENITAL HEART DISEASE

J.V. CHAPMAN, I. OBERHAENSLI, B. FRIEDLI

THE TECHNICAL ASPECTS OF DOPPLER ULTRASOUND

James V. Chapman

Introduction

The design of a two-dimensional Doppler instrument primarily for pediatric applications differs from the adult-oriented design. One must implement high frequency transducers for the high resolution sector images required in pediatric applications. This presents limitations for the Doppler modalities in terms of sensitivity and signal to noise ratio (which is the ability to detect weak signals even when there is noise present). Also, there is a limit on the peak flow velocity which can be measured at a given depth; this peak velocity limit decreases as the carrier frequency increases.

The rapid heart rates encountered in the pediatric patient also requires the possibility to perform real time color flow mapping at high frame rates. The small heart size and discrete structures in many congenital lesions also requires a high degree of spatial resolution. The complexity of congenital lesions can make the application of conventional Doppler methods difficult. The ability to perform continuous wave with the imaging probe, and to steer the cursor over the sector in real time tends to facilitate the Doppler echocardiographic examination.

A general summary of the important design requirements for a Doppler instrument would be that high carrier frequency probes can be implemented for tissue imaging and lower carrier frequencies for conventional Doppler as well as flow imaging. High color imaging frame rates are necessary for pediatric applications; fifteen to thirty five frames per second is an optimal range in our experience. The operator should have the ability to control parameters related to temporal and spatial resolution as different examinations require different priorities.

These are just a few relevant factors one must consider. In this chapter a detailed review of the physical principles of Doppler ultrasound will be presented, with a focus on the practical applications. While the primary interest of the physician is the clinical application of Doppler, an understanding of the physical and technical aspects is important. This directly affects the interpretation of the clinical study.

Ultrasound is a term used to describe acoustic waves of higher frequency than audible sound. Imaging techniques use specular reflections, which are the reflected sounds from tissue interfaces (Fig.1-1), to construct an image of the cardiac structures under investigation. Doppler ultrasound uses the backscattered signals from moving red blood cells to measure blood flow velocity.

The use of Doppler ultrasound to measure blood flow velocity began in the late 1950's, approximately the same time as the use of ultrasound for diagnostic imaging. Continuous wave Doppler instruments were initially used for the qualitative assessment of peripheral vascular blood flow. Pulsed Doppler instruments were later developed in order to study flow in a localized region. These devices were employed in the study of intra-cardiac blood flow, since flow in a specific chamber or vessel could be investigated.

Review of the Physical Principles of Ultrasound

To perform the Doppler ultrasound examination, a piezoelectric crystal is used to transmit and receive the acoustic signal as in imaging modalities. The piezoelectric crystal is said to function as a transducer, because it converts variations of one quantity to those of another quantity. For imaging and Doppler ultrasound applications, the piezoelectric crystal or element converts the electrical energy of a sinusoidal waveform to mechanical energy, and vice versa. The crystal is composed of a mixture of synthetic materials which, in response to an applied voltage, are rapidly deformed. Such rapid deformation results in the production of an alternating pressure in the surrounding medium which propagates as a sound wave.

Sound wave propagation through a medium occurs as a series of compressions and rarefactions of the particles in the medium. The time between consecutive pressure minima or presssure maxima is called a cycle, and the number of cycles taking place in one second is termed the frequency. The frequency of the emitted sound is equal to the frequency of the applied voltage. This operating frequency is also known as the resonant frequency of the transducer. The propagation velocity of the sound in a particular medium is determined by the density and the stiffness of the medium. In biological soft tissue, the average propagation velocity is approximately 1540 m/s, and 1560 m/s in blood. Since the ultrasonic wave is travelling at a relatively constant velocity, there is a small but measurable distance between the successive pressure maxima or pressure minima. This distance is termed the acoustic wavelength. The formula relating wavelength (∂), propagation velocity and frequency is:

$$\text{Wavelength } (\partial) = c/f \qquad \qquad \text{Equation 1-1}$$

where c is the propagational velocity of sound in tissue and f is the transducer frequency.

When a transmitted signal travelling through a homogeneous medium encounters an interface, a portion of that signal is reflected, a portion is attenuated (scattered or absorbed), and a portion is refracted. The angle of reflection is determined by the angle of incidence between the signal and the interface. If the incident angle is 90 degrees, the path of the reflected portion of the signal is essentially parallel to that of the transmitted signal provided that the dimensions of the reflecting surface are greater than the ultrasonic wavelength and beamwidth. The surface may then be described as a specular reflector. When the reflecting interface dimensions are smaller then the wavelength or beamwidth, specular reflection no longer takes place. Instead the sound is scattered in many directions. This phenomenon is known as backscattering and is encountered when interrogating blood flow. The red cell diameter is approximately 8 microns and is much smaller than the ultrasonic wavelength or beamwidth. Backscattering will also occur when a large but uneven interface is encountered.

Refraction is a term used to describe the bending of the incident ultrasound beam as it passes through an interface between two adjacent media in which the acoustic velocity is slightly different. This phenomenon is of minor importance in tissue or Doppler ultrasound imaging although it may infrequently be reponsible for the creation of artifacts. An artifact is a piece of information in the ultrasound display which is not representative of the structure or flow under interrogation, but is instrument generated.

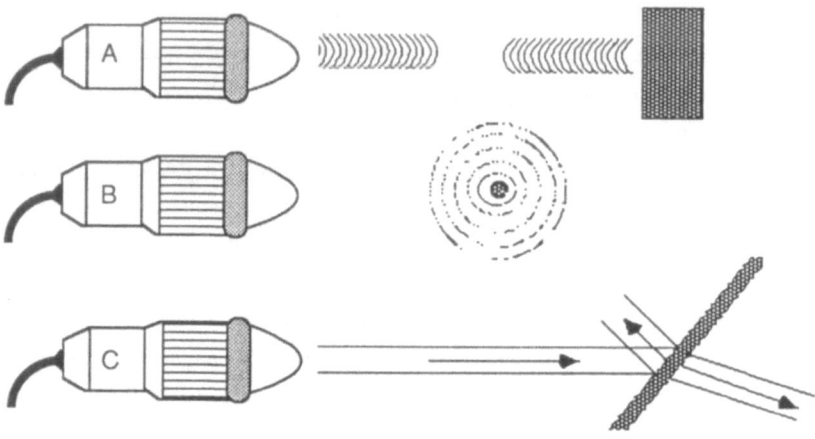

Fig. 1-1. Schematic representation of reflection (A), Backscattering (B), and reflection and refraction (C).

In a pulsed Doppler system, as in an imaging system, the piezoelectric crystal is excited only at certain intervals for a short period of time. The number of electrical pulses deforming the crystal per second is equal to the number of ultrasonic pulses emitted per second. This number is called the pulse repetition frequency and is expressed in cycles per second or Hertz. The pulseburst duration is the length of time over which one ultrasonic pulse occurs. The spatial pulse length is the distance taken up by a single ultrasonic burst.

The sound emitted by the transducer propagates as a beam. Close to the transducer surface, the beam is shaped like a cylinder with a diameter approximately equal to the transducer diameter. The acoustic energy is not uniformly distributed throughout a given beam cross-section. The beam dimensions increase with distance, and this divergence causes the beam to assume a conical shape. A considerable amount of sound may travel outside the beam boundaries; these additional small beams are known as side lobes and can generate artifacts.

The well-defined central portion of the beam which has a cylindrical shape is called the near field or Fresnel zone. The near field length can be calculated if the transducer diameter (Dt) and the ultrasonic wavelength are known:

$$NFL = \frac{Dt^2 \, f}{6}$$ Equation 1-2

where NFL = near field length , Dt = transducer diameter , and f = frequency in MHz.

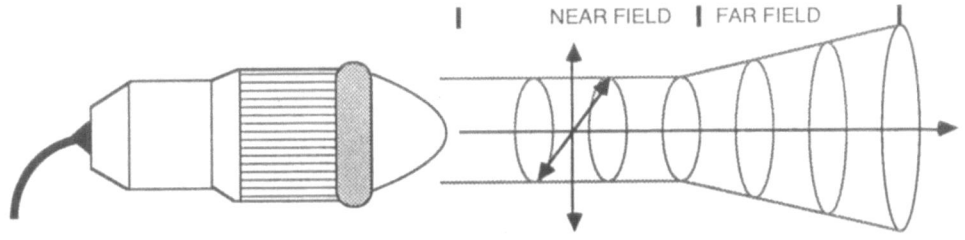

Fig. 1-2 . The near field length (NFL) is obtained from the above equation.

From this equation, one can deduce that an increase in transducer frequency (decrease in wavelength) or an increase in transducer radius will result in a longer near field. The beam diameter is determined by the ultrasonic wavelength, transducer radius, and the distance from the transducer, (Fig.1-2). The region beyond the near field is termed the far field or Fraunhofer zone. In this region, the beam has a conical configuration. The distribution of acoustic energy at a given beam cross-section is more diffuse in the far field due to attenuation effects and the widening of the beam. Weaker ultrasonic signals will be reflected by structures lying in a wide beam cross-section when compared to the signals produced by the same structures lying in narrow beam cross-section at the same imaging depth.

The selection of transducer frequency is clinically relevant because it determines the resolution and penetration of an ultrasound system to a large extent. Resolution may be defined as the ability to separate two neighbouring reflectors in close proximity to each other. Since the ultrasonic beam is three-dimensional, resolution may be described in the axial, lateral or elevational planes. Generally, the axial and lateral resolution are the most frequently discussed parameters. Axial or range resolution is defined as the minimum distance between two structures lying along the beam path which will produce two distinct reflections. The axial resolution of an imaging system can be no less than the signal wavelength.

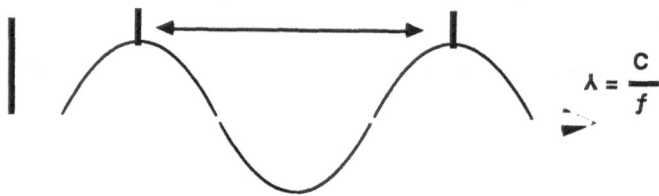

$$\lambda = \frac{c}{f}$$

Fig. 1-3. The wavelength is defined as the distance between consecutive pressure maxima or minima. The propagational velocity and transducer frequency defines the wave length. The period is the time over which a cycle occurs, and the frequency is the number of cycles which occur in a second. The frequency is the reciprocal of the period.

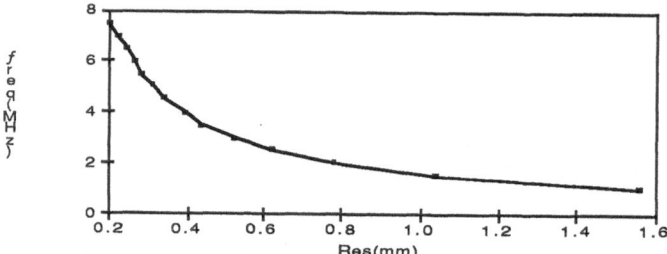

Fig. 1-4 . The wavelength sets the limits on the system's resolution and is dependent upon the transducer frequency. As the transducer frequency is increased, the resolution is improved.

The wavelength of the 7.5 MHz transducer is much less than the wavelength of the 3.5 MHz transducer, thus the axial resolution of the 7.5 MHz transducer is superior. Axial resolution can be approximated as the spatial pulse length. The axial resolution in millimeters is approximately equal to half the spatial pulse length in millimeters. The use of short ultrasonic bursts will improve the axial resolution of an ultrasound system. Lateral resolution is defined as the minimum distance between two structures lying perpendicular to the direction of sound propagation which will produce two distinct reflections. Lateral resolution is roughly equal to the beam diameter, which varies with distance from the transducer face. Lateral resolution is therefore poorer in the far field due to the increased beam dimensions in the far field.

By choosing a higher transducer frequency, the axial resolution is improved but the rate of attenuation increases. Attenuation is the loss of acoustic energy by scattering or absorption of sound. The deeper the interrogation depth, the greater the loss of energy will be due to attenuation. A general guideline for estimating the degree of energy loss is 1.0 dB/MHz/cm. In other words, biological tissue causes an energy loss of 1 dB/cm for each megahertz of ultrasonic frequency. A 2.5 MHz transducer will attenuate 25 dB at an imaging depth of 10 cm, while a 5.0 MHz transducer will attenuate 50 dB of sound energy at the same imaging depth. In general, it is more important in pediatric applications to have the best possible resolution, and since the examination depths are relatively shallow, it becomes practical to implement higher frequency transducers.

Based upon the preceeding discussion, one can conclude that a compromise is needed when choosing an operating frequency. Higher frequency transducers have superior axial resolution, longer near fields, and reduced beam divergence in the far field. At the same time however, the penetration is poor due to the increased rate of attenuation. With Doppler imaging modalities then, it is clear that a compromise must be made when choosing the tranducer frequency. Generally the highest transducer frequency which will provide adequate tissue penetration is implemented. The goal of the Doppler echocardiographic examination is to obtain accurate structural information as well as accurate hemodynamic information.

For pediatric applications high frequency transducers are required. There is a problem encountered in that the Doppler signal aliases at low velocities when high frequency probes are used. This is compounded by the fact that during color flow mapping, both imaging and Doppler must be performed for each frame. The annular array instrument we are presently using has some advantages in this respect as the carrier frequency can be shifted higher or lower depending on which part of the flow/tissue image is being constructed. In this way, the imaging resolution and the ability to measure higher flow velocities are both optimized. In the system developed at the University of Trondheim, the transducers used for pediatrics include a 3.0 MHz which performs imaging at 3.0 MHz and Doppler at 3.0 MHz , a 5.0 MHz which does imaging at 5.0 MHz and Doppler at 4.0 MHz , and a 7.5 MHz which performs imaging at 7.5 MHz and Doppler at 6.0 MHz. While several other transducer frequencies and configurations have been tested, these appear the most useful in clinical practice.

Principles of Doppler Ultrasound

The Doppler effect was first described by the 19th century Austrian physicist, Christian Johann Doppler. He described the phenomenon whereby a light transmitting source and a receiving source moving relative to one another cause a shift in the received signal frequency. This change in frequency is called the Doppler shift. The principle applies to sound wave as well as light. If the transmitter and receiver move towards each other, the received signal will be of a higher frequency than the original signal. Conversely, if the transmitter and receiver move apart from one another, the backscattered signal frequency will be lower than the original signal. In the clinical setting, piezoelectric crystals transmit and receive ultrasonic waves. The received signals are those which are backscattered from the larger solids in the blood, primarily red blood cells. The frequency shift is calculated using the following equation :

$$Fd = \frac{2FoVcos\varnothing}{c}$$

Equation 1-3

Fd = The frequency shift, Fo = The carrier frequency, V = The velocity of the red blood cells, Ø = The angle to flow, c = Propagational velocity of sound in blood.

    In the clinical applications of the technique, it is more useful to calculate the blood flow velocity rather than the Doppler shift. The blood flow velocity is calculated with the equation:

$$V = \frac{CFd}{2\,Fo\,cos\,\varnothing}$$

Equation 1- 4

V = Velocity of the red blood cells , Fd = The frequency shift , Fo= The carrier frequency. The frequency shifted signal is in the audible range (1 KHz to 15 KHz). The characteristics of blood flow with regard to turbulence or laminarity is demonstrated by such spectral parameters as the signal bandwidth and amplitude, and can be evaluated in a qualitative manner from the audio signal. Unlike frequency measurement, the velocity measurement is angle dependent, and the audio signal is the best method of ascertaining that a good angle to flow has been achieved. The calculated value may then be used to quantify the severity of several pathological conditions, both congenital and acquired. Additionally, valuable qualitative information is obtained with Doppler techniques.

    Besides the flow velocity, the direction of blood flow may also be determined. The transmitted or carrier frequency is known; if the reflected signal is of a higher frequency than the transmitted signal, then the blood flow is approaching the ultrasound transducer. If the received frequency is lower the blood flow is moving away from the transducer.

    Other factors which influence the accurate measurement of flow velocity include the carrier frequency of the ultrasonic signal, the pulse repetition frequency (prf) and the angle to flow. A higher carrier frequency may be used to measure high velocity in the near field, but is limited in peak velocity resolution in the far field by the range velocity product. This problem must be addressed in cardiac work as the depth of blood flow to be sampled is much greater than in peripheral vascular applications. The usual depths encountered lie within the 4-16 cm range in children, and within the 6-18 cm range in adult subjects. Transducer frequencies of 3.0 to 3.75 MHz seem to be best suited for scanning adults, while higher frequency transducers in the 5 to 10 MHz range are utilized in neonatal and general pediatric applications.

    It is crucial that the Doppler beam is aligned so that it is close to a parallel position to blood flow, thereby minimizing the angle Ø (Fig. 1-7). The greater the angle, the greater will be the degree of underestimation of the flow velocity. For example, if the actual flow velocity is 2.0 m/s and the beam is parallel to flow, a velocity measurement of 2.0 m/s will be obtained. But if the angle is increased to 30°, a velocity of 1.7 m/s is recorded. If the angle is increased further to 60°, a velocity of 1.0 m/s is recorded. When calculating the pressure gradient from the flow velocity, the error resulting from such underestimation will be significantly increased.

The angle to flow may be reduced using the audio signal for guidance. A signal obtained when the angle lies in the 0° to 20° degree range will have a narrow bandwidth, noise-free audio signal. As the angle is increased, a noisy wideband signal is heard. This wideband signal reflects the dispersed velocity distribution found at the peripheral boundaries of the flow. The angle may be estimated using the two-dimensional image for guidance; the cardiac structures which one assumes to be parallel to flow are used to align the Doppler beam. However, a problem often arises with this method, as the intracardiac flows and the heart itself are three-dimensional, and the image two-dimensional. The sample cell may seem to be centered in the jet, but in the unseen elevational plane, the cell may be positioned outside the jet or against a cardiac wall. Additionally, in many valvular and regurgitant lesions, the jet will be eccentric. When the velocity from an eccentric jet is being measured, but the flow is not parallel to the cardiac structure used to estimate the angle, the insertion of an angle correction factor will cause flow velocity overestimation.

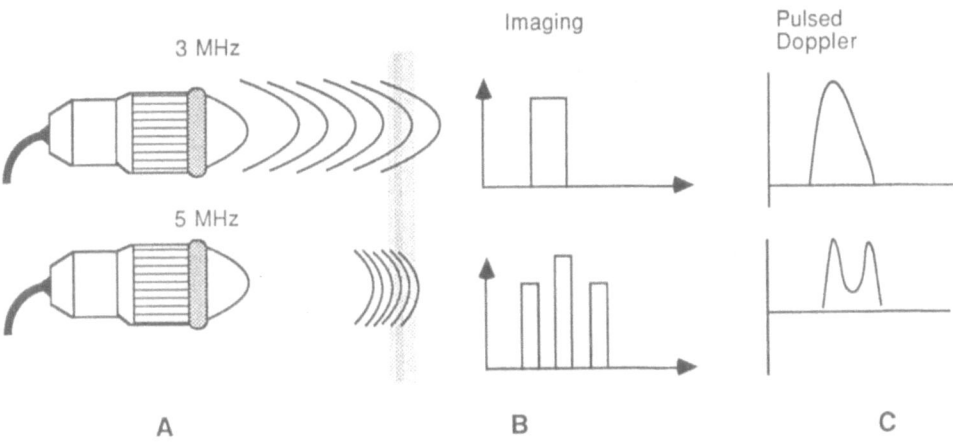

Fig. 1-5. The ability to shift the carrier frequencies higher or lower to optimize both imaging and Doppler signals is quite helpful as the higher frequencies are better for imaging and lower carrier frequencies are better for Doppler. The 5.0 MHz signal yields a higher degree of axial resolution (B), while the 3.0 MHz permits higher velocity flows to be measured (C).

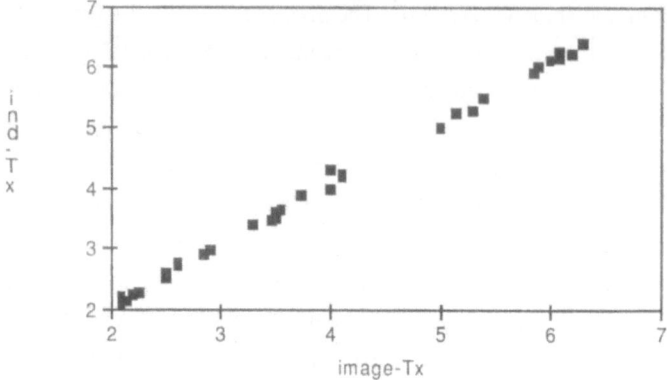

Fig. 1-6. In the initial clinical trials of a phased annular array color flow mapping device, we compared the peak velocity measurements made in a series of adult patients with both an independent 2.0 MHz transducer and a 3.0 MHz Imaging / Doppler probe. The results corresponded quite well; in difficult patients the signal to noise ratio was better with the low frequency independent Doppler probe. However, noise artifacts and penetration are generally not a problem in children.

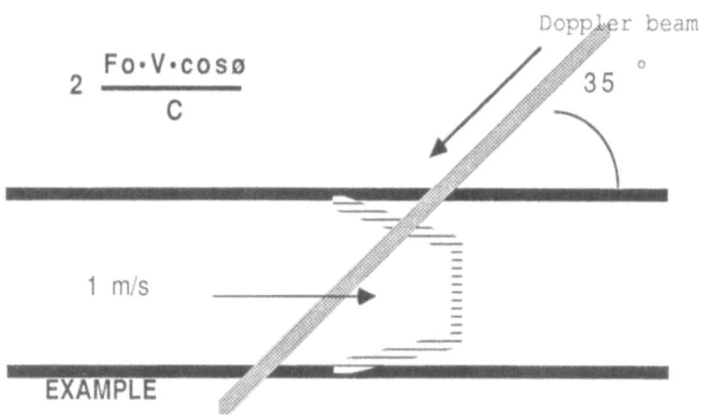

Fig. 1-7. The Doppler shift can be used to calculate blood flow velocity so long as the angle of incidence is zero or close to zero. As the angle is increased, the flow velocity is underestimated to a greater degree. The error can be corrected for in the Doppler equation if the angle can be approximated.

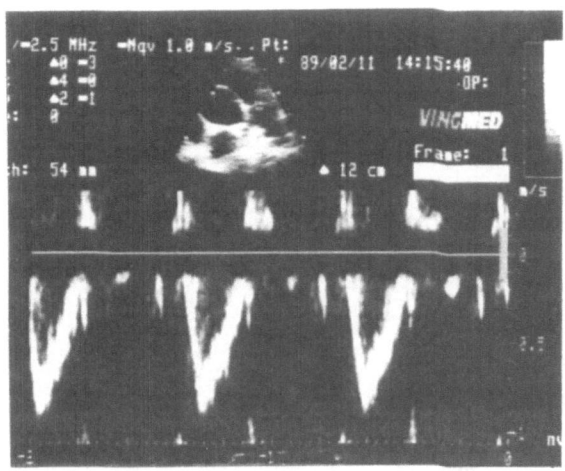

Fig. 1-8. The pulsed Doppler mode has been implemented in this example to measure the flow in a localized region of the pulmonary artery. The region of flow measured is termed the sample volume, the length of which can be increased or decreased depending upon the application. The primary disadvantage with this technique is that high flow velocities cannot be measured.

Pulsed Doppler

There are two approaches to Doppler echocardiography. One method, continuous wave Doppler, uses a transducer with a split crystal or two separate piezoelectric elements which continuously transmit and receive signals. The other method, pulsed Doppler, transmits and receives signals at specific time intervals through a single element.

With pulsed Doppler, a signal is transmitted at a specific rate (the pulse repetition frequency or prf) and for a specific length of time (the pulse burst duration). The higher the pulse repetition frequency, the higher the maximum blood flow velocity which may be measured. The transmitted signal must be received before the next one is pulsed. The pulse repetition frequency which may be used without range ambiguity occurring, decreases as the depth of interrogation increases. As the depth of interrogation increases, the value of the maximum velocity which can be measured decreases. This relation is expressed formally in the equation known as the range velocity product :

$$VmR = \frac{C^2}{8Fo} \qquad \text{Equation 1- 5}$$

Vm = Maximum measurable velocity, R = Specific range or depth, C = Propagational velocity of sound in blood , Fo= Carrier frequency.

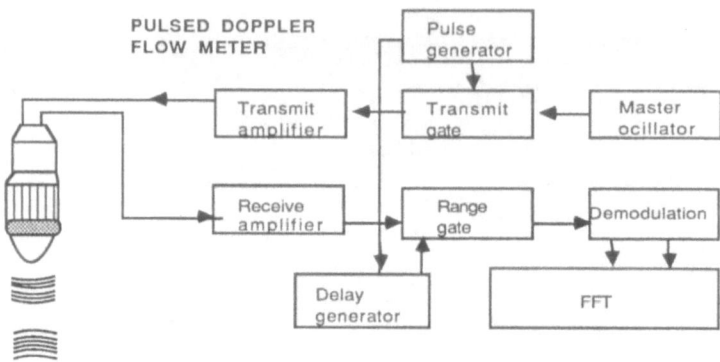

Fig. 1-9. Schematic of a pulsed Doppler flow meter. The same piezolectric element is used to transmit and receive the signal. The pulses are transmitted at specific time intervals which are controlled by the pulse generator. The signal is received at specific time intervals which are regulated by the range gate. The delay generator coordinates transmission and reception of the signals, which then undergo quadrature demodulation and spectral analysis.

The further away the reflective object (red blood cell) lies relative to the transducer, the more time it will take for the signal to be transmitted and received. It becomes necessary to lower the pulse repetition frequency (prf) when sampling at greater depths. By lowering the prf, the maximum measurable velocity is reduced. If a pulse must return prior to the transmission of the subsequent pulse, it becomes apparent that a shallow sample depth may be transmitted at a faster rate than one which is far away as the round trip distance, and therefore the travel time, is greater.

The Sample Volume

The volume interrogated by the pulse burst is referred to as the sample cell, or sample volume. Its lateral and elevational dimensions are defined by the beamwidth. Therefore, the further the distance from the transducer to the flow, the wider the lateral dimensions become as the beam profile diverges. The axial dimension of the sample volume is defined by the pulse burst duration and the amount of time the receiver gate remains open.

The advantage of pulsed mode is that if one knows at what time a signal is pulsed and when the reflected signal is received (the velocity of sound in blood is constant at 1560 m/s), the depth at which the signal is being sampled may then be resolved. Depth resolution allows localization of regurgitant flows, septal defects, flow mapping and separation of mixed lesions. The larger the sample volume dimension, the more red blood cell targets are sampled, resulting in a stronger backscattered signal strength. This serves to improve the system's ability to detect weak signals at the expense of range resolution. If however the sample volume dimensions are reduced, weaker signals may be missed although range resolution is improved.

Aliasing

The sampling theorem states that for a signal to be unambiguously reconstructed, the original must be sampled no less than twice per signal period. According to this theorem then, the maximum velocity which may be unambiguously resolved with pulsed Doppler methods is limited to half of the pulse repetition frequency. This limit is termed the Nyquist frequency or Nyquist limit. Because we are dealing with fairly large depths in cardiac applications, we are limited in the maximum velocity which may be measured by the Nyquist limit (prf/2). But because of the same factors which limit the measurable velocity, one gains the advantage of knowing from where the velocity is being sampled. We will now take a closer look at what occurs when the Nyquist limit is exceeded.

It has been stated that it is necessary for the transmitted signal to be received before the next pulse, one can use a simple analogy to explain why this is so. On film everyone has seen a spoked wheel of a motorcycle or train moving at an increasing velocity. The spokes are first noted to move in a forward motion. As the velocity continues to increase, however, the motion of the spokes appears to reverse in direction. The reason for the apparent change in direction is that the spokes are rotating so quickly that the sampling device (in this case, the movie camera) is not sampling rapidly enough to detect each spoke and an ambiguous pattern is reconstructed.

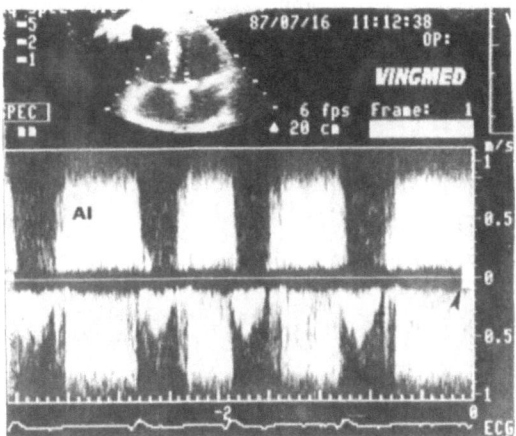

Fig. 1-10. The pulsed Doppler method permits the depth of flow to be resolved. In this example, the standard apical four chamber view is demonstrated. The pulsed Doppler sample volume is positioned in the left ventricular outflow tract, and the spectral display yields a peak systolic outflow velocity of 0.6 m/s. The diastolic flow component is from an aortic insufficiency (AI). The high velocity flow from the regurgitant jet exceeds the Nyquist limit and aliasing has occurred. This is the major limitation with a conventional pulsed Doppler system; it cannot be used to measure high flow velocities.

Assume that the wheels in Figure1-11 rotate 360° every 4 seconds. The wheel is marked with a dot to denote the starting position. Now suppose that we are looking at the wheel through a lens which opens at specific intervals, which can be adjusted. In the first series, the lens opens and the dot is seen in the 12 o'clock position. The sample rate has been set for 4 second intervals. In this period of time, the wheel rotates 360° so that when the lens opens again the dot is in the same position. As many times as this is repeated, the dot will appear to remain stationary. Now let us increase the sample rate to open every one second. The first sample shows the dot in the 12 o'clock position. The wheel rotates 90° in one second and is sampled. The dot appears in the 3 o'clock position. In the next sample, the dot is in the 6 o'clock position. Reconstructing these samples, we see that a clockwise rotation has taken place. If the sample rate is decreased to one time per three seconds, the sample first shows the dot in the 12:00 position. As the wheel rotates at one revolution every 4 seconds, it will place the dot in the 9:00 position in the second sample. The wheel rotates 270° before the next sample. The dot is now in the 6:00 position. When these samples are reconstructed the direction of the wheel's rotation appears to be counter-clockwise, although it was actually clockwise. This phenomenon is called aliasing. Aliasing is caused by the sampling mechanism's inability to sort out multiple data points in the order they originally occurred. When the Nyquist limit is exceeded with pulsed Doppler sampling, aliasing will occur. It is important that the Doppler instrument used includes a spectral unwrapping option, allowing one to display an asymmetric Nyquist limit. While the velocity on the spectral display may be resolved with spectral unwrapping, the audio signal will still alias at the Nyquist value.

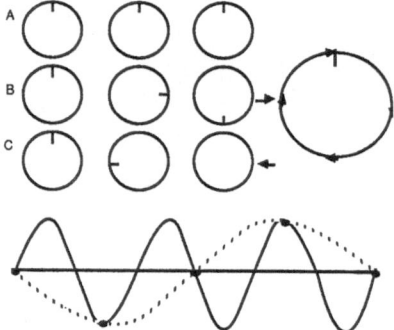

Fig. 1-11. Assume that the wheels rotate ·360° clockwise every 4 seconds. If the wheel is sampled at four second intervals, it appears to be stationary (A). When sampled at one second intervals, the correct frequency and direction are resolved (B). When the wheel is sampled at 3 second intervals (C), the wrong frequency and direction are obtained. The lower panel demonstrates how two sine waves of different frequencies can be sampled at a rate which causes them to be indistinguishable. The black dots indicate the sampling periods.

Range Ambiguity

Range ambiguity and high pulse repetition frequency techniques can be used to resolve higher flow velocities at greater depths with pulsed Doppler. With this technique, a degree of range resolution is retained when evaluating a patient with increased flow velocities. The problems of flow localization and velocity resolution can both be addressed with this technique, which is based on conventional pulsed Doppler. As in conventional pulsed mode, a signal is transmitted at a specific time interval or pulse repetition frequency (prf). The reflected or backscattered energy returns to the transducer from along the entire beam path. Because the propagational velocity of sound in tissue is constant, we can selectively sample these backscattered components by opening the receivers (range gates) at multiple time intervals. This allows the transmitted signal to travel to a given depth, and the backscattered signals to be sampled from several depth positions. There is a direct relationship between the pulse repetition frequency (prf) and the maximum velocity which may be measured. The higher the prf, the higher the maximum velocity which may be measured. But the further away the interrogation site, the lower the prf must be to allow the transmitted signal to be sampled before the following pulse is transmitted. If the next pulse is transmitted before the return of the previous transmission, multiple samples are received simultaneously and range ambiguity occurs.

Range ambiguity may be applied in the resolution of higher velocities as demonstrated in the simplified schematic shown in Fig. 1-13. By moving the sample volume closer to the transducer, the prf may be increased thereby allowing a higher limit to the maximum measurable velocity. Flow velocities from several positions are received together, but a certain degree of range resolution is retained. In this example, signals from four centemeters and eight centemeters are mixed together, but a higher velocity can be measured than if the pulse repetition frequency is set for unambiguous sampling at the eight centemeter depth.

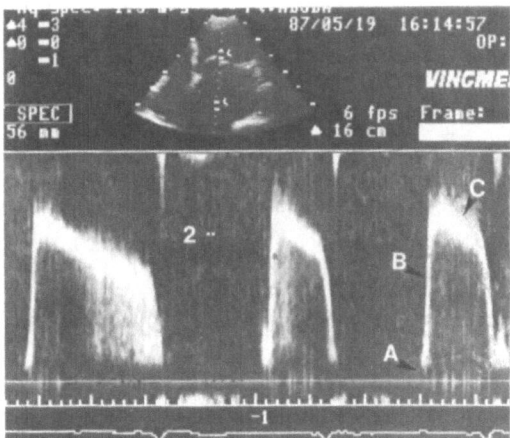

Fig. 1-12. The schematic in Fig. 1-13 demonstrates how a high pulse repetition frequency system operates. The method has been applied in this example to measure a velocity of 2.5 m/s in a patient with moderately severe mitral stenosis. Flow is sampled at multiple sites (arrows), but the only possible source of this velocity is at the orifice in this line of interrogation. A narrow bandwidth signal has been obtained. Acceleration = A and B, Diastolic filling = C.

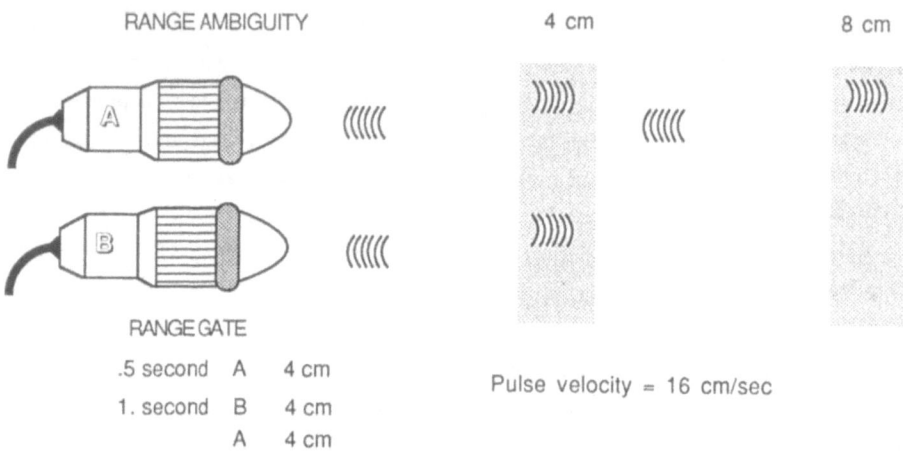

Fig. 1-13. In this example, the transducer transmits an ultrasonic signal every 0.5 second. The second sample (B) occurring 1.0 second after the initial pulse (A), receives an ambiguous signal from the first pulse (A) returning from a depth of 8 cm at the same time a signal from the second pulse (B) returns from a depth of 4 cm. This is the basic method of operation for high pulse repetition frequency mode. Reproduced from Basic Concepts in Doppler Echocardiography, J Chapman & A Sgalambro, Kluwer Academic Publishers, 1987.

Continuous Wave Doppler

To circumvent the disadvantages encountered with pulsed Doppler, the continuous mode is utilized. Continuous wave Doppler may be thought of as the extreme upper limit of pulsing. This means that a higher velocity may be measured and in fact, there is no practical limit to the velocity which may be resolved. Due to the fact that the ultrasonic signal is constantly being transmitted and received, the ability to resolve depth is lost. This does not prove problematic in that when implementing continuous wave, we are interested in the peak velocity measurement and not flow localization. Because the signal is constantly being transmitted and received, the transducer must have a split crystal, or two separate elements. This is necessary to allow the simultaneous functions of transmitting and receiving. If one attempts to transmit and receive the continuous wave signal using a single element, the receiver will become saturated, causing a significant loss in sensitivity. The same occurrence is noted to a certain degree with high pulse repetition frequency techniques when the repetition frequency is increased to a relatively high repetition rate.

The advantage of continuous wave Doppler is that very high flow velocities may be reliably measured. This is one of the most important requirements for the quantitative use of Doppler ultrasound. Continuous wave is more accurate in assessment of the beam to blood flow alignment than pulsed Doppler due to the longer sample volume length which may be considered to be the entire length of the emitted beam. One can appreciate then that pulsed and continuous wave Doppler complement one another quite well. The optimal Doppler instrument will have both capabilities available. Pulsed mode permits flow localization, while continuous mode will permit accurate measurement of high velocities.

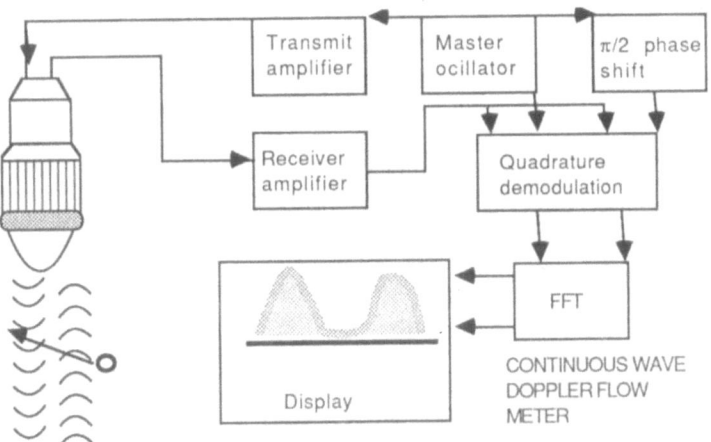

Fig. 1-14. A simplified schematic of a continuous wave Doppler ultrasound device. A dual element transducer is used to constantly transmit and receive ultrasonic signals. The master oscillator serves as a clock for both transmit pulsing and as a reference signal in the quadrature demodulation process. After the phase of the signal has been determined, it passes on for spectral analysis.

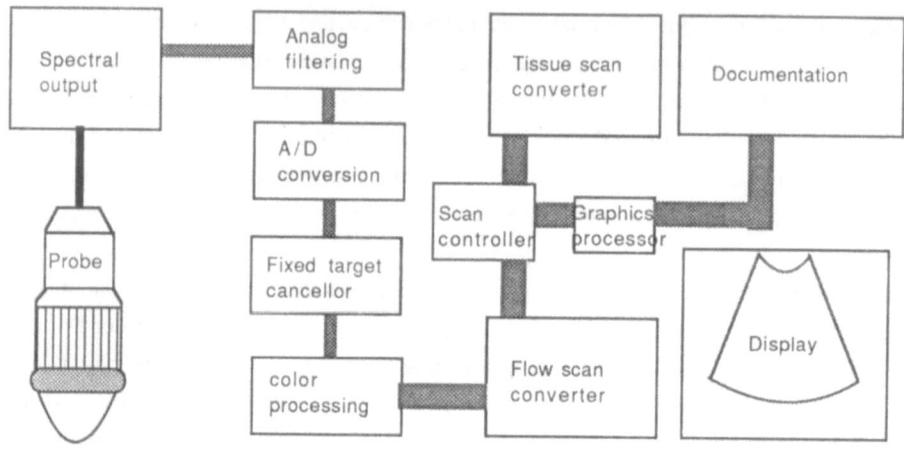

Fig. 1-15. The Doppler signal is passed from the spectral output to the analog filters to remove artifacts caused by very strong reflectors before analog to digital (A/D) conversion is performed. The digital signal is then filtered by a method called fixed target cancellation to remove signals from the cardiac wall motion, valves, etc., so that the clinically relevant blood flow information can be extracted. The Doppler signal is then analyzed, scan converted and displayed (Signal analysis is discussed in Chapter II).

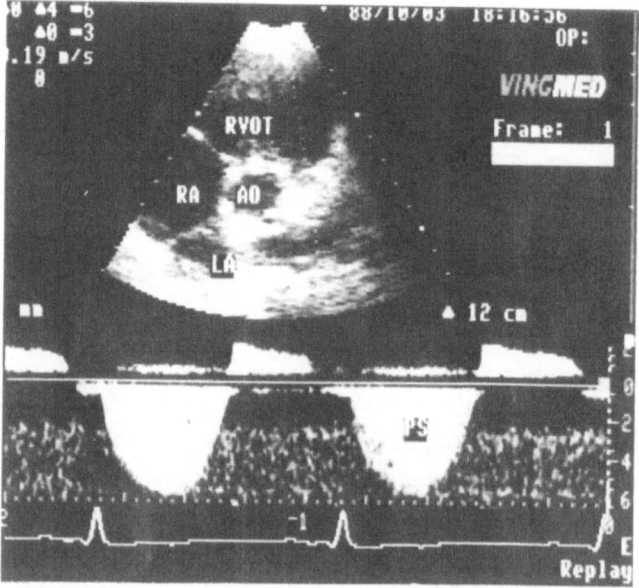

Fig. 1-16. Continuous wave Doppler permits high velocities to be measured with a high degree of sensitivity; there is however no range resolution. This is probably the single most important modality in a Doppler ultrasound system, as it is required for most quantitative measurements. In this example, the high velocity pulmonary flow in a patient with pulmonary stenosis is demonstrated: the peak velocity is 5.6 m/s. Right ventricular outflow tract = RVOT, right atrium = RA, aorta = Ao, left atrium = LA.

The Color TM Mode

In 1972, Brandistini and coworkers described a multi-gated time motion Doppler imaging system. In this modality, range gates are opened at multiple time intervals for each pulse. By increasing the number of these sample cells it is possible to improve the radial resolution of the system. The Doppler ultrasound image is then overlaid on an M-mode echocardiogram using a color coding of the Doppler signal. The color display is usually the same as that used for the color bidimensional image. Flow towards the probe is coded in red, and flow away from the probe is coded in blue. Severely aliased or turbulent flow is assigned a green color. This color map allows one to rapidly discern abnormal flows. The main advantage of color M-mode flow mapping is the high degree of temporal resolution which is obtained; no time is required to sweep the probe as in bidimensional flow imaging. This results in a more accurate frequency and variance estimation because the number of pulses per line may be increased.

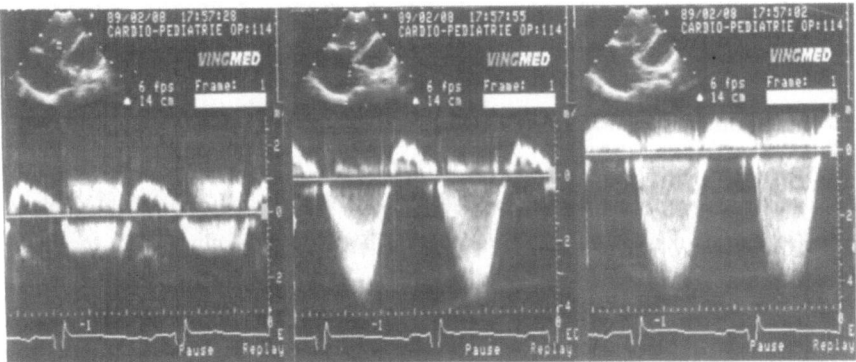

Fig. 1-17. These studies were obtained by conventional pulsed Doppler (left), high PRF Doppler (middle), and continuous wave Doppler (right), in a patient with tricuspid regurgitation. The peak regurgitant flow velocity is ≈ 4 m/s which exceeds the pulsed Dopplers Nyquist limit.

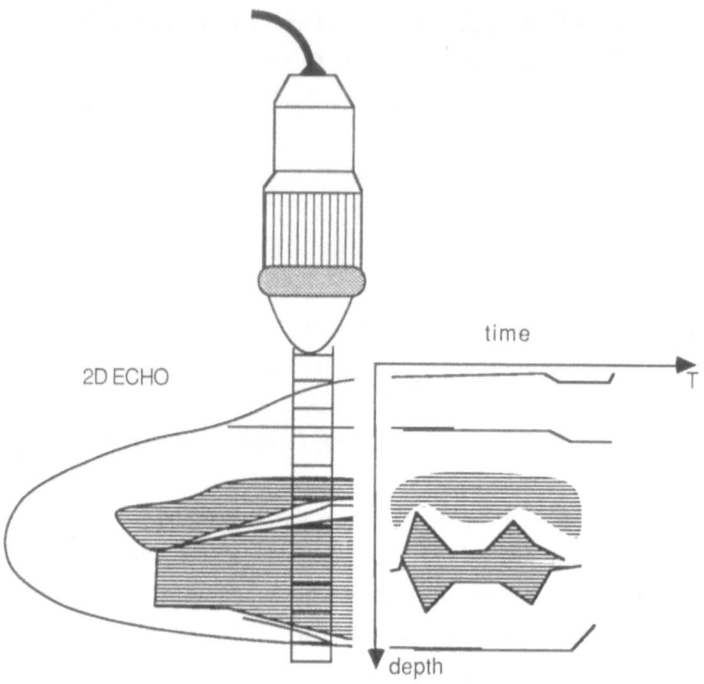

Fig. 1-18. A multigated pulsed Doppler system can be implemented to perform a color Doppler time motion (Color TM) mode. The temporal resolution is quite good, although the spatial resolution is significantly less than with bidimensional flow imaging.

Bidimensional Color Flow Mapping (CFM) Mode

If the process described for implementing a color M-mode is performed on several lines by either mechanically or electronically sweeping the ultrasonic beam, a bidimensional Doppler flow mapping image can be constructed. The various methods of performing the sweep will be discussed in detail in the following section. The received signals from the different depths in each beam direction are converted to digital information in the analog to digital (A/D) scan converter (Fig. 1-15). The memory matrix is composed of a group of pixels, with each pixel in this matrix corresponding to the ultrasonic signal's depth and beam position.

The tissue and flow imaging transmit and receive functions may be performed at the same time or separately, but either way will result in some degree of temporal mismatch (Fig. 1-27). If these functions are performed simultaneously, the mismatch will exist between the left and right sides of the sector. The reason for this is that it takes twenty to one hundred milliseconds to collect an adequate number of ultrasonic samples in each beam direction. The more pulses observed the more accurate the frequency estimation will be, but it will take a longer time period to collect the required data. If the beam is first swept for the tissue image and then swept for the flow image, the temporal mismatch will be primarily between the tissue and the flow. However, when one constructs an image in this way, it is possible to drive the carrier frequencies higher for the tissue imaging and lower for the flow imaging. The resultant image is optimized with respect to two dimensional spatial resolution besides allowing one to improve the Doppler resolution.

The color flow interrogation area consists of a certain number of lines, each with a number of range gates. The radial resolution refers to the radial or axial length that each sample volume covers along each line. When the radial resolution is increased, the length of the color flow interrogation area is decreased because the range gates cover a smaller area. As the radial resolution is decreased, the length of the color flow interrogation area increases as the range gates are expanded to cover a larger area. The larger the area of each sample volume, the better the sensitivity of the Doppler system. In addition to the increased sensitivity achieved with larger color flow areas, one may note that the color flow display is smoothed vertically, with less resolution of the color pixels. This results in decreased radial resolution (Fig. 1-23).

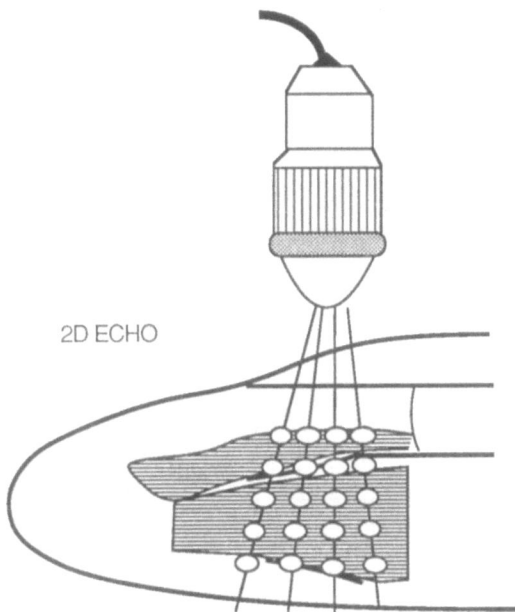

2D ECHO

Fig. 1-19. The multigated Doppler examination can be performed along several acoustic vectors to obtain spatial resolution over a large area of the heart. Each of the horizontal lines represents a range gate depth which is sampled in several positions as the ultrasonic beam is swept over the sector field.

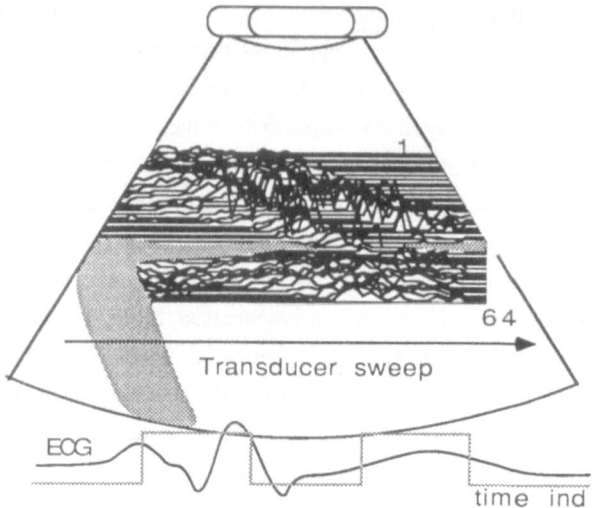

Fig. 1-20. Each of the horizontal lines (1-64) represents a sample volume depth which has been continuously sampled in several lateral positions as the beam is swept across the sector field of view. The time indicator trace (time ind) displays the length of time required to construct the two-dimensional and flow image.

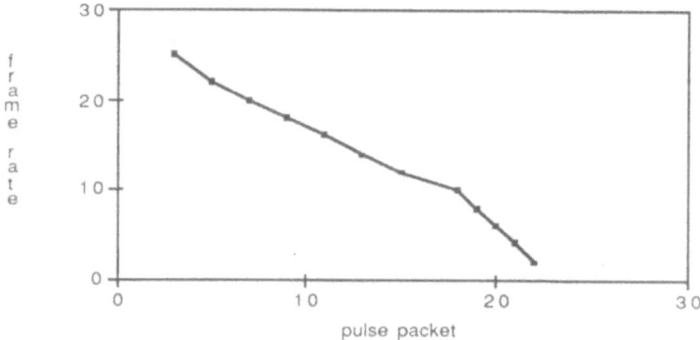

Fig. 1-21. This graph demonstrates the relationship between the frame rate and number of pulses per line (pulse packet). These parameters in turn are related to the the sensitivity , and accuracy of the frequency analysis. It is necessary for the operator to have control over these variables in order to optimize system performance.

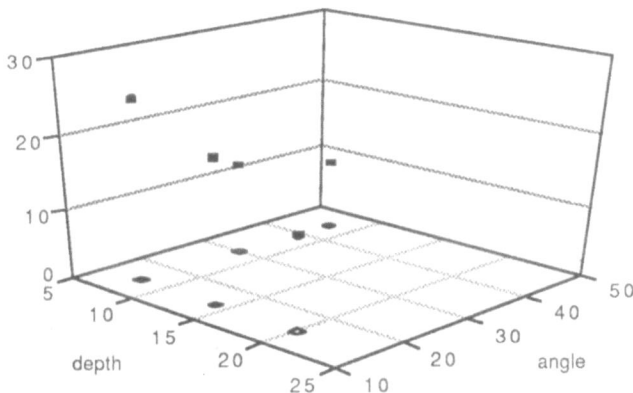

Fig. 1-22. This figure demonstrates the inter-relationship between the depth, number of acoustic beams, and frame rate. If the angle is constant at 15° and the depth is decreased, the frame rate is increased. In the elevational plane, if the depth is set at 8 cm and the angle is reduced, the frame rate is increased.

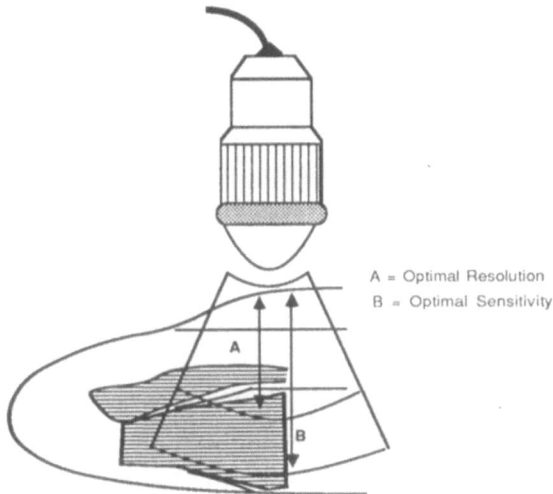

A = Optimal Resolution
B = Optimal Sensitivity

Fig. 1-23. The radial resolution is generally set up to cover the depth of the two dimensional sector, especially if the the flow signal is weak or the patient difficult to scan. The radial resolution is decreased to localize flow with a high degree of spatial resolution, such as in the separation of a valvular or paravalvular leak across a prosthetic valve. This control does not influence frame rate.

Low Velocity Reject in the Color Flow Mapping Mode

The color flow Doppler low velocity reject (LV reject) controls the threshold of the high pass filter (wall filter) in the two dimensional flow image so that strong signals resulting from slow-moving structures, ie the cardiac walls, may be eliminated. In the instrument used by the authors, the imaging frame rate is altered as the the low velocity reject is adjusted (Fig. 2-8). When the low velocity reject is decreased, the frame rate drops as the sweep rate is slowed to allow sufficient time to detect lower velocities. When the low velocity reject is increased, the sweep rate and therefore the frame rate is increased since the higher velocities require less time for detection. This change in sweep rate counteracts the motion artifacts that may occur with a rapidly moving crystal during the interrogation of low velocity flows.

Methods of Implementing a Color Flow Mapping System

The sector sweep can be performed by electronically steering the acoustic beam over the sector field of view. This is the most frequently used method of implementing a color flow mapping system. The transducer used to perform this scanning consists of a bank of piezo electric elements which are cut very thinly, with some shielding between each element. The number of these elements is directly related to the image quality: the more elements in the transducer, the better the image quality. However, the limitation on the number of elements employed is the physical size of the probe. The maximum size of the probe for a specific application is defined by the available acoustic window access. The number of elements which can be fitted within a specific aperture and the spacing required between the elements is determined by the resonating frequency of the elements. While theoretically there is no practical limitation on the frequencies which can be implemented, from a practical standpoint, it is extremely difficult to build a phased array probe with a resonating frequency over 5.0 MHz. The problem is magnified if one attempts to build these high frequency probes on a production basis. However, for probe frequencies between 2.0 and 5.0 MHz this method does offer an attractive method of implementing the color flow mapping system simply.

The ultrasonic beam is formed by electronically exciting these elements in sequence. Each element generates a wavelet which is propagated from the transducer face to the tissue medium. The Huygen principle states that when a linear array's elements are excited simultaneously, the resultant wavelets are summed to propagate in a radial direction from the transducer face, acting as a single wavefront. If the elements are excited in sequence with a delay, the wavelets combine to form a wavefront which propagates at an angle from the transducer face. By altering the firing sequence of the elements, the wavefront or ultrasonic beam is steered over the sector field.

The ultrasonic beam is steered to the left by exciting the elements on the right side of the array earlier than the other elements. To steer the beam to the right, the left elements are fired earlier.

Excitation of the elements at either end of the array earlier than the center elements allows the ultrasonic beam to be focused. By combining these two effects, a focused beam can be steered over the required sector angle. For color flow imaging the stepping of the beam is performed more slowly. This occurs because it is necessary to transmit only one pulse per acoustic vector for tissue imaging, but more pulses per vector are required for flow imaging. In most phased array color flow mapping systems, it is common to use 6 to 8 pulses per beam direction in color flow imaging. This means it takes a correspondingly longer period to collect the requisite amount of data to construct the color flow image. In the following discussion we will review the basic technical aspects for applying another method of performing color flow imaging.

The implementation of most color flow mapping systems has been based on linear phased array technology. An instrument recently designed at the Institute of Biomedical Engineering at Trondheim University is based on annular array technology which we believe is well suited for applications in pediatric echocardiography. Annular array technology offers excellent sensitivity for Doppler applications and interesting possibilities for beam focusing. The element is mechanically swept by an electromagnetic mechanism which permits a simultaneous triplex mode configuration, and high imaging frame rates to be obtained. The annular array probe consists of a series of transducer elements organized in a set of acoustically shielded rings surrounding a central element. Electronic focusing is performed by combining signals from each element to create an electronically variable focus. The beam forming process is carried out on both the transmit and receive pulses to optimize the beam characteristics for both imaging and Doppler applications. Dynamic focusing can be utilized during the receive process to sum the returning echoes from the various elements, yielding improvements in lateral resolution. Additional improvements in image quality can be obtained from focusing the sound beam over large depths during the transmit process. Variable transmit zone focusing provides an optimized spatial resolution throughout the field of view. By combining the variable focus on transmission and dynamic focusing on reception, one can achieve a highly collimated beam. This results in an expanded focal zone with greater penetration. Implementation of an annular array system based on the preceeding discussion would permit improved image quality by optimizing axial and lateral resolution and increasing sensitivity to low level echoes. The lateral resolution of an ultrasound transducer is proportional to the transducer aperture. Increasing the aperture of the probe results in improved lateral resolution and Doppler sensitivity. This method permits dynamic focusing over a wider region within the body. It should be stated that either an annular array or a phased array can be implemented with either good or poor results in terms of image quality and Doppler quality. But when reviewing the theoretical arguments of the pros and cons of each method along with criteria which had been set in terms of Doppler sensitivity, annular array was the method of choice with our group.

Annular array transducers have a concentric geometry and can focus the sound beam equally in and out of the imaging plane, which results in a small uniform dot size throughout the field of view (Fig. 1-24). A decrease in the effective transducer aperture is inherent in phased arrays when steering the sound beam to create a sector image. When the sound beam is steered off the central vector, the total transducer aperture is not fully utilized and can thereby reduce the lateral resolution and sensitivity. However, this is more of a problem in terms of Doppler sensitivity.

This problem does not occur to the same degree with the annular array technique since the transducer is mechanically positioned. The result is that the face of the crystal is always perpendicular to the travelling sound beam, circumventing this reduction in the effective aperture.

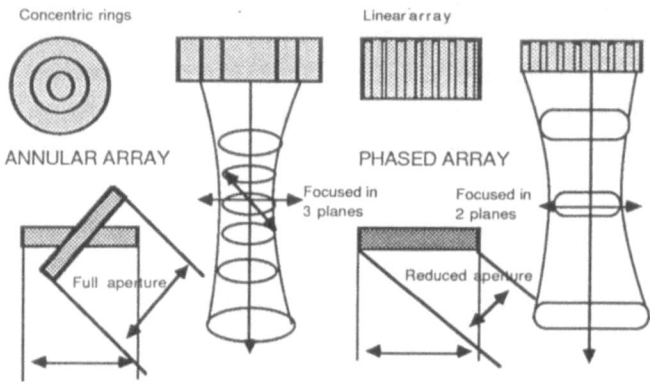

Fig. 1-24. Color flow mapping techniques can be implemented with either phased array , or more recently annular array ultrasound devices. The system used by the authors was based upon annular array technology, which offers some interesting possibilities compared to the more conventional methods.

In the annular array system, the sound beam is concentrically focused in three dimensions which tends to eliminate grating and side lobe artifacts. A phased array transducer can generate an image artifact due to the replication of the main lobe called a grating lobe. Inaccuracies in the critical time delays needed to steer the phased array sound beam can also be a factor in the generation of side lobe artifacts.

Phased array systems utilize reduced dynamic range to suppress both side and grating lobes, clinically limiting sensitivity to low level echoes which can be a limitation for Doppler applications. Annular array technology permits increased dynamic range, high tissue contrast resolution and improved differentiation of low level echoes. An electronically focused system can be used to select the optimal acoustic aperture for each scan line, which can result in improved lateral resolution simultaneously from both the near and far fields of the image. Continuously changing receive wave fronts can then be focused along each beam direction to produce high resolution images. Sliding focal zones can be used to optimize resolution from the skin line to the far field which is more difficult to obtain with a fixed focus conventional transducer.

A series of delays are implemented to control the transmit wave fronts which helps to achieve improved resolution, sensitivity and penetration. Multiple transmit focal zones along the beam can then be achieved. Variable transmit zone enhancement helps to improve the level of contrast and spatial resolution in a specific locale. The number of transmit and receive channels used will vary depending upon the clinical application, and the associated requirements.

Annular array probes have the ability to perform two-dimensional imaging, M-mode, pulsed Doppler, high pulse repetition frequency Doppler, continuous wave Doppler, and color flow mapping Doppler studies with no practical limitation on frequency, or inherent compromises when multiple modalities are implemented with the same probe. This is in part due to the large surface area of the annular array elements and the ability to obtain a wide dynamic range. In a phased array system it is necessary to perform averaging of the received signals after preamplification, requiring the preamplifiers to handle a large voltage change. Because of the large surface area of the annular array probe, a certain amount of averaging is performed at the face of the transducer (Fig. 1-25).

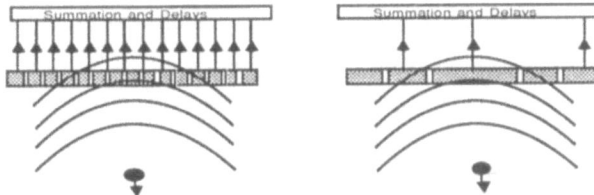

Fig. 1-25. In the phased array system (left) each element is connected to a preamplifier and the summation and delay line. This is where the averaging of the ultrasonic signal occurs. In the annular array system (right) the out of phase wave fronts are averaged at the face of the element, requiring less dynamic range.

There are certain factors which dictate the usefulness of a probe for a certain application. These factors are defined by the physical characteristics of the transducer such as the operating frequency and aperture size and by the application requirements, ie depth of target structure, required interrogation area, and window access. In this section, we shall discuss the general aspects of transducer design essential for the implementation of high frequency probes and wide aperture probes. With the exception of high frequency probes (greater than 5.0 MHz), which present certain problems for phased array systems, either phased linear or phased annular array technology can be utilized in the manufacture of such probes. The technical requirements for both technologies have previously been described, therefore we will concentrate upon the applications requirements independent of the technology selected.

The first major applications requirement which needs to be defined is the maximum interrogation depth. The axial resolution required for a specific application also needs to be defined, since a tradeoff exists between the axial resolution and the required imaging depth. Better axial resolution is obtained with higher operating frequencies, whereas better penetration is achieved with lower operating frequencies. The use of lower carrier frequencies is also advantageous when designing a probe for Doppler applications.

One method of optimizing the carrier frequency utilizes a shifting of the operating frequency; the carrier frequency is increased for imaging but decreased for Doppler applications. This shifting scheme is especially interesting for color flow imaging applications. One generally thinks of the probe carrier frequency as an absolute and well-defined value, when in fact a relatively wide band of frequencies is transmitted and received at a given operating frequency (Fig. 1-26).

The main frequency of the probe is defined by the crystal's resonating frequency and the frequency of the driving sinusoidal pulses. However, there will still be various frequency components present in the transmitted (and received) ultrasonic signal. Therefore, the use of a wide bandwidth probe is advantageous when designing a multipurpose transducer. The crystals may be driven at a higher or lower frequency depending upon the desired application.

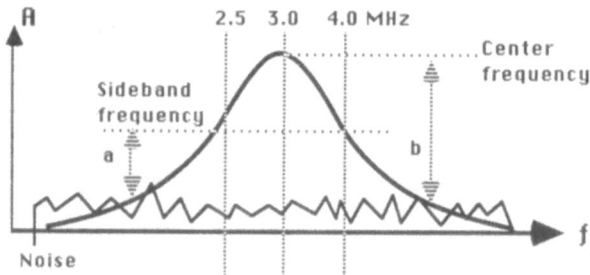

Fig. 1-26. The resonating frequency of a probe is defined by its physical characteristics, such as thickness of the piezoelectric element, and is the most efficient operating frequency for a transducer. However, several frequencies are transmitted and received for a given carrier frequency. These frequency components off the center frequency (within certain limits) can be utilized by driving the transducer at a higher or lower frequency for optimization of a given mode. The signals in the sideband are of lower amplitude and are closer to the noise level than those from the center frequency so a less optimal signal to noise ratio is obtained. This is generally not a major problem and the gains in resolution, penetration, and increases in the Nyquist limit are more important in practical terms. f = frequency, A = amplitude.

Image resolution is an important factor to consider when designing the probe. The axial or range resolution is determined by the carrier frequency, and the lateral resolution is defined by the aperture and the focusing characteristics. The larger the transducer aperture, the better the lateral resolution. However, the need to access limited acoustic windows sets a limit on the size of the transducer aperture in cardiac applications.

These factors have the same influence whether a phased annular or phased linear array system is implemented. For applications where there is no practical limitation on the window access, such as in fetal imaging, but moderate depth penetration and good resolution are needed, a wide aperture (19 - 22 mm) 3.5 or 5.0 MHz probe would be selected. While the penetration and resolution of this probe would be quite good in older pediatric patients, the aperture would be too large for optimal window access.

For intraoperative applications, a 5.0 or 7.5 MHz probe appears optimal, as resolution rather than penetration is the limiting factor. A stand-off of 2 to 3 cm is useful for imaging coronary arteries and other near field structures. The use of frequency shifting in these high frequency probes has definite advantages for Doppler applications. The operating frequency can be shifted lower to perform the Doppler investigation. By doing so, the sensitivity of the Doppler modality is increased and a higher Nyquist limit is acheived for the pulsed mode interrogation.

Frame Rate in a Color Flow Mapping System

In color flow mapping (CFM) it is often necessary to work with the highest frame rates possible. We have discussed the various limitations placed on frame rate due to depth, angle, and number of pulses per line. One may trade off one factor against another to optimize the frame rate for a specific application. When attempting to separate valvular from paravalvular prosthetic valve leakage, or evaluating the patch area in ventricular septal defect repairs, the flow image can be enhanced by improving the spatial and temporal resolution. In other words, decreasing the sample volume size will increase the spatial resolution, while increasing the frame rate by reducing the angle or depth of field will increase the temporal resolution.

The spatial or radial resolution can be altered by changing the sample volume length of the multi-gated real time Doppler. This is accomplished by lengthening or shortening the pulse burst duration, analogous to conventional pulsed Doppler mode. The advantages of leaving this control accessible to the operator are two-fold. First, the Doppler sensitivity and signal to noise ratio are improved by increasing the sample volume length, and to a certain degree the accuracy of the frequency estimation is also enhanced. Secondly, in situations as mentioned above when closely observing the morphology of a flow, the objective is to demonstrate discrete spatial changes in velocity and direction. The radial resolution is optimized by reducing the sample volume length. Frame rate is not affected by altering this parameter.

The temporal resolution is subject to the influence of more variables than the radial resolution. These parameters are depth, angle, number of pulses per line and low velocity reject. The effects and tradeoffs have been discussed previously. There has been ongoing discussion regarding the implementation of linear phased array and annular phased array systems for color flow mapping. From the clinical standpoint, the issue of how well the selected technology has been designed and implemented is more important. It is however worthwhile to touch lightly on some of the more widely discussed issues.

One issue that is often discussed is that higher frame rates are possible during color flow interrogation with a linear phased array system (PA). Another is that there will be a motion artifact with a mechanical annular array transducer (AA) due to the mechanically positioned element. We believe that it is possible to implement frame rates as high, if not higher with an annular array, and that the motion artifact is less problematic than the poor signal to noise ratio seen in some current linear phased array systems. The explanation for both of these statements is that the annular array CFM image is constructed by mechanically sweeping the beam over the sector. The sector is therefore composed of approximately 200 lines; there is a slight but continuous change in beam directions, which causes a Doppler shift to be sampled. The signal generated is low velocity, low amplitude and can be filtered. These beam positions are averaged and displayed over approximately 30 to 60 acoustic vectors. This is called the line averaging, or lateral smoothing, and is user selectable in our system. The degree of lateral smoothing employed plays a key role in determining the lateral resolution.

The methods of sweeping the transducer and constructing the image are open to several configurations. In the system used by the author, the initial method was to perform a sweep from left to right for the image, step the element to a start position, and then sweep from right to left for the real time flow image. This permits a rapid sweep to be performed, as only one pulse per line is required for the two dimensional image. The sweep for the flow image can be performed more slowly so that more pulses per line can be transmitted (Fig. 1-27). As previously mentioned, the Doppler sensitivity, signal to noise ratio, and the accuracy of the frequency shift measurement are improved by increasing the number of transmitted pulses. There are two primary disadvantages which are related to using a higher number of pulses per line. First the rotational velocity of the transducer must be reduced which in turn limits the frame rate to a range of 5-25 frames per second depending on the setup of angle, the interrogation depth, the number of pulses transmitted for color flow imaging, and the low velocity reject.

Secondly, the temporal resolution is reduced and the mismatch between the two dimensional and color flow images is increased as the frame rate becomes lower. It must be realized that color flow imaging is not in fact a real time process because it takes a certain period of time to construct the flow image. When the flow and tissue data are collected at the same time, a temporal lag occurs between the left and right side of the sweep angle due to the increased period of time each beam position must be maintained to permit an adequate number of pulses to be transmitted. Both image construction algorithms are useful. If too few pulses are transmitted in each position the sensitivity, signal to noise ratio, and accuracy of the frequency estimation are all compromised.

In fact, there can be a limitation on frame rate in a phased array system in color flow mapping mode due to this. The phased array method is performed by electronically stepping the beam in each direction as previously discussed. The receiver filters frequently implemented require a period of time before receiving from a new beam position. At frame rates up to 10 or 20 frames per second, this filter settling time is not too important. But when high frame rates of 30-50 frames per second are employed, it becomes an important limitation. Time must be allotted for the filters to settle, hence fewer pulses can be transmitted along a given beam direction. As we have discussed, a reduction in the number of pulses per vector leads to the degradation of the general quality of the Doppler signal.

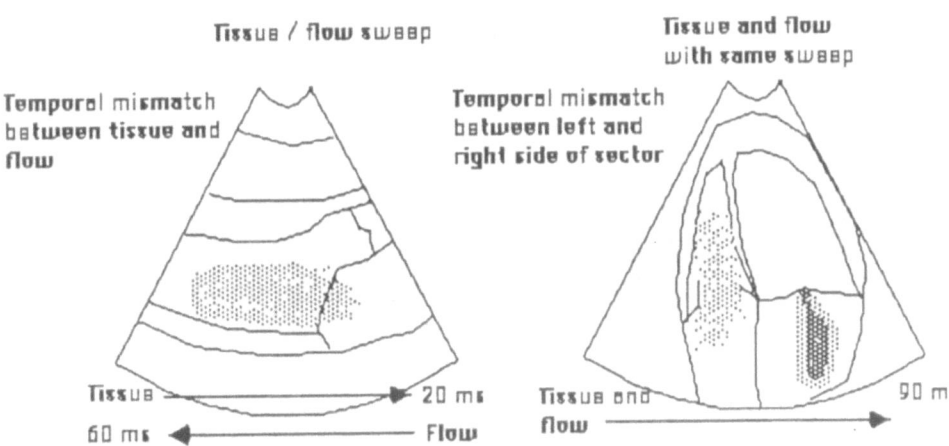

Fig. 1-27. While we generally regard two dimensional flow imaging as a real time process, it actually takes a certain period of time to construct an image. The greater the sector angle, especially the color sector angle, the greater the temporal mismatch. This mismatch will either occur between the tissue and flow image, or the left and right side of the sector, depending on the scanning algorithm implemented.

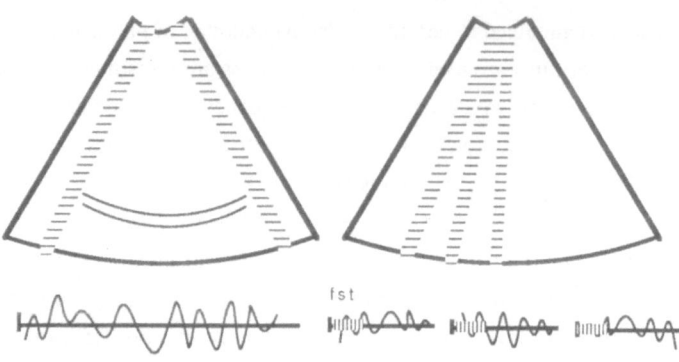

Fig. 1-28. In an annular array (left) the signal from a specific range gate depth in each beam direction is continuous. In a phased array (right) the beam is stepped so that each range gate yields a discrete sample. This can result in lost sampling time waiting for the filters to settle (fst or filter settling time) and limits the period of time available for transmitting pulses. This does not prove too problematic until high frame rates (30-50 frames per second) are attempted. Then limitations in frame rate and overall quality tend to become problematic.

   The annular array system continuously sweeps the beam across the flow interrogation area so that instead of obtaining signals at discrete intervals, a continuous signal is received. As mentioned earlier, this leads to a motion induced frequency shift, but in comparison to the frequency shift from wall motion it is a low frequency (even at flow imaging frame rates of 30-40 frames per second) and can be easily filtered. To achieve rapid frame rates with an annular array system the time sharing scheme must be modified from that previously described. Instead, the initial sweep rate is decreased and more pulses are transmitted, with the received signal being used for both the tissue and the flow image. This is analogous to the method implemented by many phased array systems, but unlike phased array, the annular array does not have a "dead time" waiting for the filters to settle, resulting in less of a limitation on the number of pulses which may be transmitted. We have demonstrated that with an annular array it is possible to work at frame rates of up 54 frames per second, while maintaining a useful sector angle, good sensitivity and signal to noise ratio, and a good definition of disturbed flow (variance) areas. The temporal resolution is also very good with a close correlation between the tissue and flow images, and the left and right sides of the sector. These factors are especially important in pediatric applications because heart rates and blood flow velocities are high. While there is no theoretical reason why these results could not be achieved with a phased array, there are some technical difficulties currently existing.

Summary

In general, pulsed Doppler is useful when measuring relatively low velocity flows for cardiac output determination, and for flow mapping of regurgitant lesions. The pulsed Doppler flow mapping technique and the regurgitant signal width and extension may be measured and used to estimate the severity of the incompetence. However, color flow mapping appears to be better suited for the assessment of regurgitant lesions than pulsed mode due to the excellent spatial orientation provided. The presence of an eccentric regurgitant jet can be detected with flow imaging, where as an eccentric jet may be difficult to track with pulsed Doppler alone. In situations requiring the resolution of high velocity flows, continuous wave Doppler is necessary. Once the value of the peak flow velocity is known, various qualitative measurements can be performed.

The severity of stenotic lesions can be accurately measured with continuous mode. In the setting of tricuspid insufficiency, the value of the peak regurgitant velocity can be used to calculate the right ventricular and pulmonary artery pressure. Although there is no practical limit to the maximum measurable velocity with continuous mode, no spatial or range resolution is provided. Consideration of the advantages and drawbacks of each of the Doppler modalities in the setting of a specific lesion allows one to construct a useful applications matrix for most cardiac pathologies.

When proper care is given to the selection of the Doppler modality used for a specific application, quite accurate hemodynamic information may be obtained. The reproducibility, ease of application, and potential for follow-up examination make the use of Doppler ultrasound attractive in the routine clinical environment. Further technological advances in the areas of data acquisition, data analysis, transducer design, and high frequency transducer development will serve to enhance the use of Doppler echocardiography in pediatric and adult cardiology.

References

1. Doppler JC. Uber das farbige Licht der Dopplersterne und einiger anderer Gestirne des Himmels. Acten der Koniglich Böhmischen Gesellschaft der Wissenschaft. Prag 1842 11; 465.

2. Angelsen B. Analog estimation of the maximum frequency of Doppler spectra in ultrasonic velocity measurements. Report 76 21W, Div. of Eng. Cybernetics, Nor. Inst Tech, Univ of Trondheim, 1976.

3. Baker DW, Rubenstein SA, Lorch GS. Pulsed Doppler echocardiography: Principles and applications. Am J Med 63:69, 1977.

4. Hatle L, Angelsen B. Doppler Ultrasound in Cardiology: Physical Principles and Clinical Applications, second ed, Lea & Febiger, Philadelphia, 1985.

5. Chapman JV. Applications of pulsed and continuous wave Doppler. J Natl Soc Cardio Pulm Tech 1982,13:4.

6. Brandistini M. A digital full range Doppler velocity meter. IEE Trans on Ultrason 1978;287.

7. Omoto R. Color Atlas of Realtime Doppler Echocardiography. Shindan To, Tokyo, 1984.

8. Chapman JV. Evaluation of a phased array color Doppler system (abstr), Int Cong Cardiac Doppler, p. 121, 1985.

9. Chapman JV. Brun P, Meguira A. Initial clinical evaluation of a phased annular array color flow mapping system (abstr), Int Cong Cardiac Doppler, p. 161, 1986.

10. Chapman JV, Sgalambro A. Basic Concepts in Doppler Echocardiography, Martinus Nijhoff, Dordrecht, 1987.

11. Sahn DJ. Real time two dimensional echocardiographic Doppler flow mapping. JACC 1988;77:736-44.

CHAPTER II

CLINICALLY RELEVANT TOPICS IN SIGNAL ANALYSIS

James V. Chapman

Frequency Analysis

The Doppler signal consists of several frequency components, some of which are relevant to blood flow measurement, others which are not. A method of extracting this useful information while suppressing the extraneous data is required. Two of the more important issues when deciding on an analysis algorithm to be used are the amount of time available to perform the analysis, and the requirements for the accuracy of the frequency estimation. In conventional Doppler applications spectral analysis is the method of choice as the time is available to perform a quite accurate breakdown of the various frequency components. Autocorrelation is most frequently used in color flow applications as it may be implemented very rapidly, however, there are limitations in the accuracy of the frequency estimate.

The Fourier transform is the most common technique of performing spectral analysis, yielding information pertaining to the various frequency components and their relative intensity within the Doppler-shifted signal. But before entering into this discussion, it is relevant to review the manner in which directional information is derived from the complex Doppler signal.

Quadrature Demodulation

Before spectral analysis is performed, the signal undergoes quadrature demodulation. Modulation describes the process by which information is coded onto a carrier wave by varying the amplitude, frequency, or phase of the carrier wave. Conversely, demodulation involves the extraction of the information. In Doppler signal analysis, one is interested in determining the direction of blood flow from the returning ultrasonic signal. The way in which this is performed is called quadrature demodulation; the received signal is detected in two channels by the use of quadrature reference signals. Quadrature signals are simply waveforms having the same frequency but differing in phase by ninety degrees. The master oscillator drives the transducer periodically by sending an electrical impulse to the transducer face. A signal is simultaneously sent to the master oscillator for later use as a reference signal. This reference channel is known as the direct channel. The oscillator sends a second signal which has been shifted ninety degrees in phase to a second channel, known as the quadrature channel. The incoming Doppler signal is subsequently compared to the reference signals in the direct and quadrature channels in order to resolve the phase and direction of the frequency shift. By using a quadrature demodulation system in combination with a spectral analyzer, accurate and useful information regarding the direction and distribution of the flow velocities may be obtained.

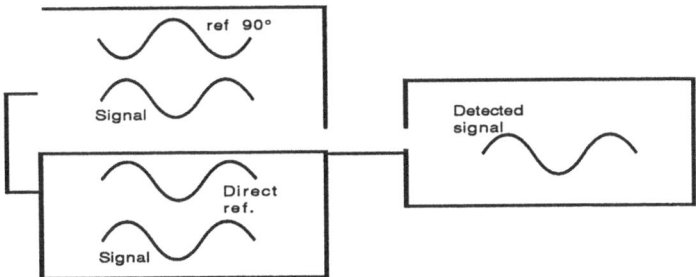

Fig. 2-1. This schematic illustrates the function of quadrature demodulation. A signal is sent to a direct channel for comparison with a reference signal which was generated by the oscillator. A signal is also sent to another channel shifted 90° in phase. The signal phase is compared and the corresponding signal phase is allowed to pass .

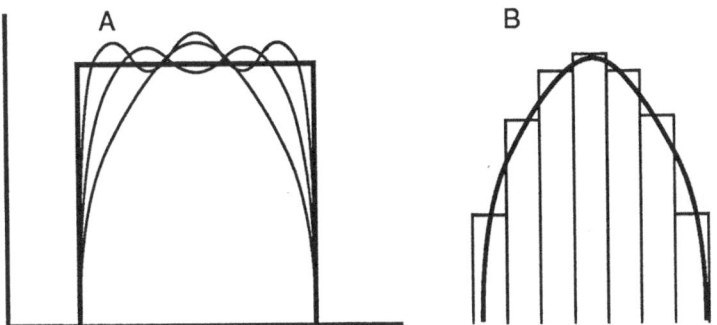

Fig. 2-2. The Fourier theorem states that the mathematical description of any discontinuous phenomenon can, for purposes of analysis, be transformed by a complex procedure into a mathematical description of a continuous phenomenon (A).Wiener proved this theorem by demonstrating that any continuous progression can be resolved into discontinuous sequences (B).

The Fourier Transform

The calculation of the Fourier transform is a rather complex process performed on samples of the Doppler shifted signal. Because these are discrete, i.e. representing a finite period, a discrete

Fourier transform is implemented. A general description of the conversion of the nonperiodic signal to the time and frequency domains is given by the following paired equations;

$$f(t) = \frac{1}{2\pi} \int_{-\infty}^{\infty} F(w)e^{-iwt}\, dw$$

$$F(w) = \int_{-\infty}^{\infty} f(t)e^{-iwt}\, dt$$

Equation 2-1

f (t) is the time description of the signal, F (w) is the frequency description. As mentioned, this equation is valid for a non periodic signal and demonstrates that a waveform f (t) can be constructed by adding an infinite number of sinusoidal signals of a frequency and amplitude as demonstrated in Figure 2-2.

For analyzing Doppler signals from blood flow, which are periodic, it becomes necessary to modify the above equations to replace the continuous functions F(t) and F(w) (with sample period ∞ to -∞), with a number of periodic samples F(k) and F(n). These equations are rewritten to solve for a periodic signal;

$$F(k) = \frac{1}{N} \sum_{N=0}^{N-1} f(n)\, \exp\left(\cdot i\frac{2\pi nk}{N} \right)$$

$$F(n) = \sum_{K=0}^{N-1} f(k)\, \exp\left(i\frac{2\pi nk}{N} \right)$$

Equation 2-2

The power of the signal at each sample point (n) is calculated ;

$$P_i = \left(a_i + jb_i \right)^2 + \left(a_i - jb_i \right)^2$$

Equation 2-3

The power (P) at each point is the sum of positive and negative frequency components (a) and (b). This set of equations is used to calculate the power spectrum and yields information regarding the density and distribution of Doppler scatterers.

The accuracy of the frequency determination is to a large extent defined by the scatterer transit length. As the sample volume length (range gate) is decreased, the transit time error increases.

The frequency broadening caused by the transit time error is generally negligible in conventional Doppler applications, but can cause inaccuracies. If the range gate length is greater than 5 wavelengths, the resulting error is less than 10%. The wavelength of a 5 Mhz transducer is 0.3mm. The acceptable maximum error (10%) for a 5 MHz transducer would be achieved by a sample volume length greater than 1.5 mm. The normal sample volume length is usually greater than this in pulsed mode and if the dimensions are greatly reduced, the decreased signal to noise ratio is more often a problem than the frequency broadening. These technical factors are important as they can affect the accuracy of the collected frequency data, and the analysis can not be more accurate than the data being analysed.

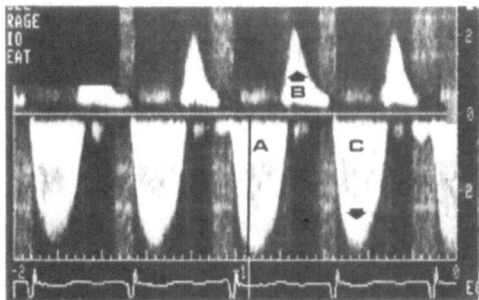

Fig. 2-3. The information relating to the blood flow in this spectral trace include : bandwidth (A), and direction. The pulmonic regurgitation flow trace is above the baseline (B), and therefore towards the transducer. The systolic outflow is below the baseline indicating that flow is away from the probe (C).

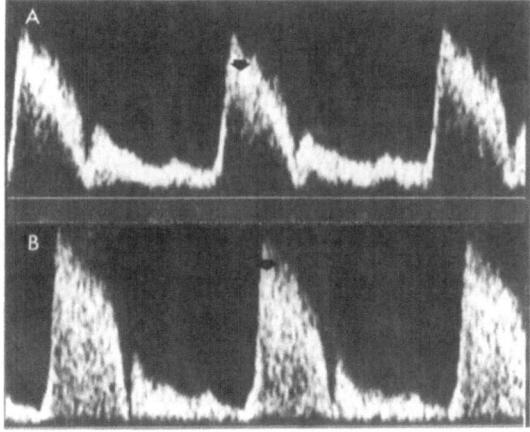

Fig. 2-4. These traces were obtained from the right and left carotid arteries in the same patient. The left artery is normal and a narrow spectral bandwidth is noted. The right carotid artery has a 50% occlusion and a widebandwidth signal (due to the stenosis) is noted.

The discussion of the Fourier transform calculation and spectral analysis has been general in nature and a detailed examination is beyond the scope of this chapter. From a practical standpoint, there are various means of performing the discrete Fourier transform. Either a Fast Fourier Transform (FFT) or a Chirp-Z algorithm may be employed in the computation of the Fourier Transform. The FFT is a digital approach to computing the Fourier transform, while the Chirp-Z algorithm represents a combined analog and digital approach. There are some design advantages in the use of the Chirp-Z algorithm, such as a wider dynamic range, faster computation time, and lower cost. The FFT's now available meet the same requirements, with the added potential advantage of being fully digital.

Whichever approach is used, the purpose is the same: the complex Doppler waveform is broken down into its basic frequency components. One may think of the FFT as an electronic prism which separates the individual frequencies contained in the Doppler signal, just as the conventional prism separates white light into its various components.

The Spectral Display

The output from the FFT analyzer is displayed as an x-y plot on the viewing monitor. Time is represented on the abcissa, frequency or velocity is displayed on the ordinate, and the intensity of the signal is indicated by varying shades of grey. An intense signal will be represented by shades of grey which are close to white, while a relatively weak signal will be displayed in darker shades of grey, in the format used here (Fig. 2-3, 2-4).

The y-axis is usually divided into 64 or 128 points, each possessing a defined velocity or frequency value. The range of frequencies above and below the zero baseline which may be obtained is termed the frequency window. If one is analyzing a low velocity flow, it is helpful to select a lower frequency window so that the 64 or 128 points are used to display the low velocity information. In effect, this yields a larger spectral waveform for analysis. Conversely, if one is measuring a high velocity flow, it is necessary to select a higher frequency window so that adequate space is allotted for displaying the frequency shift. The frequency resolution of these measurements is inversely related to the computation time of the spectral analyzer.

Since the spectral analysis is displayed on an x-y plot, changes in the frequency or velocity distribution and their relative intensity may be observed in time. Note that only the relative density of scatters may be extrapolated from the time-varying spectrum, as shown by the varied shades of grey (Fig. 2-5). A more accurate interpretation of the distribution of scatters may be obtained from the power spectrum. This will be discussed later in more detail.

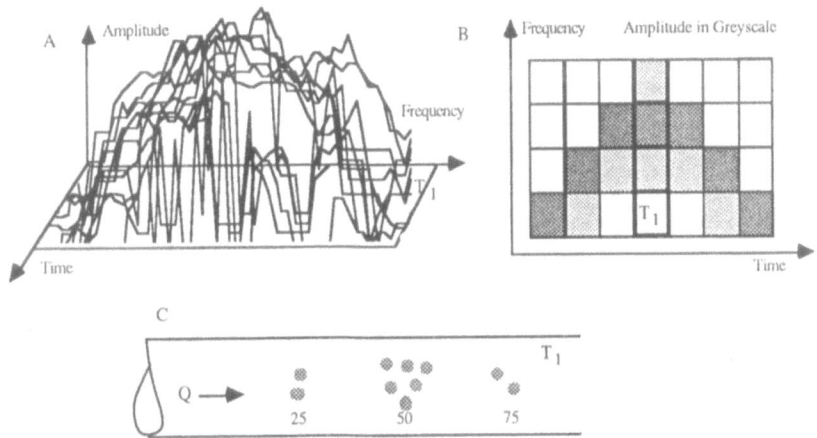

Fig. 2-5. The spectral analysis yields information regarding the signal frequency and amplitude, as demonstrated in the three dimensional time variable plot (A), and the more conventional spectral display (B). The flow in this case has velocities in the 25, 50 and 75 cm/s range. Most of the scatterers are in the 50 cm/s range. This means that there will be more reflected energy in this frequency range than is measured from the 25 or 75 cm/s range. This is denoted on the spectrum by a darker grey scale assignment to the frequency bin assigned to flows in the 50 m/s range at (T_1) an instant in time.

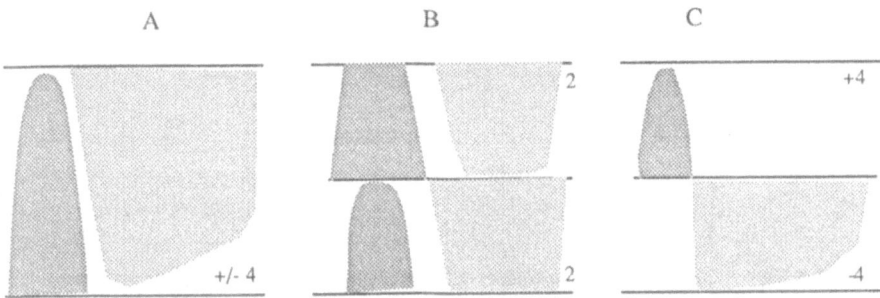

Fig. 2-6. The Doppler spectrum can be configured in several ways; in example A the Nyquist limit has been positioned in the center of the display and the baseline at either velocity boundary. In B the Nyquist limit is positioned at either boundary and the baseline is centered with spectral wraparound occurring. These displays are representative of a high pulse repetition mode in which the maximum velocity resolution is limited. When continuous wave Doppler is used (C), the frequency window may be expanded up to allow high velocity flow in either direction to be measured without requiring a baseline shift.

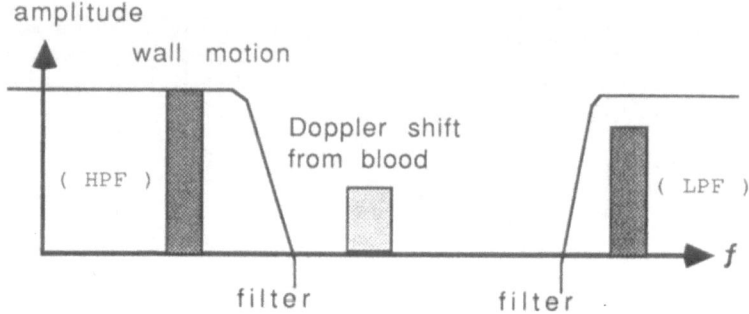

Fig. 2-7. *The highpass filters (HPF) remove the low velocity flow components from the Doppler signal, and are operator defined. The lowpass filters (LPF) remove high frequency noise from the signal, and are generally preset .*

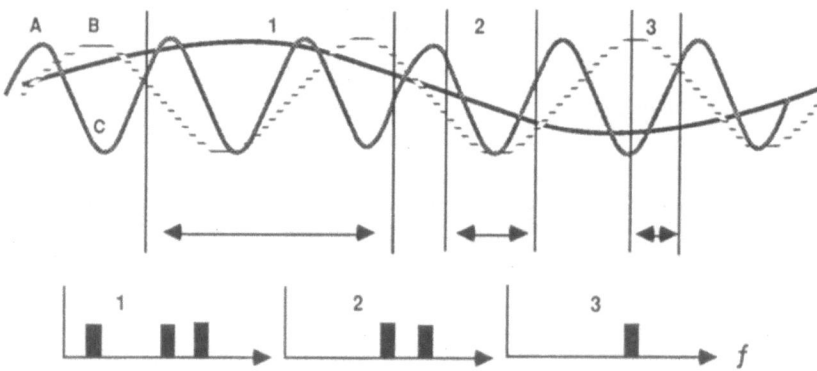

Fig. 2-8 *In this figure the low velocity reject is set in three steps to remove increasingly lower velocities. The signal is sampled for a certain period of time and frequencies which show little or no change in frequency are cancelled. This method is known as fixed, or slow moving target cancellation. As the low velocity reject is reduced to measure low velocity flow, the frame rate drops. This is due to the fact that the flow must be observed for a longer period to measure low velocity flow, but is generally not a problem as this type of flow pattern is found in the presence of structures which are not highly dynamic.*

Filtering

It is necessary to perform filtering of both low and high frequency signals from the spectral analyzer in the practical setting. If this is not done, so much external and internal noise is generated that the receivers can be saturated. Low pass filters are used to remove high frequency noise generated from external sources as well as those from the system itself. These filters are sometimes noted in the spectral display as bands in the upper velocity range (4-6 m/s). The filters "roll off" and are not an absolute cut off, therefore velocity traces often exceed the filter limits. Low pass filters are usually not accessible to the operator and are preset based on various operating parameters.

The high pass filters are frequently referred to as wall motion filters, and are operator selectable. These are used to remove low frequency signals generated by cardiac wall motion and valve motion. They generally operate between 100 Hz to 1400 Hz and are one of the most important factors in obtaining accurate measurements of peak velocities. The value of these filters in terms of the velocities rejected depends on the carrier frequency of the probe. For example, a high pass filter value of 1300 Hz rejects velocities under 0.5 m/s when using a 2.0 MHz transducer, and under 0.35 m/s with a 5.0 MHz transducer.

In most continuous wave applications it is best to use the maximum high pass filter setting available to prevent saturation of the receivers by high intensity low velocity noise. The poorer the signal to noise ratio in a particular case, the more important high pass filtering becomes. When one considers that the amplitude of a reflected signal originating from wall motion is many times stronger than that originating from the red cell scatterer, the importance of removing that signal component becomes obvious. In Fig. 2-7, we see a schematic representation of high and low pass filtering of a Doppler shifted signal. The proper selection of filters is an integral part of optimizing the spectral analysis and display for clinical applications.

Spectral Broadening

The term spectral broadening refers to the range of frequencies present along each spectral computation line. This is in turn related to the velocity distribution of scatterers travelling through the sample cell at a specific point in time. The more frequencies stored in these vertical bins (Fig. 2-5), the wider the spectral bandwidth. In laminar flow states, the scatterer velocity and direction is fairly uniform so the resulting spectral trace will be narrow bandwidth.

In a turbulent flow state with rapidly varying scatterer velocity and direction, one will find that the spectral trace is wide bandwidth. We can therefore use the spectral characteristics to describe various flow characteristics such as laminarity or turbulence (see chapter III). But the clinician must keep in mind that a wide band signal does not necessarily mean that the flow is turbulent, or even abnormal. The presence of aliasing, for instance, generates a wideband signal, but depending on the transducer frequency and pulse repetition frequency, aliasing may be recorded in normal flow states .

The spectral bandwidth is essentially the same parameter as variance (See color flow mapping discussion). But regardless of which technique is used, there are possible sources of spectral broadening not related to physiologic occurrences, but are rather instrument related. Fig. 2-9 demonstrates the effect of the sample volume size on the frequency bandwidth.

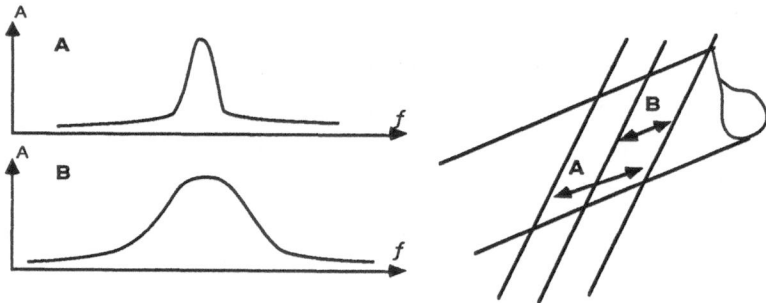

Fig. 2-9. There are both technical and physiologic reasons for the occurrence of spectral broadening. It may be due to the presence of turbulent flow, or it may in fact be due to aliasing, a transit time effect error, or some other technically related factor. Example (A) represents a narrow band signal due to a long transit time and example (B) represents a wide band signal due to a shorter transit time. Amplitude = A, frequency =f.

Signal Analysis in Color Flow Imaging

The analysis of the Doppler signal for color flow imaging must be performed very rapidly due to the amount of information which is used to construct the color flow image. The need to maintain a high frame rate is an opposing requirement. In conventional Doppler applications, a spectral analyzer breaks down a complex mixture of signal frequencies into more basic units. These units consist of a range of frequencies; the smaller the range, the better the frequency resolution is said to be. The frequency resolution and the analysis time are inversely related. For example, a computation time of 10 msec yields a frequency resolution of 100 Hz. With a computation time of 5 ms, the frequency resolution is 200 Hz. Conversely, the spectral envelope definition is better with the 5 msec analysis time, than with a 10 ms analysis time. For cardiac Doppler applications, this is generally an acceptable trade-off for frequency resolution. For color flow mapping applications, the use of complex spectral analysis is not a practical method of frequency analysis because it is much too slow .

An autocorrelator is the most commonly used method of frequency analysis in color flow imaging, offering the advantage of being very fast. However, the uncertainty of the analysis can be increased by this short analysis time, resulting in a decreased accuracy of the estimate. In fact, a discrete break down of the frequency components is not yielded with autocorrelation, but the mean frequency shift is derived instead. This explains to a certain degree why aliasing can be absent in a color image but present on the pulsed Doppler examination of the same flow, even if the pulse repetition frequency is the same. Spectral analysis provides a range of velocities from baseline to the Nyquist velocity, while the autocorrelator only predicts the mean velocity. The value of the mean velocity can be much lower than the peak velocity.

The color flow mapping technique involves rapid sampling and analysis of the multi-gated Doppler signal from several acoustic vectors. The received signal is a continuous train, the timing of which is used to determine the sample position in the scan converter. If a phased array system is used, a small amount of time is required for the filters to stop ringing after each change in position. This results in a reduced sampling time which can in turn decrease the accuracy of the frequency estimate. An annular array transducer is continuously swept and therefore is not subject to this limitation. However, transducer motion may result in some inaccuracy in the frequency estimation instead.

In color flow mapping, ultrasonic pulses are repeated several times along each line to form a pulse packet. The greater the number of pulses per packet, the more accurate the frequency and variance estimation. At least three pulses per line are required to extract the mean frequency and at least five pulses per line are required to estimate variance. A prime requirement in color flow imaging is that the returning signals must be processed rapidly. As mentioned conventional spectral analysis is too slow to be applied for flow imaging applications, although the frequency estimation is quite accurate. Autocorrelation is employed for flow mapping because it is a relatively rapid method of signal analysis, trading off frequency resolution for processing speed. As previously mentioned, instead of a spectrum of frequencies only the mean frequency is extracted along with variance, and signal amplitude.

In Fig. 2-11, the angle (∂) is equivalent to the mean frequency and the fluctuations in bandwidth (Bw) are equivalent to the variance. The third parameter which is extracted is the signal amplitude. The system used by the author maps the mean frequency, variance and amplitude onto the color scale. This method of evaluating the Doppler signal results in a better signal-to-noise ratio as well as a better separation of low velocity turbulence and low grade aliasing. As illustrated in this figure, noise, aliasing and disturbed flow may be defined in terms of frequency, bandwidth, and amplitude or intensity. One must keep in mind that the velocity extracted by autocorrelation represents a mean velocity and is related to the most dense distribution of velocities within a flow structure.

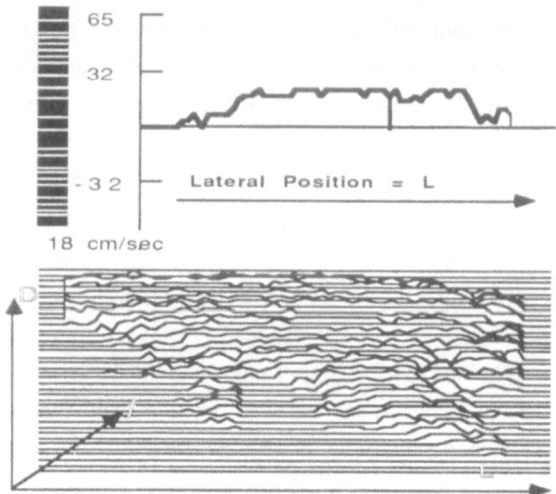

Fig. 2-10 . The flow profile can be reconstructed by displaying the mean velocities measured at a specific depth in various horizontal positions across the flow circuit (A). Because the information lags temporally between spatial positions, a correction factor must be incorporated into the analysis system. This process is carried out at several depths in a color flow mapping system (B) and can be displayed in a three-dimensional format with a coordinate system based on depth, lateral position, and mean frequency. D = depth, f = mean frequency, L = lateral position.

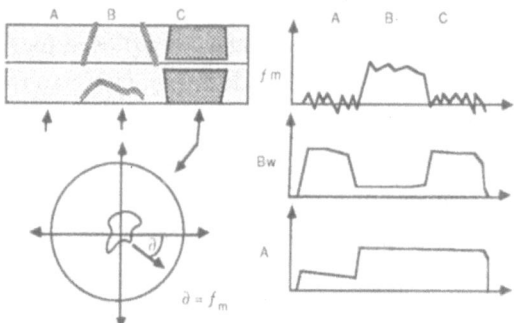

Fig. 2-11. The characteristics of blood flow such as (A) noise (B) mild aliasing or laminar flow and (C) severe aliasing or turbulent flow can be evaluated from observations based on the mean frequency, bandwidth, and amplitude of the signal. The plot in the lower left demonstrates the mean frequency (∂) which varies due to the wide bandwidth nature of the received signal.

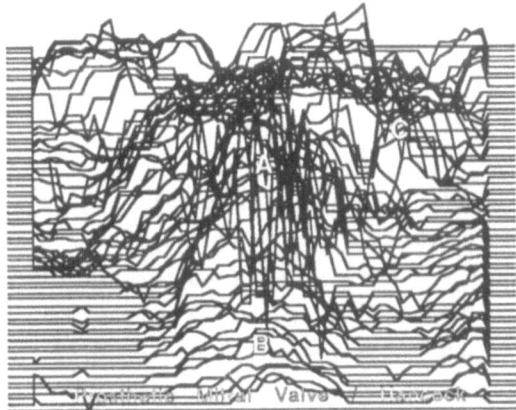

Fig. 2-12. A three-dimensional display of normal inflow through a prosthetic mitral valve (A) which has aliased, resulting in a great deal of fluctuation in the signal's mean frequency. The flow is more organized and has a lower mean frequency downstream from the valve (B). In the jet periphery (C), there is a fluctuation in the mean frequency due to the presence of low velocity vortices.

The Mean Frequency and Variance

The mean frequency is a weighted average of the backscattered signal as a function of the frequency distribution of targets within the observed sample. As previously stated, the mean frequency can be significantly lower than peak frequency value. This should be considered if one attempts to quantify blood velocity by color flow imaging. The most relevent analysis for clinical use is performed on the power spectrum, which permits the mean frequency to be calculated :

$$fm = \frac{A_1^2 \, f_1 + A_2^2 \, f_2 + A_n^2 \, f_n}{A_1^2 \quad A_2^2 \quad A_n^2}$$

Equation 2-4

for a discrete time period, where A = the square of the signal power and f = the frequency. One can appreciate that the longer the data collection time, the more accurate the frequency estimation becomes, but at the expense of increasing the required sampling and analysis time. The accuracy of the frequency analysis can be expressed:

$$fa = \frac{1}{ta}$$

Equation 2-5

where ta is the data collection time. In color flow mapping applications the tradeoff is generally made in favor of a more rapid data collection and analysis time.

The dispersion of frequency scatter around the mean frequency is termed variance and corresponds to the spectral bandwidth of conventional Doppler. This is generally used to describe disturbed flow but can be caused either by physiologic factors such as turbulent flow, or technical factors such as aliasing. The variance (v) can be calculated:

$$v = \frac{(f_1 - f)^2 A_1^2 + (f_2 - f)^2 A_2^2 + (f_n - f)^2 A_n^2}{A_1^2 + A_2^2 + A_n^2} (Hz)^2$$

Equation 2-6

where f1...fn are the individual frequency components and f is the mean frequency. There is a higher degree of accuracy in the variance estimation with a larger number of samples.

This has been a review of the signal analysis in color flow mapping in general terms. The way in which the data are analyzed and the colors are assigned will vary with different manufacturers' instruments.

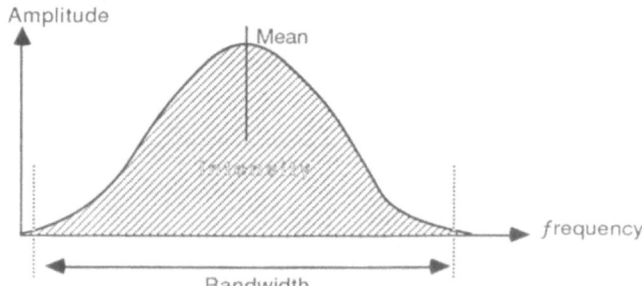

Fig. 2-13. A schematic representation of the signal from a single sample volume. The frequency bandwidth, the mean frequency shift, and the signal power are three important parameters which are obtained from the power spectrum.

Color Flow Mapping Display Algorithms

An interesting possibility in color flow mapping applications is the detection and display of blood flow disturbances. It is relevant to the discussion of quantitative methods in regurgitant lesions, to contrast areas of severe frequency broadening. The etiology of this broadening may be either severe aliasing due to high velocity flow components, or the presence of disturbed flow. While in the case of severe aliasing it may be impossible to determine the underlying cause of frequency broadening, it is possible in less severe aliasing situations (less than prf). This is accomplished by assigning the color map as a function of mean frequency (Fm), bandwidth (Bw), and amplitude (A). This permits separation of low level aliasing which is an instrument induced phenomenon, and actual physiologic events in the setting of disturbed flow.

The autocorrelation function can be demonstrated in a polar plot. (Fig. 2-11, 2-14). The angle (∂) between consecutive sample points corresponds to the mean frequency, the amplitude is defined by the magnitude of the horizontal vector, and the separation between the points (x,) defines the signal bandwidth. For this reason it is practical to set up the color scale based on the vector indication plot (c) The angle between consecutive points can then be used to display frequency information, and positions towards the origin are used to designate increasing bandwidth or variance. A color map can then be implemented which displays the mean frequency in shades of red for flow towards the transducer and blue for flow away from the transducer. As the degree of variance increases, the sample point approaches the origin, and more green is added until the color assignment becomes a mosaic pattern. In the color map we have implemented, the color is changed to a solid green. We have concluded that this color map provides the best indication of disturbed flow regions. The amplitude, which is related to the power of the backscattered signal, is indicated by the brightness of the color.

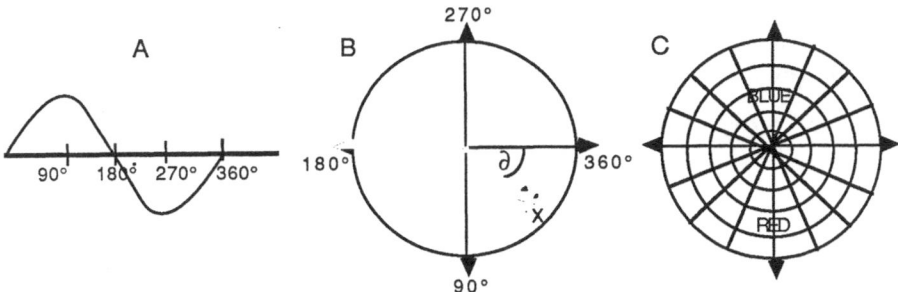

Fig. 2-14. The sine wave (A) can be displayed in a plot of its polar coordinates (B). A color scale configured as a wheel is one practical means of displaying the real time Doppler information (C).

There are basically two requirements of a color map. First, the flow map should yield a spatially accurate display of flows and the mean velocity of those flows. Secondly, the flow map must characterize the laminarity or turbulence of the interrogated flow, and indentify the presence of abnormal blood flows. One factor which should be considered is the information being color encoded: velocity, variance, and/or power. When variance is not used, the frequencies can be mapped onto various hues and shades of colors to help differentiate flow velocities.

It is the opinion of the author that whatever color map is used for the display, there is a great deal of interesting data which is being neglected. The subtle variations in colors and brightnesses, especially in real time, lead to a situation of information overload. Therefore, the color map should facilitate rapid and accurate indentification of abnormal flow as a primary concern. It is more useful to transfer the data offline to a quantitative analysis system (this is discussed later). The other factor to consider is the configuration of the color scale. If we look at the wheel again, it can be broken in either of two places to construct a color bar with a symmetric Nyquist display. The first is to set the baseline in the center position with the Nyquist limit at either extreme. The other possibility is to set the Nyquist limit in the center and the baseline at either extreme. There are advantages in setting up the scale stated in the latter description, so that for instance, velocities over the Nyquist limit in either direction can be measured without requiring a baseline shift (Fig. 2-15).

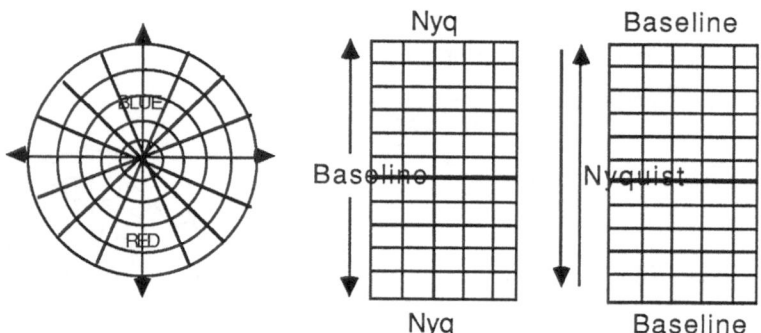

Fig. 2-15. A symmetric color bar can be set up by opening the color wheel at either the baseline or the Nyquist limit .

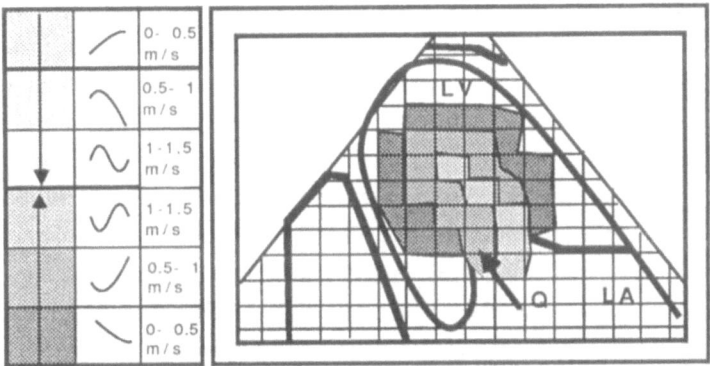

Fig. 2 -16. When the color scale is set up so that the baselines are at either end and the Nyquist limit is in the center, velocities which exceed the Nyquist limit are mapped onto the colors reserved for flow in the opposite direction. This in fact allows for an asymmetric Nyquist display in either direction, without requiring a baseline shift. The velocity value for each color represents a range of velocities which introduces an inaccuracy into the absolute velocity measurement obtained from the real time Doppler.

Methods of Quantifying Color Flow Signals

We have discussed various factors which may influence the accuracy of velocity measurements from color flow imaging, and the fact that the autocorrelator yields the mean Doppler frequency. In this section, methods of extracting the velocity information from color Doppler will be presented. But one should note that no matter how accurate this velocity quantitation is, it will be different (lower velocity, and less accurate) from the spectral analysis peak velocity. The information contained in the color Doppler signal relates to frequency (or velocity) and amplitude (or power). Each display picture element (pixel) then contains the mean frequency and the signal amplitude of a received signal from a discrete sample cell. One method of analyzing the content of the real time flow image utilizes video densitometry. With this method, the color flow images are stored on video tape and replayed through an offline computer which permits digitization, and either a greyscale or colorscale transfer function to be performed. This digitized information may then be displayed as a numeric value or graphically. The interest with such methods is that it is possible to measure stenotic or regurgitant flow areas based on the spatial velocity distribution. If this measurement is combined with mean velocity or velocity time integral, it would theoretically be possible to calculate flow volume. The direct data transfer system used by the author, and circumvents problems associated with quantifying video processed images. A Vingmed

CFM-700 (Vingmed AS, Horten, Norway) is interfaced with an Apple Macintosh II (Apple Computers Inc, Cupertino, USA), allowing the Doppler signal and two-dimensional color flow images to be transferred from the system memory to the computer at very rapid rates. Down loading 90 frames of R Ø data (32k or 64k per frame) is accomplished in less than 10 seconds. Capabilities of this system permit the operator to quantify pixel velocity, customize color maps and construct single line and three-dimensional flow velocity profiles. CFM measurements transferred for analysis are presented in Fig. 2-10 and 2-12. The three dimensional frequency plots of a laminar and an aliased flow are demonstrated. The subtle variations in frequency as a function of spatial position are clearly visualized in this type of display, though it is somewhat difficult to interpret in real time. For detailed analysis of the flow structure based on the Doppler shifted information though, the digital manipulation of the data is much more precise than measuring color encoded images. The horizontal lines represent velocity profiles at a specific sample volume depth. In some respects this represents a series of uniplanar flow profiles at several depths. However, before this horizontal line can be considered representative of the profile, a correction of the temporal skew which is caused by the image sweep must be factored into the analysis (Fig. 2-10). The time distortion in a flow profile from left to right (or vice versa is due to the delay caused by sweeping the beam across the area of interest. The color Doppler pixel velocity and amplitude can be used to characterize specific components of the flow structures in regurgitant and stenotic jets. The peak pixel velocity, averaged pixel velocity, and the frequency shift area can be measured, but the value of the velocity is probably more useful in terms of demonstrating relative changes or differences in flow velocities and perhaps for flow volume calculations than absolute peak velocity measurements for gradient calculation. These methods of analysis have demonstrated a good correlation of orifice area by real time Doppler and those derived by the continuity equation in vitro. It has also been demonstrated that the presence of serial obstructions can be evaluated by digital techniques. It is reasonable to assume that these methods will be useful in the evaluation of various regurgitant and shunt lesions by color flow imaging. Further, as previously stated, if the program permits angle correction and time distortion correction, it is possible to construct representative flow profiles. We feel that for detailed analysis of the color flow image, digital flow mapping offers several interesting possibilities.

References

1. Atkinson P, Woodcock JP. Doppler Ultrasound and its Clinical Measurement. Academic Press, London, 1982.

2. Hatle L, Angelsen B. Doppler Ultrasound in Cardiology, Lea & Febiger, Philadelphia, 1985.

3. Chapman JV, Sgalambro A. Basic Concepts in Doppler Echocardiography, Martinus Nijhoff, Dordrecht, 1987.

4. Chapman JV. Clinical evaluation of the Doppler power spectrum. Eur Rev Biomed Tech 1986; 8:3.

5. Chapman JV, Brun P, Meguira A, Torp H, Angelsen B. A new method of indicating disturbed flow in a color flow mapping system (abs). Heart and Vessels 1987, supp 3.

6. Angelsen B, Kristoffersen K, Torp H. Diagnostic information in the color flow image (abs). Heart and Vessels 1987, supp 3,1-52.

7. Omoto R. Color Atlas of Real Time Two Dimensional Doppler Echocardiography. Shindan-To-Chyro, 1984.

8. Perronneau P, Diebold B, Guiglimi JP, et al. Structure and performance of mono- and bi-dimensional pulsed Doppler systems. In: Color Doppler Flow Imaging, J. Roelandt (ed), Martinus Nijhoff, Dordrecht, 1986.

9. Kyo S, Kondo Y, Takamoto S. Effect of scanning direction and frame rate on the area of flow image in phased array color Doppler echocardiography (abstr). J Am Coll Cardiol 1988,11; 2: 98A.

10. Tamura T, Sahn DJ, Krabill K. Low velocity sensitivity in color flow mapping: Power mode versus dynamic range reallocation for display (abstr). J Am Coll Cardiol 1988, 11; 2: 98A.

11. Linker DT, Johansen E, Torp H, et al. Practical considerations and design of a digital system for acquisition of two-dimensional ultrasonic tissue and flow data. Echocardiography 1988, 5; 6: 485-494.

BLOOD FLOW MEASUREMENT BY DOPPLER ULTRASOUND

James V. Chapman

Introduction

The heart is a basically a pump, and to function optimally, the flow of blood through the heart must be organized to maintain an efficient flow environment. There are many factors which influence the characteristics of blood flow in the circulatory system, such as pressure dynamics, peripheral resistance, viscosity of blood, and the dimensions and geometry of the flow circuit [1]. When the measurements required for the calculation of the cardiac output can be obtained, accurate measurement of flow volumes are possible. There are often clinical situations when relative measurements of changes in flow are adequate, i.e. optimization of pacemaker function, pharmacological studies, and exercise stress testing. The Doppler methods for measuring flow velocities are very well suited for this type of application.

In the following chapter we will review the principles of blood flow relevant to the application of Doppler ultrasound measurements. This discussion will focus on three primary topics. First, the characterization of flow structure, i.e. the turbulence or laminarity of flow, secondly, on the determination of the flow profile, and finally, on the measurement of volumetric flow and the Qp/Qs ratio.

Laminar Blood Flow

The Poiseuille's model is used to describe the rules which govern fluid motion in a tube, but can be adapted to describe the flow of blood in the circulatory system. The ratio of the pressure gradient to flow is a function of the flow circuits' cross-sectional area and the viscosity of the fluid (Fig. 3-1).

The ratio of pressure gradient to flow can be defined as the vascular resistance. The dimensions of the vessel have a significant effect on vascular resistance, as changes in resistance are inversely proportional to the vessel radius. The viscosity of blood and vessel length are relatively constant in the circulatory system and these two parameters have a lesser impact on the vascular resistance. The value of blood viscosity reflects the internal friction between adjacent blood layers (lamina). As mentioned previously, Poiseuille's law refers to a steady laminar flow in a rigid cylindrical tube, however it is a valid model in the study of hemodynamics. The pulsatile flow in the cardiovascular system can be understood by extension of the principles applied in the steady state flow model. The pressure and flow pulse waves can be dealt with as steady flow upon which pulsations are superimposed[2,3].

In the physiologic setting, blood flow is usually laminar which implies that the flowing blood streams in a series of concentric cylindrical lamina moving in a direction parallel to the tube walls (Fig 3-2). The highest velocity is found in the core layer; the velocity diminishes in each concentric layer with increased distance from the core layer. At the vascular wall, a stationary fluid layer is encountered. This symmetrical distribution of velocities with increasing distance from the core layer results in the development of a parabolic flow profile. The decrease in velocity from the vessel core to the wall is referred to as the velocity gradient. Each cylindrical layer exerts a forward force on the adjacent layer which is flowing at a slower velocity. This stress is called shear stress and is defined as the moving force per unit area between adjacent lamina.

The slower moving lamina exerts a drag or backward force on the faster moving inner lamina. In order to maintain a steady flow, the shear force must overcome this viscous resistive force. The shear stress and the velocity gradient are greatest at the vessel wall and zero in the center axis of the vessels cross-sectional area. The greater the velocity gradient, the greater the shear stress.

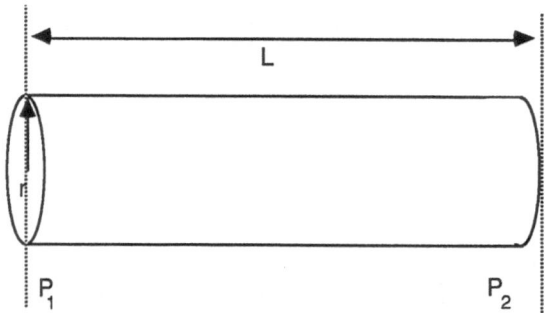

$$F=\left(P_1 - P_2\right)\frac{\pi\, r^4}{8\, L \times n}$$

$$R=\frac{8}{\pi}\times\frac{L \times n}{r^4}$$

$$R=\frac{P_1 - P_2}{F}$$

Fig. 3-1. This figure and set of equations demonstrates the relationship between pressure (P), flow (F), and resistance (R) for flow in a cylindrical tube based on Poiseuille's law for steady state flow of a Newtonian fluid in a rigid tube. The principles apply in blood flow as well, even though blood flow is pulsitile and blood is a non-Newtonion fluid.

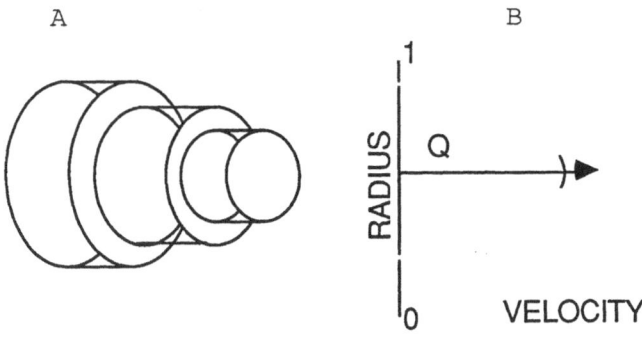

Fig. 3-2. Flow moves in concentric organized layers in a laminar flow state (A). The flow velocity is highest in the center of the flow cross-section (B).

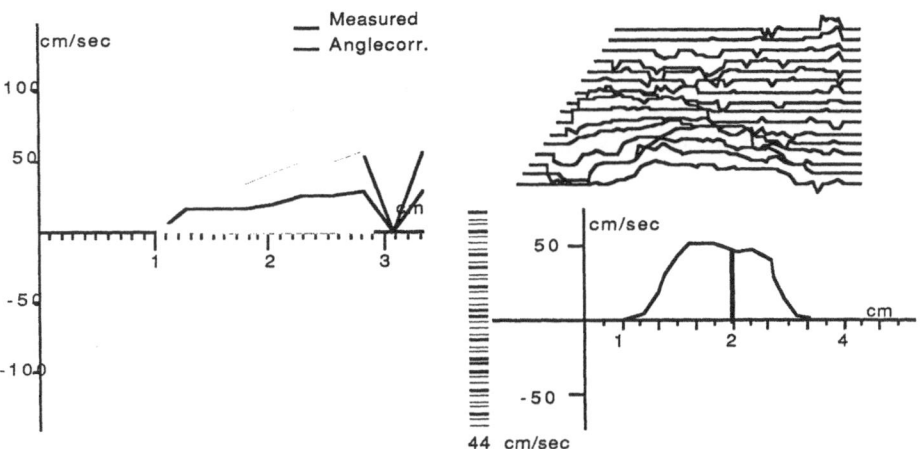

Fig. 3-3. This series of figures demonstrates the flow profiles measured from a normal aortic outflow. The lower right figure is a single line flow profile demonstrating the mean velocity on the abcissa, and vessel diameter on the ordinate. Above this, one notes a series of flow profiles obtained from the multigated Doppler. The traces on the left demonstrate a flow profile with and without correction of the temporal skewing caused by the sector sweep.

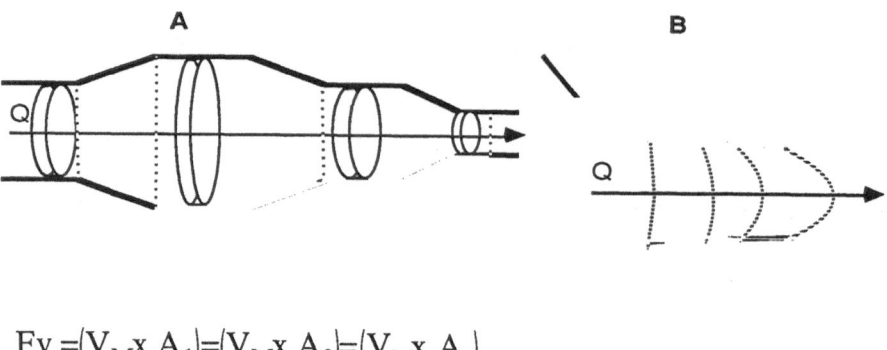

$$Fv = \left(V_M \times A_1\right) = \left(V_M \times A_2\right) = \left(V_M \times A_n\right)$$

Fig. 3-4. The principle of conservation of mass predicts that in a closed flow circuit the volumetric flow rate at one point must be equal to that at another point (A). The distance of the flow into the vessel affects the flow profile. The flow profile is flat at the vessel entrance, becoming more parabolic distal to the inlet (B).

There is generally a linear relationship between the velocity gradient (shear rate) and the applied shear stress. This is true of water and other fluids. The existence of a linear relationship implies that viscosity is a constant value, being an inherent physical property of the liquid and independent of the shear rate. These fluids are referred to as Newtonian or ideal fluids.

In non-Newtonian fluids, viscosity is not constant but depends upon the shear rate. Blood is not a Newtonian fluid, for at low shear rates the viscosity rises exponentially with a further fall in shear rate. In very small flow circuits with a diameter less than 0.5 mm, the viscosity diminishes with decreasing tube diameter. Under physiological shear rates, the hemodynamic behavior of blood resembles that of a Newtonian fluid. The SI (International System) unit of viscosity is the Pascal-second (Pa.s) which is equivalent to the Newton per square meter (N/sq-m). The viscosity of blood with a hematocrit of 45% at 37 degrees Centigrade is 0.04 P (0.004 Pa.s).

The Flow Profile

We have already presented the general description of the parabolic flow profile, and stated that the flow profile can be defined as the distribution of flow velocities in specific lamina, which decreases in velocity in the outer layers. The discussion of flow profiles is relevant to the clinical application of Doppler, especially when measuring flow volume. An ideal model of parabolic and flat velocity profiles has been described in this section. But in the physiologic setting, the ideal situation is not always encountered. The profile will vary temporally and spatially. When measuring the cardiac output at any of several positions in the heart one must assume a flat profile exists. However, if the profile is observed at various points distal to the vessel inlet, distinct changes are noted. The profile will be blunt at the level of the inlet, becoming more parabolic distal to the inlet. If the vessel is curved, such as the aortic arch, the profile may be skewed to differing degrees. The run off to the subclavian arteries further complicates matters. The flow profiles are in fact more complex than one might imagine. When measuring the profile across the mitral valve for instance, one can make the measurement at the annulus or at the tips of the leaflets. Samstad and coworkers have demonstrated that the mitral velocity profile varies at different positions, that it varies with time, and it varies between patients. From the practical side, it would appear that the degree of error is tolerable, at least for the evaluation of relative changes in the cardiac output. However, we believe that this can be a limiting factor in the accurate determination of flow volume in many instances. As described in Chapter II, the Doppler imaging information can be displayed in a three dimensional format, which in fact represents a series of horizontal flow profiles at several radial positions (Fig.3-3).

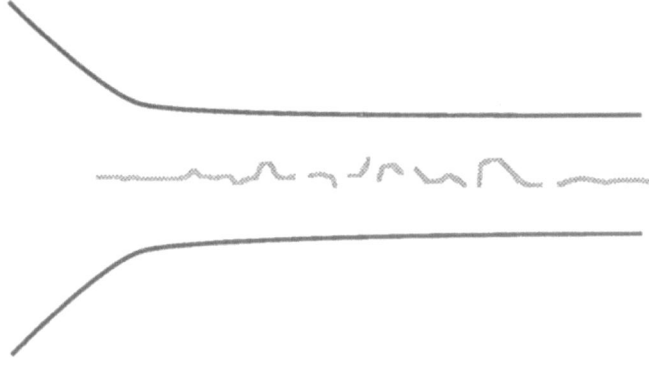

Fig. 3- 5. In a steady state flow situation, the flow will change from laminar (A) to turbulent flow (B) with increasing Reynolds numbers. Relaminarization (C) may occur at some location distal to the point where the turbulence began to develop. In laminar flow the layers of fluid do not mix as they do in turbulent flow.

Turbulent Flow

As a laminar flow's velocity increases, a break down in the organization of the flow structure occurs. The layers of flow mix, and there is an exchange of energy in the plane transverse to the flow plane. There are two primary components in a turbulent regime, one which is slowly varying in the parallel plane, and one rapidly varying in the radial plane. The flow profile is flat in comparison to that noted in a true laminar flow situation.

The transition of laminar flow to turbulent flow occurs when a certain threshold, which is defined by the vessel diameter, flow velocity, density and viscosity of the fluid are exceeded. The Reynolds number is a valueless unit which is used to predict the critical threshold at which laminar flow becomes turbulent. The following equation relates these parameters: vessel diameter (D), mean flow velocity (V), and viscosity (u), yielding the Reynolds number;

$$RE = \frac{\text{Inertial forces}}{\text{Viscous forces}} \text{ or } RE = \frac{V\ D}{u}$$

Equation 3-1

There is a transition between laminar and turbulent flow, which in the physiologic setting is frequently encountered. For our purposes, the term will be used to define a flow structure which is primarily disorganized. An example of this type of flow is noted in aortic regurgitation, where there is a core jet of an organized flow with peripheral eddies and vortices, which are disorganized or turbulent in nature.

In a steady flow state, the turbulent flow will reorganize at some point distal to the obstruction (Fig 3-5). This may or may not happen in the physiologic state. It is not uncommon to have turbulence from one site conducted to another site downstream. For instance, one may find turbulent flow in the main pulmonary artery of a patient with a normal pulmonary valve which was generated from a ventricular septal defect below the outflow tract. This phenomenon is termed the series effect.

Volumetric Flow Measurements

Doppler ultrasound in conjunction with standard imaging techniques provides a method of measuring the volumetric flow noninvasively. If the measurements are made very carefully, observing rigid criteria for selection of the study subjects, quite accurate measurements of absolute volumetric flow can be made. There are many limitations in the accuracy of these absolute measurements which will be discussed later, but even in these cases clinically interesting information regarding relative changes in cardiac output can be extrapolated. Before starting a discussion of the applications methods for the measurement of the cardiac output, we will review the underlying basis for these measurements.

In the setting of blood flow through a vessel with a cross-sectional area A, the rate of blood flow (Q) through an element of the cross-section is defined:

$$Q = (V)(A)$$

Equation 3-2

where V is the blood velocity at that given cross-section. The total rate of flow is then calculated as the sum of all the contributions across the vessel cross-section:

$$Q = \sum[(V)(A)]$$

Equation 3-3

If the increments of cross-sectional slices become very small, we can replace A with dA, and rewrite the equation as follows:

$$Q = \int VdA$$

Equation 3-4

Measurement of the frequency shift permits one to calculate the blood flow velocity, as stated in the Doppler equation. Blood flow can be calculated in various ways, which are suggested by Equations 3-2 and 3-3. These equations imply that the spatial velocity distribution in the vessel (the velocity profile) is first determined and then the flow contributions from the various area elements are computed and added together to give the total flow rate in the vessel. However, in the measurement of blood flow the average velocity can be computed and this spatial average velocity can be multiplied by the cross-sectional area to calculate the total rate of flow (Fig. 3-6).

The calculation of cardiac output is based upon the assumption that a flat velocity profile exists at the sampling site. If this assumption is valid, then the Doppler measurement of volume becomes feasible. If a flat velocity profile is present, then the mean and maximum frequency (or velocity) are approximately the same. The flow volume at a given vessel cross-section is defined as the product of the spatial mean blood flow velocity and the cross-sectional area of the vessel. In order to calculate accurately the volume of blood flow by Doppler techniques, the angle between the Doppler beam and the blood flow must be zero, or close to zero, degrees.

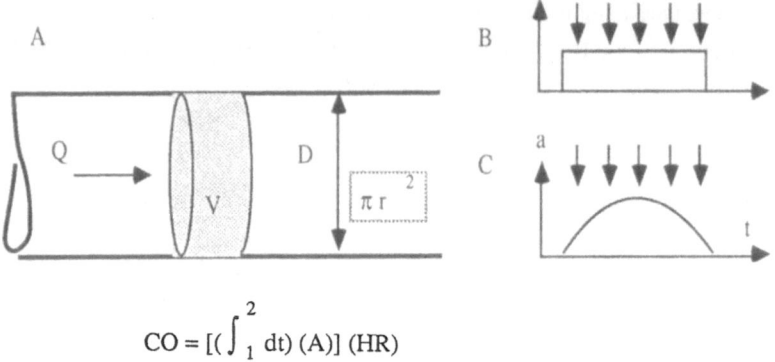

$$CO = [(\int_{1}^{2} dt) (A)] (HR)$$

Fig. 3-6. The flow volume for a steady state flow can be calculated by multiplying the cross-sectional area by the flow velocity (B). When pulsatile flow is encountered (C), the mean velocity is inserted into the equation as velocities measured at different times will vary. CO = cardiac output, V = velocity, dt = flow time, A = flow area, HR = heart rate.

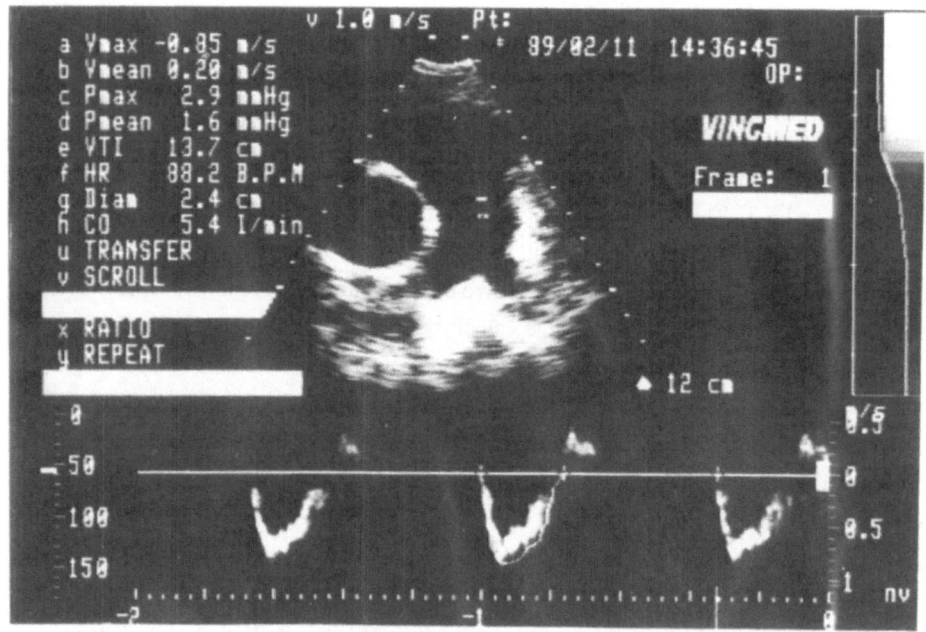

Fig. 3-7. The cardiac output can be estimated at the pulmonary valve using pulsed Doppler, as demonstrated in this example. The diameter of the pulmonary artery was measured at the same level as the sample volume, and was used to calculate the cross-sectional area. The velocity time integral (VTI) is multiplied by the cross-sectional area to obtain the stroke volume. The stroke volume is then multiplied by the heart rate to calculate the cardiac output.

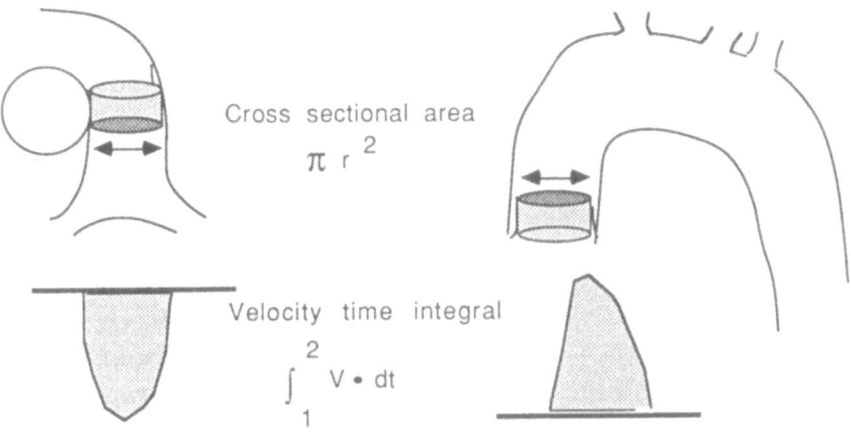

Fig. 3-8. *The cardiac output can be measured at either the pulmonary artery (left), or the aorta (right) in most patients. The cross-sectional area is derived from the two dimensional diameter measurement (arrow), and the Doppler is used to measure the velocity time integral.*

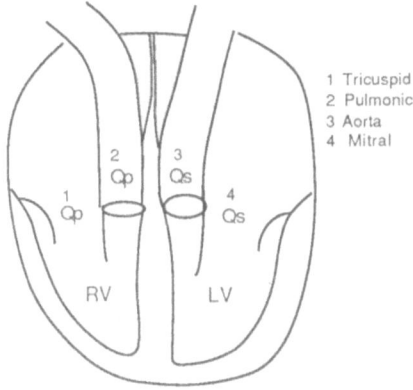

1 Tricuspid
2 Pulmonic
3 Aorta
4 Mitral

$$Qp / Qs = \frac{V{\cdot}A_p}{V{\cdot}A_s}$$

Fig. 3-9. *This figure demonstrates the manner in which the Doppler derived measurement of the cardiac output can be used to calculate the Qp/Qs ratio in a patient without shunting or regurgitations. The pulmonic flow can be measured from either the tricuspid or pulmonary positions, and the systemic flow can be measured from the mitral or aortic positions.*

The Clinical Measurement of Blood Flow

There are several sites in the heart where the cardiac output can be measured. The site selected for the measurement is dependent on the examination windows available and the specific information required. The sites most commonly applied are, in order of importance, the aortic, pulmonic, mitral, and tricuspid.

The Aortic Site

The volume of left ventricular outflow is usually measured at the level of the aortic valves maximum cusp separation. We prefer this position for practical reasons, first, it is not always possible to measure the flow velocity and the diameter measurement (used to calculate the flow circuit's cross-sectional area) from the same position. The aortic cusp serves as a position marker so that flow information can be measured from the suprasternal notch (from which a good beam to flow alignment can be obtained), and the diameter measured from the parsternal long axis view (from which a good window for the diameter measurement can be obtained). Another important factor is that this is the position in the flow circuit at which the flow profile is most likely to be flat.

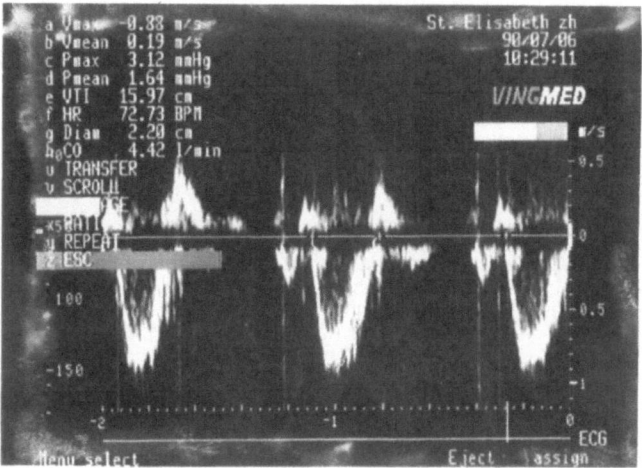

Fig. 3-10..In this study, the cardiac output is measured from the aorta in a healthy young adult. The sample volume is positioned at the level of the aortic cusp from the suprasternal notch and the diameter used to calculate cross-sectional area is measured from the parasternal long axis view.

The Pulmonic Site

The right ventricular outflow volume is usually measured at the level of either the infundibular ring, or the maximum cusp separation, or in the main pulmonary. We feel that the exact site of measurement in the right ventricular outflow tract is not as important as in aortic measurements because A) the flow velocity and the diameter can usually be made from the same position and B) the flow profile is somewhat less variable than in the left ventricular outflow tract. The left parasternal position at the second or third intercostal space is the most frequently applied window for this measurement. It is often necessary to turn the patient to an extreme left lateral position so that the lateral wall of the pulmonary artery can be measured. Fig.3-11 demonstrates a typical study used for the measurement of the cardiac output at the level of the main pulmonary artery in a healthy adolescent.

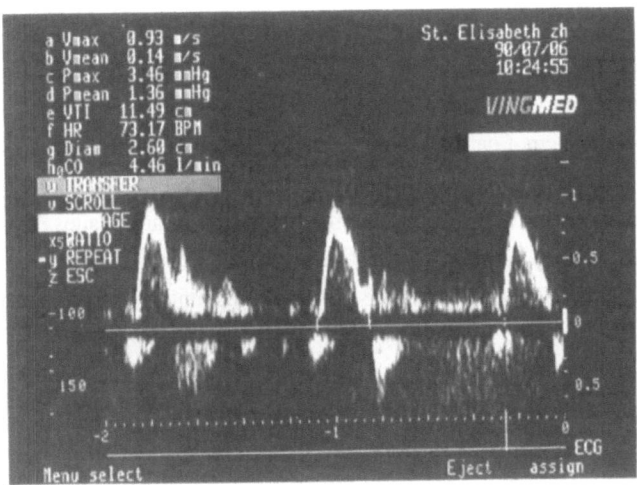

Fig. 3-11. In this study, the cardiac output is measured from the pulmonary artery in a healthy adolescent. The sample volume is positioned in the main pulmonary artery, permitting measurement of both the diameter and the flow velocity from the same position.

The Mitral Site

The measurement of flow across the mitral valve is affected by the same factors discussed previously for the semilunar valve sites. Additionally, the fact that the flow circuit is elipsoid and the area changes temporally must be considered. The apical position is generally the most useful window for measuring the velocity of blood flow across both the atrioventricular valves. The diameter of the mitral anulus can be used to calculate the cross-sectional area, though the geometry of the orifice is then assumed to be circular, introducing error into the calculation.

To circumvent these problems in the mitral flow calculation, several methods have been proposed for the correction of the temporal changes in the flow circuit's cross-sectional area. The short axis of the mitral valve is measured from the left parasternal window, which removes the assumption of a circular geometry. However, due to the fact that the orifice at the level of the valve tips is much more variable than at the level of the annulus, correction of these temporal changes is required. The TM mode echocardiogram of the mitral valve can be recorded, the separation of the leaflets measured at small time intervals, integrated, divided by the diastolic flow period, then divided by the maximal leaflet excursion to correct temporal changes in the flow area. In practice, this measurement can be quite difficult to apply, and there are several potential sources of error which might be introduced i.e. error in the flow measurement, errors in the 2D measurements, errors in the TM measurement, and the fact that these measurements must out of necessity be performed at different times.

Measurement of the Qp/Qs Ratio

The ratio between pulmonary to systemic blood flow, or Qp/Qs ratio, can be used to evaluate the hemodynamic significance of cardiac shunting at various levels in the heart. In a normal heart, the pulmonary flow can be measured at either the tricuspid or pulmonary artery sampling sites, and the systemic flow can be measured at either the mitral or aortic sites. The pulmonic flow and systemic flow are approximately equal, however, due to the inherent inaccuracies in flow volume calculations small discrepancies are frequently encountered, even when there is no shunting present.

In the abnormal situation where there is a shunting of blood flow, the sampling sites for measurement of the pulmonic to systemic flow are dependent on the level of the shunt [3,4,5]. In the case of an atrial septal defect, Qp is measured at either the tricuspid or pulmonary site, and Qs is sampled at either the mitral or aortic sites. If the shunt is at the ventricular level, Qp is measured at the pulmonary or mitral site, and Qs is measured at either the tricuspid or aortic site. This is due to the fact that the shunting of blood from the left ventricle increases the volume of blood in the right ventricle passing through pulmonary circulation. Therefore, more blood flows across the pulmonic valve than the tricuspid valve which means that the trans tricuspid flow does not reflect pulmonary flow. However, the tricuspid flow does represent the flow to systemic circulation and can be used for the Qs measurement. The aortic site can also be used to measure Qs in these patients. In the setting of patent ductus arteriosus the flow to the pulmonary circulation is increased at the level of the pulmonary artery branch. Therefore the trans mitral and aortic flows represent pulmonary circulation. Pulmonic valve and tricuspid flows can be used to measure systemic flow.

The accuracy of the Qp/Qs ratio is limited by the factors previously reviewed in the discussion of volumetric flow measurements. In our experience, even when the Qp/Qs ratio's absolute value is inaccurate, relevant semi-quantitative information can be extrapolated. Another means of qualitatively assessing the shunt severity is to compare the Qp flow's mean velocity or velocity time integral to that obtained from the Qs measurement site. While differences in the flow circuit's cross-sectional areas are ignored, it is possible to differentiate no-shunt situations from hemodynamically significant shunts.

When discussing the accuracy of the Doppler derived measurement of the Qp/Qs ratio in comparison with invasive techniques, it must be mentioned that the invasively derived "gold standards", i.e. thermal dilution or oximetry, are also subject to inherent inaccuracies.

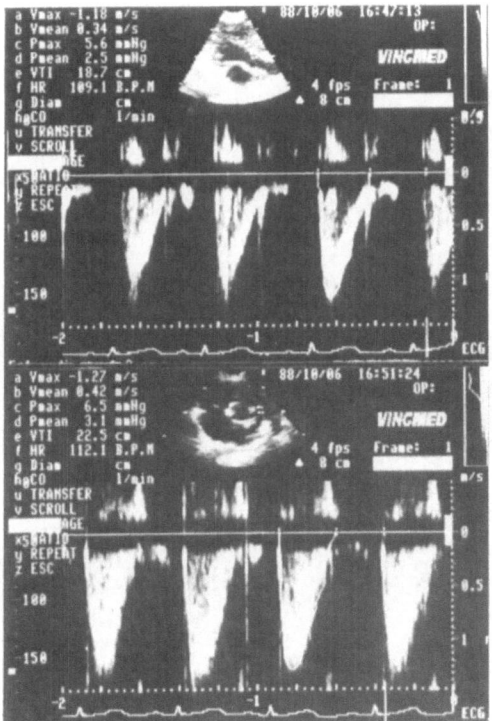

Fig. 3-12. The aortic flow velocity time integral and the pulmonary flow velocity time integral can be compared to obtain a qualitative assessment of the presence of blood flow shunting. The Qp/Qs ratio calculated from these data is 1.2 : 1.0, we consider ratios greater than 0.5 : 1.0 to indicate a shunt.

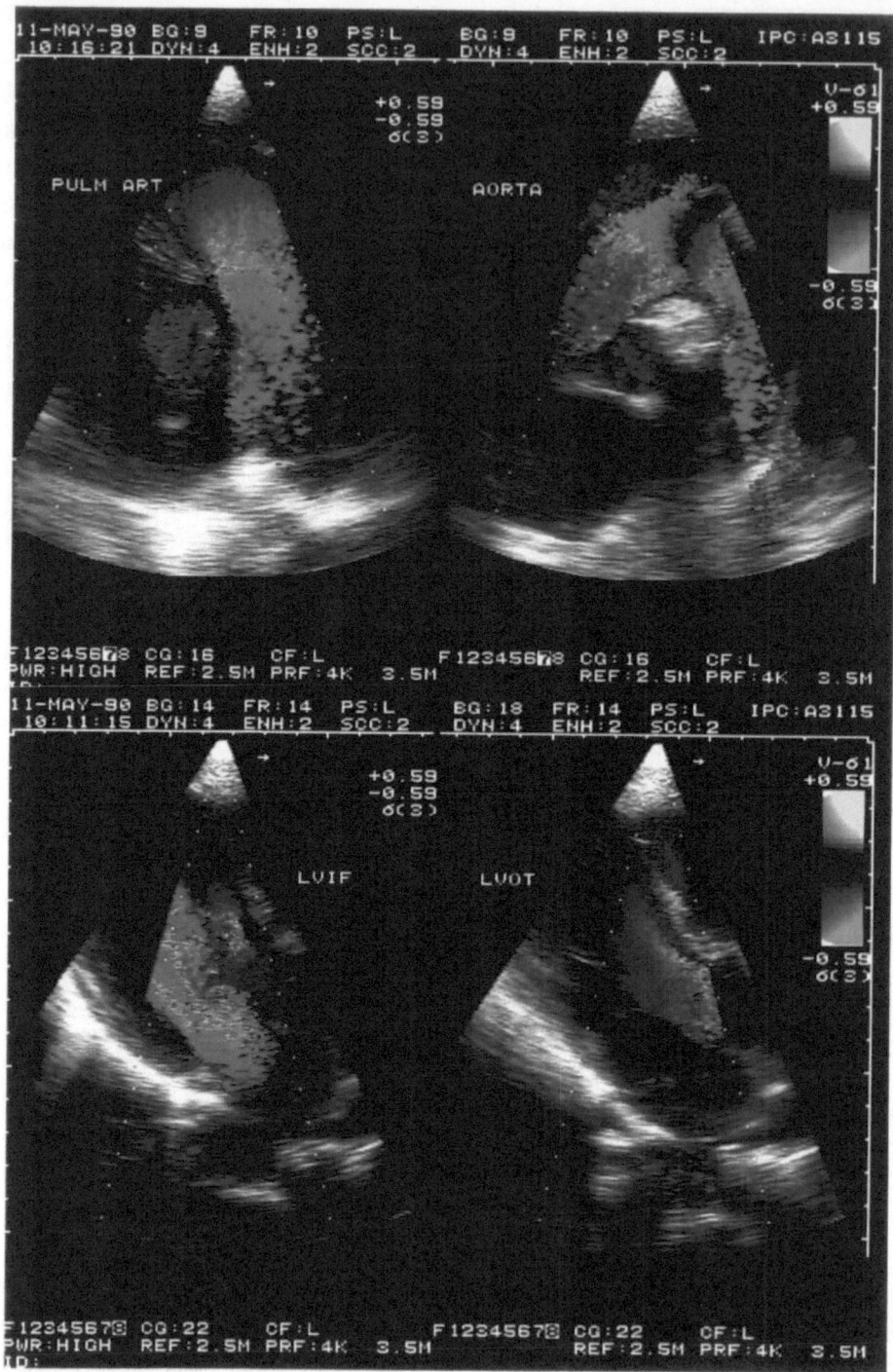

Color Plate 3-1. This series of images is from a healthy 14 year old boy. The aliased blood flow in the the main pulmonary artery (A) , and in the aorta (B) is due to the low Nyquist limit rather than abnormal flow. The left ventricular inflow (C) and outflow (D) are demonstrated in diastole and systole, respectively.

References

1) Shepard JT, Vanhoutte PM. Components of the cardiovascular system. In: The Human Cardiovascular System pp 1-62, New York, Raven Press, 1979.

2) Grossman W. Blood flow measurement: The cardiac output. In: Cardiac Catheterization and Angiography pp 89-102, Philadelphia, Lea and Febiger, 1980.

3) Brun P, Meguira A, Strauss A. Intracardiac Flow Dynamics. pp 37-55, In: Basic Concepts in Doppler Echocardiography, Chapman J, Sgalambro A. Editors, Dordrecht, Martinus Nijhoff, 1987.

4) Ihelen H, Amilie JP, Dale J. et al. Determination of Cardiac Output by Doppler echocardiography. Br. Heart J. 51, 54-60.

5) Skjaerpe T. Measurement of Cardiac Output, pp 128-140, In Cardiac Doppler Ultrasound. Houston A., Simpson I. Editors, London, Wright, 1988.

THE NORMAL EXAMINATION TECHNIQUE

James V. Chapman

Introduction

As with two-dimensional imaging, the optimal application of the various Doppler techniques necessitates that the investigator approaches the examination in a systematic and organized manner. Unlike two-dimensional imaging in which a suboptimal examination technique will result in suboptimal, but still interpretable images being obtained, in Doppler applications a suboptimal examination may result in erroneous measurements. This fact defines a fundamental difference between imaging and flow measurements, it is inherently more difficult to standardize the Doppler examination in terms of routine transducer positions. If one wishes to image the aortic valve, a parasternal window is used. It may be necesssary to move the probe around somewhat to optimize the image. But when the best visualization of the valves is obtained, it is fairly straightforward. Either one obtains a useful image, or one does not. For the measurement of flow velocities across the aortic valve however, it may be necessary to use the apical window, the subcostal window, the suprasternal window, the right parasternal window, or some variation thereof. While the flow may be measured from each of these windows, the true peak velocity might only be measurable from one of them. Therefore, a situation is encountered in which measuring the flow velocity is inadequate; it must be further demonstrated that an accurate measurement has been made. Slight errors in the measurement of velocity can translate into a significant error in the Doppler derived pressure gradient measurements.

We have reviewed some of the fundamental principles of blood flow in the previous chapter. The various clinical and technical factors related to the use of Doppler to measure flow velocities and to characterize various flow parameters, such as turbulence or laminarity of blood flow, were also discussed. One often thinks in terms of visualizing the heart with ultrasound, and observing blood flow with Doppler ultrasonic methods. In fact, one is observing the reflection or backscattering of acoustic energy from cardiac tissue or blood flow, which is quite different. While these methods yield information which can very closely approximate the anatomy and physiology, one must be aware of factors which can affect the clinical interpretation of the ultrasonic data.

The Characterization of Blood Flow by Doppler Ultrasound

From the previous chapter, we can make the following general statements about laminar flow: A) the flow is generally moving in the same direction (neglecting small changes at the boundary layer), and B) the flow profile may be either flat or parabolic. We would therefore expect the pulsed Doppler tracing to be narrow bandwidth, as this reflects the velocity distribution of flow crossing the sample cell. However, this also depends on the size of the sample cell, as larger sample cells will pick up backscattered signals over a larger area. For instance, if one interrogates the normal flow with a small sample cell in the center of the flow, a narrow bandwidth signal will be obtained. If the sample volume length is increased, the eddies at the boundary area of the flow are also sampled resulting in a spectral broadening. If we then extend this discussion to continuous wave Doppler, it becomes apparent that pulsed Doppler will usually yield a narrower bandwidth signal than continuous wave Doppler from the same beam direction in the same flow. However, if the sample volume is decreased too much, the transit time effect can result in spectral broadening as well. If the velocity of blood flow exceeds the Nyquist limit, aliasing occurs. This is manifested as spectral broadening, and indeed, when severe aliasing occurs a very wideband signal is noted even in the presence of organized flow.

Color flow imaging can also be used to characterize blood flow. The same factors influencing the spectral bandwidth (or variance) in a conventional pulsed Doppler systems applies to the color flow mapping mode (which is a multigated pulsed Doppler system). These include sampling and analysis rates, sample volume dimensions, and the presence of aliasing. In the setting of laminar flow measured with color flow mapping, the flow image will be either red or blue, although if aliasing is present the red, blue, and green may be mixed together. An important point to keep in mind is that to a color flow imaging system, wideband signals have a high degree of variance regardless of their etiology. There have been many descriptions of turbulent flow based on Doppler ultrasonic findings in the literature. Variance and mosaic flow patterns are terms which have been used to describe disturbed flow based on Doppler derived measurements, but can be due to aliasing.

Based on the previous description of turbulent flow, one can make the following general statements; A) The flow is disorganized with backscattering targets travelling at different velocities and in different directions, B) the flow profile is generally flat and C) there are various transition states where the flow structure may have both laminar and turbulent flow characteristics. Note that high velocity was not stated as a criteria, as low velocity disorganized flow can also be encountered. If the high velocity jet across the stenotic aortic valve were a turbulent flow, one would be unable to apply the Bernoulli equation to calculate pressure gradients. The Bernoulli equation relates the pressure drop and velocity in a laminar flow state. This is an interesting point; we are using terms which imply very specific criteria to describe flows which do not strictly adhere to these criteria.

With the application of color flow imaging, the complexity of characterizing flow is in some ways compounded. Most color flow mapping systems incorporate an algorithm for displaying disturbed flow areas. We prefer the term disturbed flow indicator rather than "mosaic" flow pattern for two reasons. First, as we have stated in the previous chapter, it is our opinion that the mosaic flow map is inferior to a direct shift to solid green for the demonstration of abnormal flows. Secondly, we wish to point out once more that the colors, or mixtures thereof, have no inherent value. What is important is that one collects and analyzes the Doppler information in such a way that the accuracy of the data is optimized (within the constraints of the techniques described in Chapter I and II), and the color map implemented optimizes the display of this information. In the system we are using, flow towards the probe is encoded red, flow away is encoded blue, and green is used as the disturbed flow indicator.

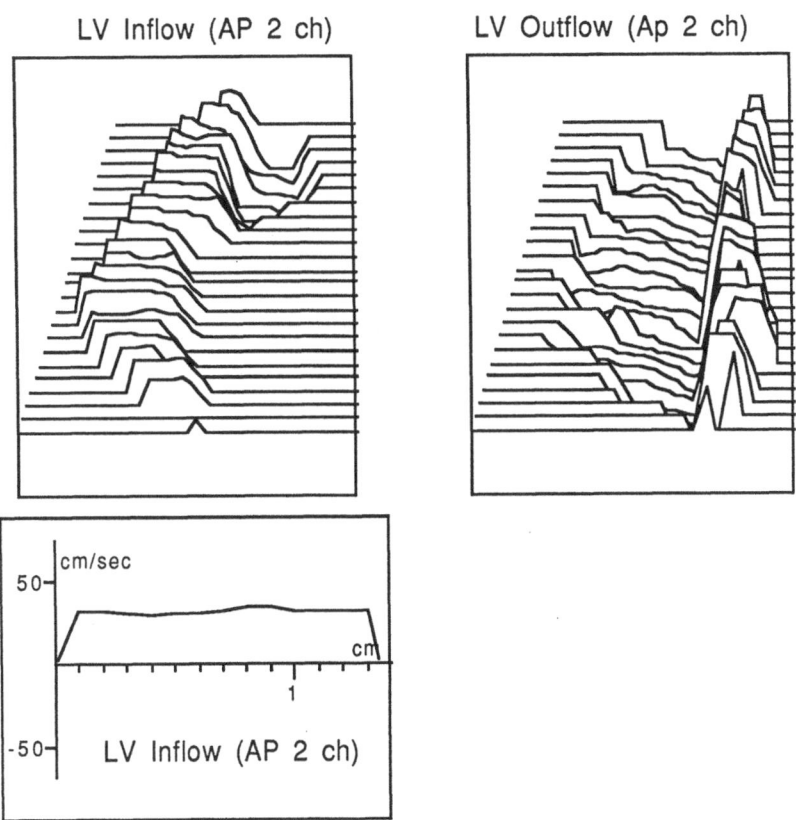

Fig. 4-1. *A multigate Doppler recording of left ventricular inflow (upper left) and outflow (upper right) obtained from the apical two chamber view. Note the organized flow characteristic of the normal laminar flow pattern. A single gate is used to demonstrate the flow profile at a specific depth (lower left) and for quantitative measurement of the mean velocity.*

One sometimes encounters what appears to be disturbed flow regions in normal flows. A common example of this is seen when observing normal diastolic filling in the left ventricle. The forward flow through the mitral valve is encoded in red,while a bolus of flow occurring shortly after the onset of transmitral flow directed towards the outflow tract is encoded in blue. Between these flows, one notes the disturbed flow indication in green. This is due to the fact that at the interface of these two flows (transmitral and recirculation towards the outflow tract) the sampled signal represents flow in both directions and it is interpreted as disturbed flow. One can draw certain conclusions regarding the flow structure, but it is important to consider first all the factors which influence the color encoding when doing so.

The Normal Doppler Examination

   In the following section we will review the various blood flow recordings obtained at different positions in the heart and vessels. The normal interrogation sites include the aortic and pulmonary valves, the left ventricular and right ventricular outflow tracts, the mitral and tricuspid valves, the ascending, descending and abdominal aorta, the superior vena cava, inferior vena cava, and the hepatic veins. The interatrial and ventricular septum can routinely be evaluated in pediatric patients, however there should be no flow at these sites in normal patients. We will present a review of normal flow velocities in patients of different age groups in this chapter.

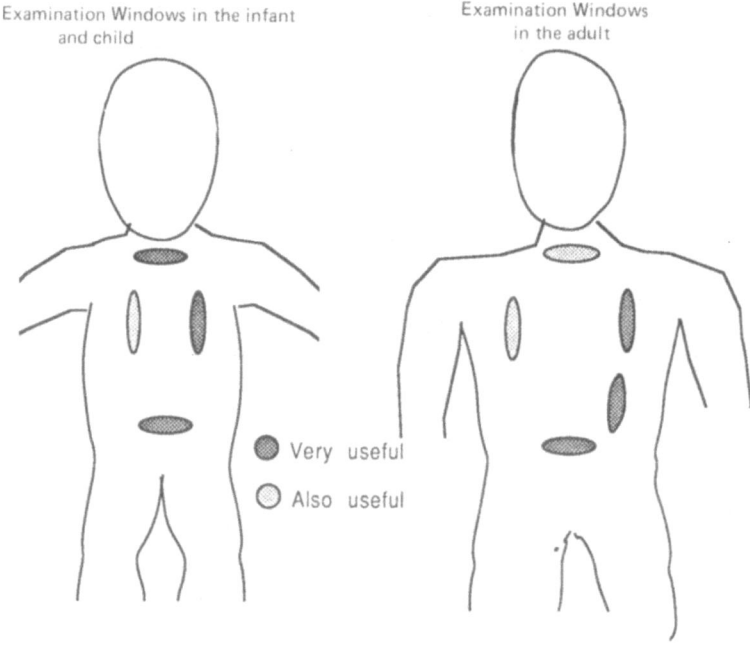

Fig. 4-2. These schematics demonstrate the useful Doppler interrogation windows implemented in the examination of both the pediatric and adult patient. The same windows are used in both, however the apical window is generally more important in adults, and the suprasternal notch window is more useful in children.

The Acoustic Windows and Transducer Positions

The Doppler ultrasound method of measuring blood flow requires that a good alignment between the Doppler beam and flow be obtained. The investigation therefore necessitates the use of several transducer positions. The most useful views in pediatric applications are the parasternal window, the subcostal window, the suprasternal window, and the apical window. In adult patients the left and right parasternal and apical windows are frequently used, the subcostal and right parasternal windows are used less often. The spatial complexities of congenital heart disease necessitate the use of non-standard views.

The use of multiple windows should ascertain that the peak velocity has been recorded. The schematic in Figure 4-2 demonstrates the areas of the heart which can be interrogated by Doppler ultrasound. The pulmonary artery and tricuspid valve can be examined by Doppler from the left parasternal position (LPS) and a good beam-to-flow alignment can be obtained. Color flow mapping can be used to study these flows as well as the mitral valve and left ventricular outflow tract, which do not offer good beam-to-flow alignment from this window. The subcostal window can be used to obtain measurements from the pulmonary artery and tricuspid valve for quantitative measurements, and the interatrial and ventricular septum are usually quite well visualized. The apical window is usually used to study the atrioventricular valves, the left ventricular outflow tract, the left ventricle, and the aorta. The suprasternal notch position is the primary site for visualizing the aortic arch, from the valve to the thoracic aorta, the superior vena cava can also be visualized and flows measured from this window. The right parasternal window is primarily used to evaluate the aortic valve and ascending aorta, however this view is generally more useful in the setting of aortic stenosis. One should not limit the study to these windows alone, as the important requirement is that the velocity be accurately measured.

For infants, the body position is not really very important; the child can be supine, or held by the mother or an assistant. We prefer to place older children and adults in a left lateral position. It is sometimes helpful to have the patient supine with the knees flexed for the subcostal view. When performing the suprasternal notch view the patient should be placed in a supine position with a pillow behind the shoulders and slight hyperextension of the neck. With pediatric patients, we generally save the suprasternal and subcostal examination for the end of the study when possible. These windows are frequently uncomfortable, and the patient often becomes agitated at this point in the examination. As penetration with high frequency probes is not usually a problem in the pediatric patient, and lower frequency probes can be used for adults, almost every flow in the heart can be examined using one of the windows described in this chapter.

Evaluation of Left Ventricular Outflow and Transaortic Blood Flow

Left ventricular outflow can frequently be interrogated from the apical window in both children and adults [1,2]. The pulsed mode recording is obtained by placing the sample volume in the left ventricular outflow tract below the aortic valve. In normal adults, a systolic flow signal is recorded with a peak velocity in the 0.7 to 1.1 m/s range. The maximal flow velocity is slightly higher in children, and flow velocities up to 1.7 m/s are often encountered. The morphology of this flow velocity curve differs from the aortic flow pattern in two respects. The value of the peak outflow velocity is less than the value of the peak aortic velocity, and the peak outflow velocity occurs later in systole. The result is a more "rounded" flow pattern when compared to the flow pattern recorded in the ascending aorta.

As the sample volume is moved closer to the aortic valve, the closing valve spike and then the opening valve spike originating from cusp movement through the sample volume is detected. It is not uncommon to record mitral flow in diastole along with systolic left ventricular outflow. This flow contamination is due to the proximity of the inflow and outflow circuits. The mitral flow signal can be differentiated from the signal of aortic insufficiency on the basis of timing and peak velocity. The signal of aortic regurgitation begins immediately after aortic valve closure, but mitral flow does not begin until after isovolumic relaxation. The peak mitral velocity is significantly lower than the peak regurgitant flow velocity. The color flow analysis of left ventricular outflow may be performed from the apical window or from an intermediate transducer position between the apex and the left sternal border. By late diastole, a flow bolus in shades of blue is visualized in the left ventricular cavity. When left ventricular ejection occurs, there is movement of this bolus into the outflow tract. The peak outflow velocity may exceed the Nyquist value, resulting in color aliasing.

The aortic valve flow is generally best recorded from either the apical or suprasternal notch position in both the pediatric and adult patient. With the transducer in the apical position a systolic flow away from the transducer is sampled (Fig.4-6). There is a rapid flow acceleration with a slightly prolonged deceleration.

The opening and closing of the aortic valve is recorded if the cusps enter the pulsed Doppler sample volume. From the suprasternal notch position the same flow characteristics are noted. As the systolic outflow approaches the transducer from this window, a positive signal is obtained. The spectral bandwidth is narrow during acceleration, with a slight spectral broadening during deceleration. The high pass filters should be set high enough to remove the low frequency signals generated by valve and wall motion. The parasternal transducer position is of limited use to interrogate the blood flow through the aortic valve, as there is a poor beam-to-flow alignment. The subcostal window can sometimes be used to measure aortic flow in the pediatric patient, but is of limited use in adult patient.

The entire ascending aorta can be examined from the suprasternal notch position. The left clavicular window is a good alternative in children. However, in most children the ascending aorta can be well visualized from either window. Using pulsed Doppler, the sample volume is positioned in different regions of the aortic lumen.

Aortic Blood Flow

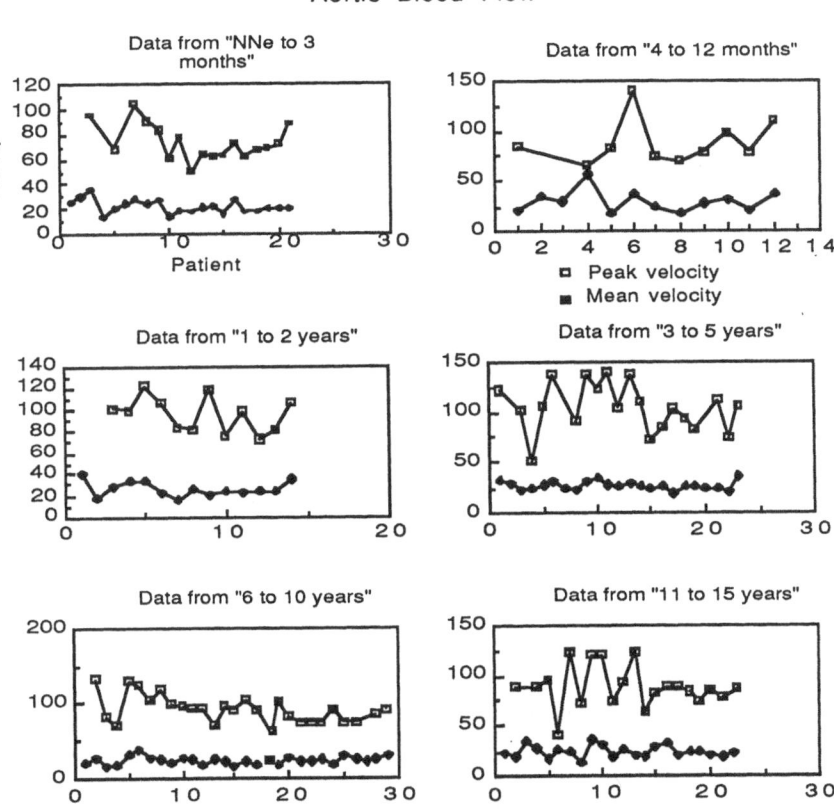

Fig. 4-3. These tables demonstrate the trans-aortic blood flow velocities measured in normal subjects. Various age groups , from the neonate (nne) to fifteen years, were studied. The open boxes represent the peak velocities, and the solid boxes represent the mean velocity.

Quite different flow velocities can be sampled at different sites. The systolic flow tracing will register above the baseline, as the flow is towards the transducer when recorded from this window. Flow in the ascending aorta may also be sampled from the suprasternal, or right parasternal windows, and infrequently from the subcostal window, but in most normal subjects the best recording is usually obtained from the suprasternal window. The bidimensional image permits visualization of the ascending aorta, which is located on the left side of the sector, the transverse aorta which is located at the top of the sector, and the descending aorta which is located on the right side of the sector. The aortic valve can sometimes be visualized from the suprasternal window in children; this occurs far less frequently in adults.

To perform the pulsed Doppler interrogation of the ascending aorta, the sample volume is placed in the lumen just distal to the valve. The transducer angulation is changed slightly until a narrow bandwidth signal is obtained. If an optimal beam-to-flow angle cannot be achieved from this position, the right parasternal window should be used. The transducer is placed in the second or third right intercostal space and angled medial and inferior so that the ascending aorta is visualized. The peak aortic flow velocity ranges from 0.7 to 1.6 m/s in normal adults; the normal range is slightly higher in children. The characteristic normal ascending aortic flow pattern obtained by color flow mapping from the apical window is demonstrated as a red flow bolus in the ascending aorta moving towards the suprasternal notch in systole. The flow profile usually appears flat as the flow crosses the valve, becoming more parabolic as the distance from the valve becomes greater. A skewing of the flow profile towards the inner bend of the ascending aorta can often be noted (fig. 4-4).

The pulsed mode is most often implemented to record the flow in the descending aorta. The sample volume is positioned in the lumen of the descending aorta distal to the subclavian artery, although one often samples diastolic run off into the left subclavian artery and left common carotid artery as well. The peak flow velocity in the descending aorta is usually slightly less than that in the ascending aorta and the curve itself is more "rounded".

With the color flow mapping technique, the systolic flow in the descending aorta is seen as a blue flow bolus moving away from the transducer; the flow profile may appear to be skewed to the outer wall of the descending aorta.

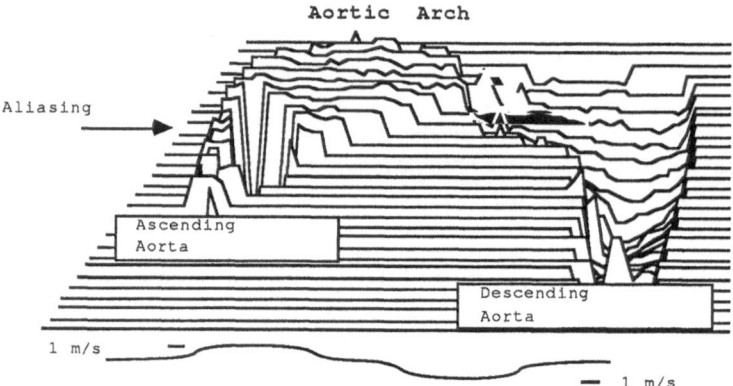

Fig. 4-4. A multigate Doppler study of the ascending and descending aorta obtained from the suprasternal notch of a subject with normal aortic flow. Each horizontal line depicts the mean velocity at a specific depth, the calibration is demonstrated below. Aliasing is noted at the level of the valve in the ascending aorta.

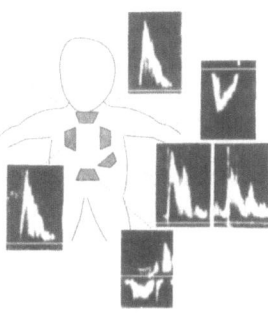

Fig. 4-5. This figure demonstrates the flow velocity tracings which can be sampled from the various windows. Clockwise from the top: the ascending aortic flow (suprasternal notch), pulmonary flow (left parasternal window), the mitral and tricuspid flow (apical window), the pulmonary flow (subcostal window), and the aortic flow (right parasternal window).

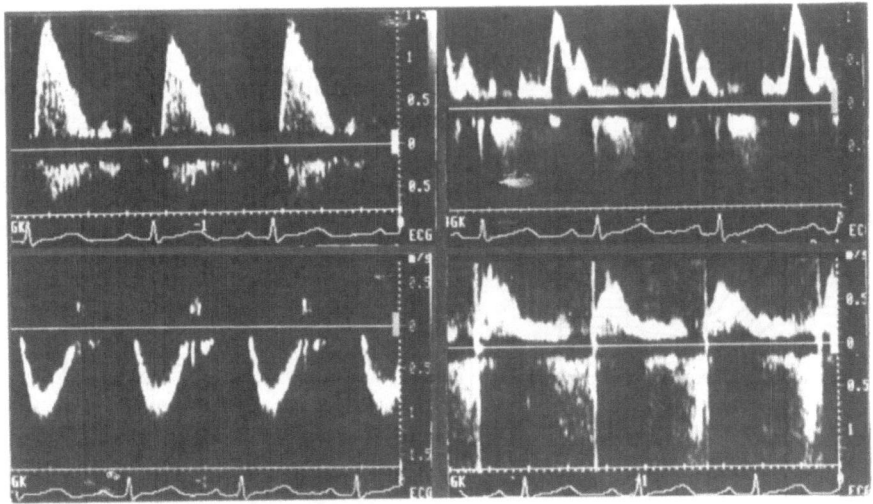

Fig. 4-6. These recordings from a normal eight year old girl demonstrate the aortic (A) mitral (B), pulmonary (C), and tricuspid (D) flow. A small regurgitation is demonstrated behind the tricuspid valve. The mitral and tricuspid flows are biphasic, and a beat-to-beat variation in the peak velocity of the tricuspid flow is demonstrated. The peak velocity of aortic flow occurs earlier than that of the pulmonary flow, giving the pulmonary flow velocity curve a more rounded appearance.

Evaluation of Pulmonary Artery Blood Flow

Pulmonary flow can be examined from the left parasternal window in both children and adults, and the subcostal imaging window is also frequently used in children [3,4]. The pulsed Doppler recording is obtained by positioning the sample volume slightly downstream from the pulmonary valve. A negative flow velocity curve is recorded in systole. The peak flow velocity in adults will be in the 0.6 to 1.3 m/s range, although the maximal velocity may exceed this range in normal children.

The pulmonary flow velocity curve has a more rounded contour than the aortic flow trace, and the peak pulmonary velocity occurs later in systole. The morphology of the pulmonary flow curve is altered with changes in sample volume placement within the arterial lumen. When the sample volume is positioned too close to the vessel wall, a marked systolic flow reversal can be recorded. When the sample volume is positioned in the center of flow, the audio signal is clear and the contour of the flow pattern is well deliniated.

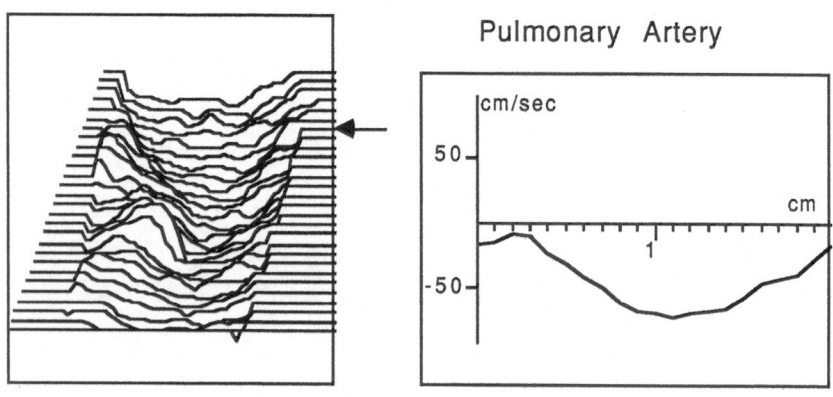

Fig. 4-7. A multigated Doppler study of right ventricular outflow in a normal subject. The peak velocities occur at the level of the valve. The flow is organized, with a slightly skewed profile noted. A positive flow component is demonstrated in the main pulmonary artery, and represents a flow eddy (left). A single range gate (arrow) is extracted to permit measurements of the mean velocity (right).

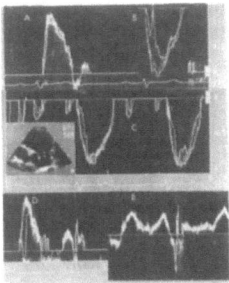

Fig. 4-8. This study was obtained from a 4 month old baby. The left ventricular outflow was measured from a low parasternal window (top) and the right ventricular outflow was interrogated from a right parasternal position (bottom).

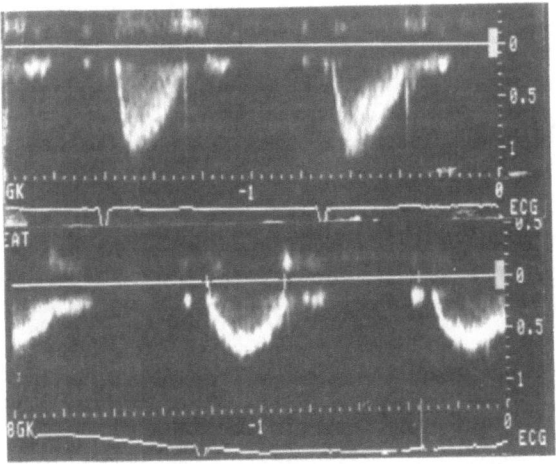

Fig. 4-9. The aortic (top) and pulmonary (bottom) flow velocity traces obtained by pulsed mode interrogation from the subcostal window in a seven year old child. Narrow bandwidth signals have been obtained in each trace. The peak velocity is lower in the pulmonary artery than in the aorta.

After recording a well-defined pulmonary flow curve, the right ventricular ejection time and the pulmonary acceleration time can be measured. The right ventricular ejection time is the period in which systolic pulmonary flow takes place; it is the interval from the beginning to the end of pulmonary flow. The pulmonary acceleration time is defined as the time interval required from the onset of flow to the peak flow velocity. It is measured as the period of time elapsed between the beginning of the flow trace and the peak of the flow trace. Generally, the pulmonary artery acceleration time is greater than 110 ms in normal adult subjects, but is usually shorter in pediatric patients. In the presence of elevated pulmonary artery pressure, the acceleration time is decreased. The value of these time interval measurements may vary from beat to beat, and a mean value should be calculated to minimize error.

In normal individuals, a weak diastolic regurgitant flow signal can often be detected when the sample volume is positioned in the right ventricular outflow tract, slightly proximal to the pulmonary valve. This low velocity flow can often be recorded only in mid- to late-diastole. The presence of this insignificant pulmonary insufficiency signal is often described as physiological. The position in which a signal from physiological insufficiency is sampled is confined to a very discrete region behind the pulmonary valve.

The color flow mapping study of pulmonary flow is generally performed from the parasternal window in the pediatric and adult subject, and the subcostal window is often useful for interrogating this flow in children. A flow bolus encoded in shades of blue is seen in the pulmonary artery during systole. The flow profile in the right ventricular outflow tract may appear to be skewed, becoming flat as the flow crosses the pulmonary valve, a parabolic flow profile may be visualized at a distance from the flow inlet. The core flow velocity may exceed the Nyquist value, and color aliasing may be observed in the center of the flow bolus.

The physiological pulmonary insufficiency detected with conventional pulsed mode can also be demonstrated with color flow imaging. The regurgitant flow is represented as a small red flame originating from the valvular level. The flow is localized to a discrete area behind the pulmonary valve, extending for approximately 1.0 cm into the right ventricular outflow tract. The orientation of the jet changes throughout diastole.

Evaluation of Mitral Blood Flow

The pulsed mode examination of mitral flow is most commonly performed from the apical window [5,6]. The sample volume is positioned in the mitral annulus and moved to the tips of the leaflets to measure the highest flow velocities. The normal mitral flow is biphasic; there are two components of transmitral flow, passive filling and a component occurring with atrial contraction. The passive filling component has a higher peak velocity than the atrial flow component, lying in the range of 0.6 to 1.3 m/s in adults, and velocities of up to 1.8 m/s are often noted in children. The passive filling component is also known as the E wave, while the atrial component is known as the A wave; if the "A" wave is of higher velocity than the "E" wave, one should suspect left ventricular dysfunction, hypertension, (or an acute myocardial infarct). The pulsed Doppler recording of mitral flow is a fairly sensitive indicator of alterations in the left ventricular filling pattern. The biphasic nature of left ventricular inflow is dependent upon the cardiac rhythm. In the presence of atrial fibrillation, the A wave will obviously be absent.

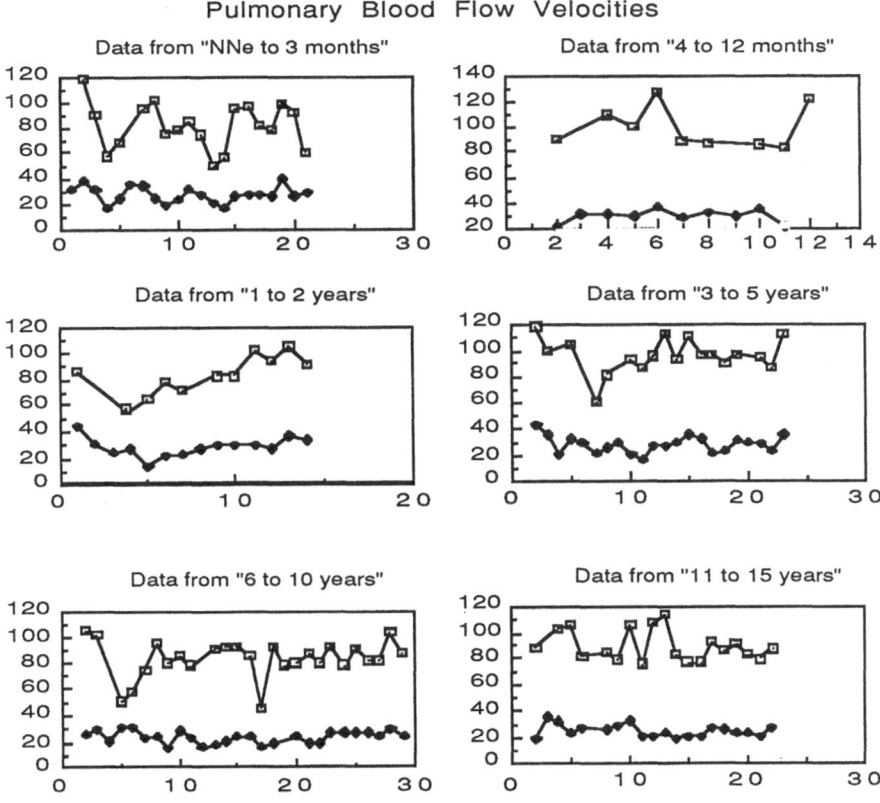

Fig. 4-10. These tables demonstrate the peak and mean pulmonary valve flow velocities measured in the same subject as the aortic flow.

The color flow analysis of left ventricular inflow from the apical examination window demonstrates a diastolic flow bolus in shades of red moving towards the cardiac apex. The flow is directed along the posterior left ventricular wall and flow adjacent to the wall is clearly visualized in normal subjects. Following atrial contraction, an increase in the flow bolus dimensions is noted. Flow eddy formation in mid- to late-diastole may be observed in patients with low heart rates. The eddies will be depicted in shades of blue. In late diastole, the flow direction reverses, and flow is towards the left ventricular outflow tract.

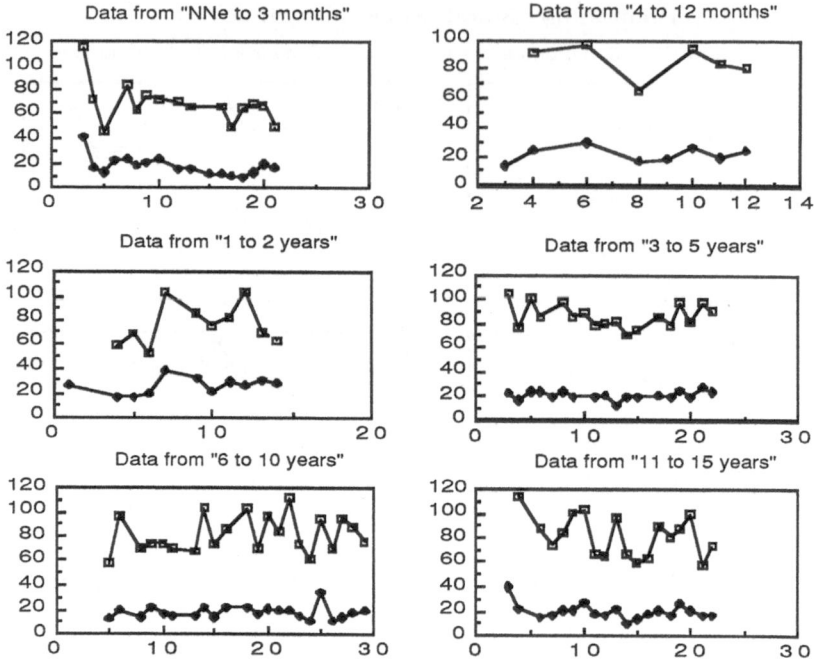

Fig. 4-11. Normal trans-mitral flow velocities from same patient groups

Evaluation of Tricuspid Blood Flow

The pulsed Doppler recording of tricuspid flow is obtained from either the apical or left parasternal imaging window in both children and adults. The sample volume is placed slightly distal to the tricuspid valve, and a positive biphasic diastolic flow pattern is recorded. The passive filling component normally has a higher amplitude than the atrial flow component. The peak flow velocity is generally less than the mitral peak velocity, lying in the 0.3 to 0.7 m/s range, in children the velocity is higher (up to 1.0 m/s). Tricuspid flow varies with respiration; this characteristic can help to distinguish tricuspid flow from mitral flow .

In the study of normal tricuspid flow, a high incidence of physiological tricuspid insufficiency has been reported. The regurgitant flow can frequently be detected when the sample volume is positioned proximal to the tricuspid valve. The signal intensity is usually quite weak because of the small regurgitant flow volume.

Color flow analysis of tricuspid flow is performed from the either the parasternal or apical windows in both children and adults. A diastolic flow bolus in shades of red will be seen in the right ventricular cavity. The flow is usually more clearly delineated from the parasternal window, probably because of the reduced interrogation depth. When physiological insufficiency is present, a small systolic jet in shades of blue appears at the level of the tricuspid annulus. The jet extension is about localized proximal to the valve in physiological insufficiency and the jet width is narrow.

Evaluation of Pulmonary Venous Flow

The blood flow in the pulmonary veins can be interrogated from the apical transducer position in children and adults. In adults, the left upper pulmonary veins can often be interrogated, the lower pulmonary veins less so. In children the lower pulmonary veins are also frequently visualized. The normal flow velocity is low (<1m/s), and is a continuous flow with a late diastolic peak. The flow is best studied with pulsed Doppler, with a positive trace being obtained from the apical window. The high pass filters are reduced so as not to reject the low velocity pulmonary venous flow inadvertently.

Evaluation of the Superior and Inferior Vena Caval Flow

Flow in the superior vena cava may be studied by pulsed Doppler interrogation from the right supraclavicular, suprasternal (in children and adults), or subcostal windows (in children). The supraclavicular window frequently provides the best beam-to-flow alignment. The normal flow pattern in the superior vena cava and the hepatic veins consists of four components; there are two anterograde and two retrograde flows. The retrograde flow occurs following the P wave and the T wave of the electrocardiogram. These two components are termed the a wave and the v wave, respectively. The anterograde systolic flow is called the x wave, and usually has the highest velocity. The anterograde diastolic flow component is called the y wave. When recording at a small angle to flow, the peak velocity of the x wave ranges from 0.5 to 1.3 m/s in normal adults. This value is often higher in children and adolescents.

Flow in the inferior vena cava may be detected from the apical, parasternal, or subcostal window. The velocity pattern is similar to that of the superior vena cava. The velocity of flow in the caval veins increases with inspiration, although it is easier to demonstrate this when recording flow in the superior vena cava.

The color flow analysis of flow in the superior vena cava is performed from the right supraclavicular or suprasternal window. A flow bolus in shades of blue is visualized in diastole, frequently a short period of flow reversal after atrial contraction is noted. Systolic flow is depicted in shades of blue, and the flow reversal occurring after the T wave may not be visualized. Flow in the inferior vena cava is difficult to image with color analysis due to the near perpendicular beam-to-flow alignment.

Evaluation of Blood Flow in the Hepatic Veins

The blood flow in the hepatic veins is usually measured using the subcostal window in both children and adults. The veins are easily imaged in most patients and a good alignment to the flow is obtained. The flow is triphasic with two negative components, a systolic and a diastolic wave. The positive component is the A wave, resulting from atrial contraction. The magnitude of the flow velocity increases with inspiration and decreases with expiration. When recording this low velocity flow, it is necessary to decrease the high pass filters so as not to reject the desired information. It is usually better to use a larger sample volume so that the hepatic vein lumen is insonified, even if the vessel moves. In the color flow study, the flow, or the hepatic vein is blue during systolic with a small reversal of flow during atrial component encoded in red. This reversed flow ussually occurs over only a few frames, unlike the large reversal of flow noted during systole in patients with severe tricuspid regurgitation.

Measurement of Normal Blood Flows

The normal velocities in children depend of course on the size of the child, but heart rate has a significant impact on the velocity of blood measured at different time periods. The rapid contraction of the ventricle in small infants can generate a significant amount of wall motion artifact, so in these patients it is especially important to set the high pass filters high enough to remove artifact without rejecting clinically relevant information. Pulsed Doppler can be used to measure normal velocities in most patients. High pulse repetition frequency mode or spectral unwrapping of an aliased signal is sometimes required, usually when high frequency probes are used. There is frequently a beat to beat difference in velocities, and to improve the accuracy of the measurement several complexes should be measured. Another method which can be used is to temporally compress the Doppler traces in a digital memory and visually select a mean value from several complexes. Then the time base can be expanded so that accurate time and velocity measurements can be made. Tables containing normal values for various age groups are included in this chapter.

The normal flow in adults tends to be less variable, and the flow velocities are generally lower than those encountered in children. Pulsed Doppler can be used and the high pass filters need not be set as high in adults since the wall motion is less dynamic.

Regurgitation in Normal Valves

There have been several reports on the frequency of small regurgitations in normally functioning pulmonary and tricuspid valves [7]. There have also been reports of left-sided leaks, but with a much lower incidence. It has been our observation that as Doppler instrumentation has been refined over the last 8 or 9 years, the incidence of pulmonary and tricuspid insufficiency has increased. From our experience with transesophageal Doppler, we suspect that the incidence of mitral as well as aortic regurgitation is probably slightly more frequent than supposed. However, one must define the criteria by which a flow is termed regurgitant, as there is invariably some back flow caused by valve closure. This is especially the case in atrioventricular valves. Our criteria for defining a physiologic regurgitation is that the spectral Doppler recording from the regurgitation can be measured for more than half the time of valve closure, and the velocity will exceed 1.5 m/s on the right-sided valves and 2.5 m/s on the left-sided valves. These regurgitant flows are localized proximal to the valve, and can be difficult to record due to the artifact generated by the valve motion. These regurgitant flows are of interest, particularly for the tricuspid valve, as they can be used to estimate right-sided pressures.

Physiologic pulmonary insufficiency is the most frequent regurgitant flow encountered in normal subjects. It is sampled by placing the pulsed Doppler sample volume behind the tricuspid valve. A wideband signal, which can be of either weak or strong intensity, is sampled in the later half of diastole. In the setting of normal pulmonary artery pressure the velocity of flow will be less than 2.0 m/s. If the velocity exceeds the Nyquist limit, it will be necessary to implement either high pulse repetition frequency or continuous wave Doppler. The presence of an elevated velocity is evidence of pulmonary hypertension. The second most frequent regurgitant flow is from the tricuspid valve. The frequency of insufficiency is to a large extent dependent on how agressively one separates back flow from regurgitation. The large pliable leaflets appear to generate reverse flow eddies as they close more often than the other valves. This flow is most frequently measured from the left parasternal window, second or third intercostal space with a posterior medial angulation of the probe. The signal is wide bandwidth and one often records strong spikes caused by valve opening and closure. If the right ventricular pressure is not increased, the regurgitant flow will be under 2.50 m/s. We do not measure the tracing unless more than two thirds of systolic flow have been well recorded.

The presence of physiologic mitral regurgitation and aortic regurgitation are seen far less often . In our opinion, in the case of the mitral valve, this "regurgitation" is more often a back flow related valve closure. We have seen a significant number of small regurgitations in otherwise normally functioning valves by transesophageal examination in the adult patient. This could be due to a clearer imaging of back flow facilitated by the use of high frequency probes and a shallow interrogation depth. The most useful windows for sampling mitral regurgitation are the left parasternal or the apical window. The sample volume is positioned proximal to the valve behind the posterior leaflet. The jet is often eccentrically directed along the posterior leaflet and this is a good interception point. The high velocity reject should be increased as the valve motion tends to generate a high degree of noise.

In the case of the aortic valve, the apical window is the most useful for interrogating the outflow tract. Increasing the size of the sample volume can help to localize the small regurgitant jet more quickly. In color flow mapping applications the regurgitant jets sometimes occur on only two or three frames. A digital memory and cineloop function are quite helpful in extracting the regurgitant flow sequence. A gated ECG can also be used to isolate the frames which demonstrate the regurgitant flow.

References

1. Mowat DHR, Haites NE and Rawles JM. Aortic blood velocity measurements in healthy adults using a simple ultrasound technique. Cardiovas. Res. 1983 ; 17, 75-80.

2. Wilson N, Goldberg SJ, Dickinson DF, and Scott O. Normal intracardiac and great artery blood velocity measurements by pulsed Doppler echocardiography. Br. Heart J. 1985 ; 53, 451-458.

3. Hatle L, and Angelsen B. Doppler Ultrasound in Cardiology: Physical Principles and Clinical Applications, 2nd edn, pp. 74-76. Philadelphia: Lea and Febiger.

4. Gibbs JL, Wilson N, Witsenburg M, Williams GJ, and Goldberg SJ. Diastolic forward blood flow in the pulmonary artery detected by Doppler echocardiography. J. Am. Coll. Cardiol. 1985 ; 6, 1322-1328.

5. Kitabatake A, Inoue M, Asao M, et al. Transmitral blood flow reflecting diastolic behaviour of the left ventricle in health and disease. A study by pulsed Doppler. Jpn. Circ. J. 1982 ; 46, 92-102.

6. DeZuttere D, Touche T, Saumon G, et al. Doppler echocardiographic measurement of mitral flow volume : Validation of a new method in adults. JACC 1989 ; 11:343-50.

7. Berger M, Hecht S, Van Tosh A, Lingham U. Pulsed and continuous wave Doppler echocardiographic assessment of valvular regurgitation in normal subjects. JACC 1989 ; 13 :1540-5.

CHAPTER V

OBSTRUCTIVE LESIONS IN CONGENITAL HEART DISEASE

James V. Chapman

Ingrid Oberhaensli

Beat Friedli

Introduction

In the setting of stenosis and obstruction, several Doppler modalities can be used to obtain quantitative information concerning the lesion. The relevant measurements from a clinical perspective are the mean and maximal pressure gradient, and the valve area determination. These values can be derived by Doppler ultrasound with a high degree of accuracy and offer distinct advantages over invasive methods.

As a rule, conventional Doppler modes, i.e. pulsed and continuous wave Doppler modes, are implemented for these quantitative measurements. The requisite flow velocity information for the calculation of the the pressure gradient and the valve area contains high velocity components with a low signal strength. Therefore, a high sensitivity continuous wave Doppler mode is necessary in order to perform the quantitative analysis of the degree of obstruction. The echocardiographer currently using Doppler techniques in patients with acquired heart disease will note that the methods applied in acquired and congenital lesions are much the same. However, due to differences in anatomy, heart rate, and flow dynamics certain factors become more relevant in the setting of congenital heart disease. In this chapter, we will discuss the various means of investigating obstructive lesions with Doppler technique, and the clinical rationale for the implementation of these methods.

Determination of the Pressure Gradient

As blood flow approaches a rapidly narrowing flow circuit, the path is said to be obstructed. Such an obstruction can be fixed or temporally constant, as in a valvular stenosis, or dynamic in nature, as in hypertrophic obstructive cardiomyopathy. Because the flow volume across the narrowed portion of the circuit must equal the volume across the nonobstructed portion, an increase in flow velocity occurs (Fig 5-1). This increased flow velocity is directly related to the pressure drop across the obstructed flow circuit and the value of this velocity can be measured by Doppler echocardiography.

The direct relationship between the frequency shift, Fd, and the maximum blood flow velocity, Vm, is expressed in Equation 1-3. When obstruction is present, an increase in blood flow velocity will occur. By accurately recording the peak transvalvular flow velocity, the pressure gradient existing across the valve can be estimated noninvasively [1,2,3].

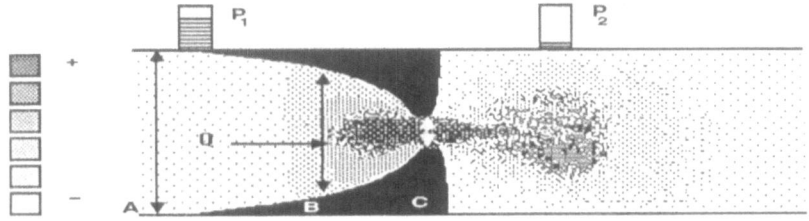

Fig. 5-1. The velocity of a flow increases when approaching a narrowing of the flow circuit . This is because the volume of flow at points A, B, and C must be equal, and if the flow cross sectional area is reduced, the velocity of flow must increase proportionally to maintain this volume. The continuity equation is based upon the principle of conservation of mass. The velocity of the blood flow is directly related to the pressure drop across the flow circuit, and the Bernoulli equation can be implemented for the noninvasive measurement of pressure gradients in various clinical settings.

It has been demonstrated that the modified Bernoulli equation can be used to determine the transvalvular pressure gradient [P1 - P2]. The modified Bernoulli equation is :

$$P1 - P2 = 4\,(Vm)^2$$

Equation 5-1

where Vm is the maximum red cell velocity across the valve, P1 is the pressure proximal to the valve, and P2 is the pressure distal to the valve. Some confusion may arise regarding the derivation of this simplified equation. The Bernoulli equation is written as follows:

$$P_2 - P_1 = 1/2\,(p)\,(V_2^2 - V_1^2) + p \int_1^2 (dv/dt)\,ds + R(v)$$

Equation 5-2

where V1 is the peak velocity proximal to the valve, V2 is the velocity distal to the valve, p is the density of blood, and S is the distance over which flow acceleration takes place. The first term represents the convective acceleration, the second represents the flow acceleration, and the third represents the contribution due to viscous friction. The term for flow acceleration is negligible except in high acceleration states such as valve opening or closure. The term for viscous friction, R(v), is also omitted as the ultrasonic beam should be directed to the center of blood flow to interrogate the peak velocity. Viscous friction effects are insignificant in the center of flow, but must be considered when examining flow proximal to the vessel or chamber walls.

Equation 5-3 may then be rewritten, leaving out the terms for flow acceleration and viscous friction:

$$P - P = 1/2 (p) (V_2^2 - V_1^2)$$

Equation 5-3

If V2, the velocity distal to the obstruction site, is assumed to greatly exceed V1, then V1 may be eliminated from equation 1-4. This is a reasonable assumption in cases where the obstruction is localized to one site, as in valve stenosis.

Equation 5-3 may then be rewritten:

$$1/2 (p) \cdot V_2^2$$

Equation 5-4

The constant for the density of blood , denoted as p, is 1060 kg/cubic m. Half of this value (1/2p) is 530 kg/cubic m. This value is stated in units of kg/cubic m, and the pressure drop calculated using such units would be expressed in nts/sq m. This must be converted to mm Hg, since these are the units of pressure utilized in angiography. The conversion is: 1 nt/sq m = 0 .0075 mm Hg so 1/2p in units of mm Hg is (530)(.0075) or 3.975 mm Hg. This value may be rounded off to 4.0 and inserted into equation 5-4.

$$4 \cdot V_2^2$$

Equation 5-5

V2 represents the maximum flow velocity distal to the the obstruction. The accuracy of the modified Bernoulli equation in measuring the peak pressure gradient in a wide range of pathologic conditions has been well documented in both adult and pediatric study groups . Our own study of 99 patients with left ventricular and right ventricular outflow obstruction demonstrated a very good correlation with invasively measured peak pressure gradients. These patients included both those in which the obstruction was the primary lesion and those in which the obstruction was one aspect of a more complex anomaly.

In simple obstructions, an independent Doppler transducer is useful, but in the more complex cases it is essential to use a duplex two-dimensional/Doppler probe as part of the investigation. Ascertaining that the correct flow has been interrogated without an image for guidance is quite difficult in a patient with a complex anomaly. In addition, flows are much closer spatially due to the smaller anatomic dimensions in the pediatric patient. The presence of more rapid heart rates in the pediatric patient results in less temporal separation of flow as well.

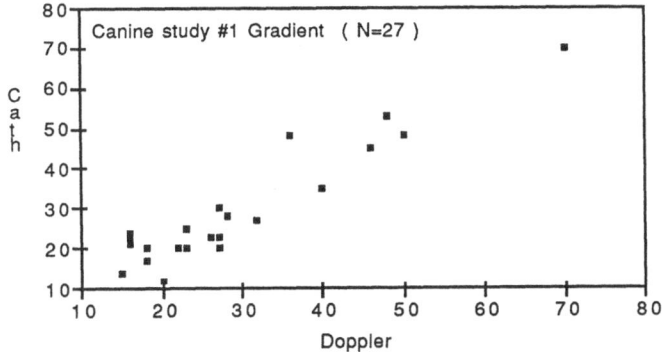

Fig. 5-2. In a series of pressure recordings obtained simultaneously wth CW Doppler and catheterization methods in an animal preparation, we demonstrated a good correlation between the two methods. For the purpose of this study, the instantaneous peak gradients were compared.

Limitations of the Modified Bernoulli Equation

When the flow velocities at positions 1 and 2 are of approximately the same value, because either the proximal flow velocity (V1) is high or the distal velocity is low, the more complete form of the Bernoulli equation should be implemented. The rationale for eliminating the term for convective acceleration was that V2 greatly exceeded V1, and such an assumption does not apply in this case. As an example, in the setting of valvular aortic stenosis with normal cardiac output, the left ventricular outflow velocity (V1) is approximately 1.0 m/s. Therefore, a peak velocity of 3.0 m/s distal to the aortic valve yields a peak gradient of 36 mm Hg. When V1 is included, a peak pressure gradient of 32 mm Hg is obtained. If V2 remains the same but V1 is increased to 2.0 m/s, the effect of including V1 in the Bernoulli equation is substantial. The peak pressure gradient is now estimated to be 20 mm Hg when V1 is considered. Generally, the more complete form of the Bernoulli equation (Eqn 5-3) should be applied in the setting of coarctation, multiple obstructions along a flow circuit, and when cardiac output is increased or decreased [5]. Whenever the proximal velocity (V1) is greater than 1.0 m/s, or V2 is less than 2.0 m/s, then the Bernoulli equation should not be used without inclusion of the term for V1 (Fig. 5-3).

The clinical utility of using continuous wave Doppler ultrasound to assess the pressure gradient has been well established. The greatest source of error lies in the underestimation of the maximal flow velocity when a parallel alignment to the interrogated flow is not achieved. When the peak velocity is underestimated, the peak pressure gradient determined by the modified Bernoulli equation will be lower than the actual gradient.

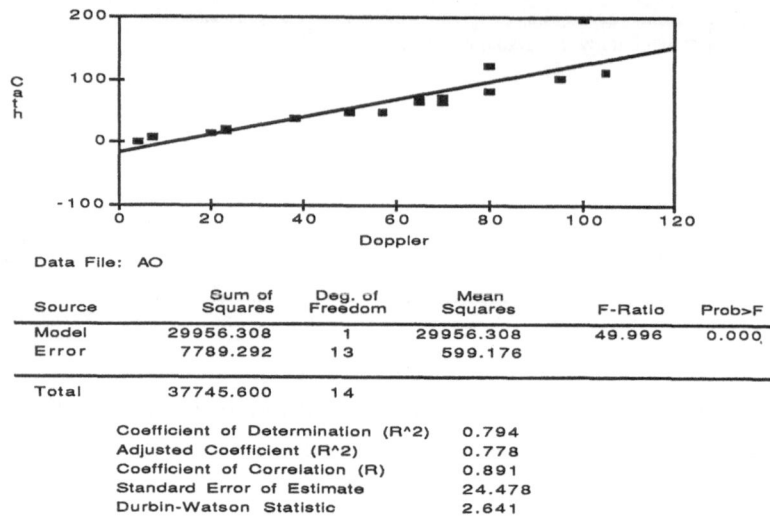

Data File: AO

Source	Sum of Squares	Deg. of Freedom	Mean Squares	F-Ratio	Prob>F
Model	29956.308	1	29956.308	49.996	0.000
Error	7789.292	13	599.176		
Total	37745.600	14			

Coefficient of Determination (R^2)	0.794
Adjusted Coefficient (R^2)	0.778
Coefficient of Correlation (R)	0.891
Standard Error of Estimate	24.478
Durbin-Watson Statistic	2.641

Fig. 5-3. In this series of 14 consecutive patients with valvular aortic stenosis, the invasively and noninvasively obtained gradients were in close agreement (r=.89).

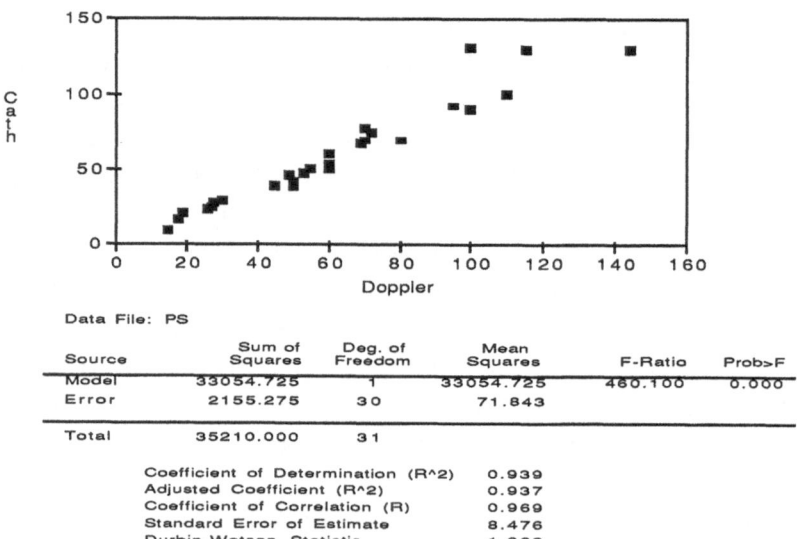

Data File: PS

Source	Sum of Squares	Deg. of Freedom	Mean Squares	F-Ratio	Prob>F
Model	33054.725	1	33054.725	460.100	0.000
Error	2155.275	30	71.843		
Total	35210.000	31			

Coefficient of Determination (R^2)	0.939
Adjusted Coefficient (R^2)	0.937
Coefficient of Correlation (R)	0.969
Standard Error of Estimate	8.476
Durbin-Watson Statistic	1.822

Fig. 5-4. In the setting of pulmonary stenosis, a very good correlation between catheterization and Doppler derived gradients was obtained (r=.97).

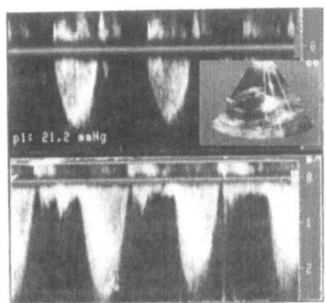

Fig. 5-5. In this patient with mild pulmonary stenosis, the peak flow velocity across the valve is 2.6 m/s, yielding a peak outflow gradient of 27 mm Hg. The peak infundibular gradient is 21 mm Hg, indicating that the transvalvular gradient is 6 mm Hg. This study was obtained from the parasternal transducer position (inset). The infundibular (top) and valvular (bottom) flow velocity traces are demonstrated. The infundibular flow was recorded with pulsed Doppler, while the outflow was recorded with high pulse repetition frequency (HPRF) mode. To calculate the actual valvular gradient, flow velocities need to be sampled from localized regions in the flow circuit. Both conventional pulsed mode and HPRF mode offer range resolution; HPRF mode permits the measurement of relatively high velocities.

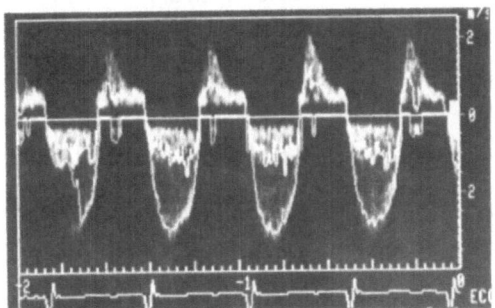

Fig. 5-6. The spectral analysis-derived peak and mean velocity analog curves are demonstrated. The peak flow velocity is 3.0 m/s, and has a weaker signal strength than the mean velocity of approximately 1.3 m/s. In a disturbed flow, the mean and peak velocities may be markedly different in value and signal strength. If the Doppler system employed does not have a high degree of sensitivity, the signals in the high velocity range could be missed. In this example, inserting the mean value rather than the peak value of the flow velocity into the modified Bernoulli equation would result in the underestimation of the peak gradient by more than 25 mm Hg.

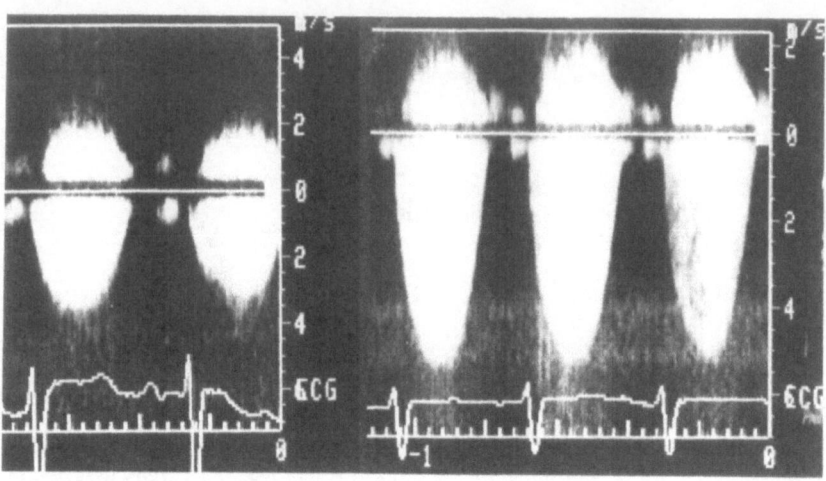

Fig. 5-7. If the beam-to-flow alignment exceeds 10 degrees, a significant underestimation of the gradient will occur. In example A the angle to flow is approximately 30 degrees and a large underestimation of the true peak velocity (B) results. Any error in the value of the peak velocity is squared in the calculation of the pressure drop, thereby creating a greater error in the estimation of the pressure drop. Note that the spectral envelope appears as though it is well delineated in both recordings. However, the audio signal in example A was less intense and of a wider bandwidth than the audio signal in example B. One should interrogate the flow from different angles while carefully listening to the audio signal until the narrowest bandwidth audio signal is obtained.

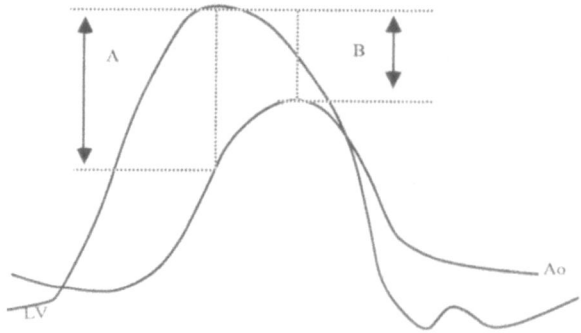

Fig. 5-8. The Doppler method for measurement of the pressure drop yields the instantaneous pressure drop across the obstruction (A) rather than the peak-to-peak or mean value generally measured at catheterization (B).

An overestimation of the peak velocity and the peak pressure gradient will result when an erroneously large angle is assumed to exist between the ultrasonic beam and the interrogated flow. There is no reliable visual method of ascertaining the beam-to-flow angle since the flow is not parallel to the vessel or chamber walls, and the flow is three dimensional. The best method of obtaining the true peak flow velocity is to use the audio signal to guide the beam into a parallel alignment with the blood flow. An audio signal which contains mostly high frequencies indicates a good alignment to flow, and the recorded flow velocity curve will have a clearly defined envelope. Using this technique, continuous wave Doppler ultrasound may be used to noninvasively estimate the peak pressure gradient.

The modified Bernoulli equation yields a physiologic pressure gradient, while the catheterization peak gradient represents the peak-to-peak gradient measurement (Fig. 5-8). Variations in heart rate and cardiac output must also be considered when the Doppler derived pressure gradient is compared to the catheterization gradient. In the setting of some lesions such as subvalvular aortic stenosis, pulmonary stenosis, or coarctation of aorta, the obstruction can be tunnel-like. There has been some question as to whether or not the modified Bernoulli equation is applicable in this type of obstruction, as the inclusion of the terms for acceleration and viscous friction become more important. Simpson and coworkers have demonstrated in vitro that with the segment lengths and cross-sectional areas encountered in the clinical settings, i.e. subvalvular aortic stenosis, subvalvular pulmonary stenosis, and muscular ventricular septal defects, the modified Bernoulli equation is still a reliable predictor of the instantaneous pressure gradient across the total outflow obstruction.

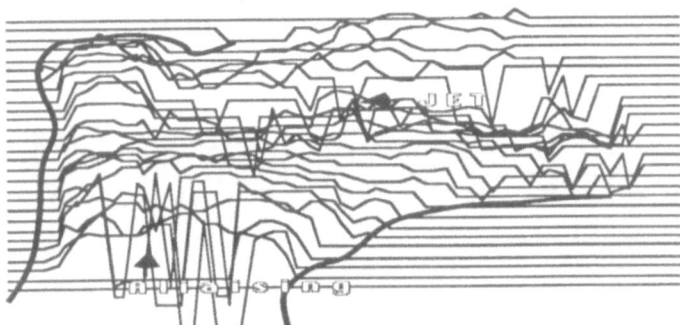

Fig. 5-9. This three dimensional frequency plot was obtained from a patient with moderate aortic stenosis. The systolic jet across the narrow valve opening is seen as an area of fluctuation in frequency. As the outflow in the aorta aligns with the Doppler beams, aliasing occurs. This also results in a fluctuation in frequency.

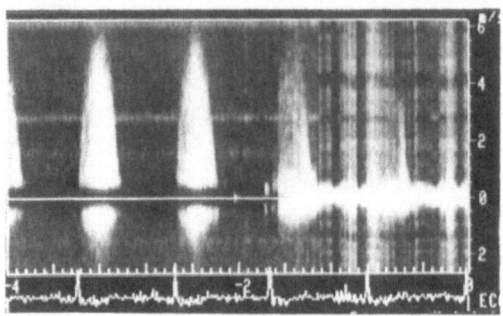

Fig. 5-10. High pass filtering is used to remove high intensity but low velocity signals such as wall motion from the Doppler signal. As seen in this tracing of aortic stenosis from the right parasternal position, the high pass filtering can affect the velocity measurement in the high velocity range. In the first two beats the filters are set at approximately 1300 Hz and the strong low velocity components are eliminated. The peak flow velocity envelope is clearly visualized. In the following two beats, the high pass filtering has been set quite low, and the resulting saturation of the receivers causes the high velocity but low amplitude signals (which are clinically relevant) to be dropped out.

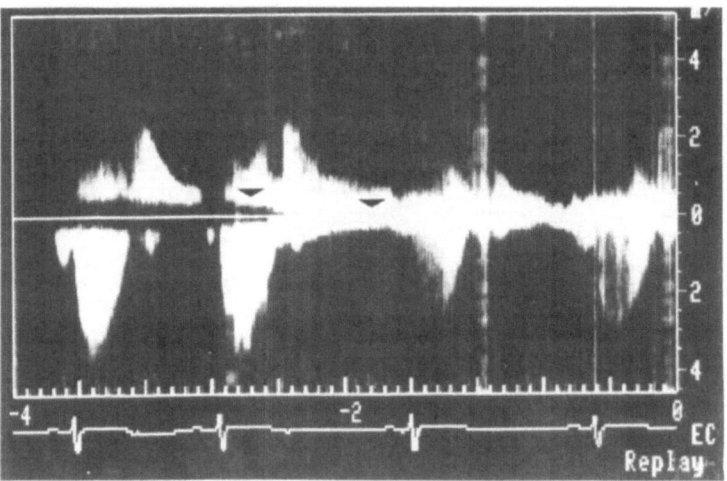

Fig. 5-11. In a patient with mild pulmonary stenosis and regurgitation, both forward and reverse flow velocity traces are dropped out when the high pass filters (also called wall filters or low velocity reject) are reduced from 1200 to 300 Hz (arrows) respectively. High velocity flows which could be measured by the examiner are often missed because an inadequate degree of low velocity reject is employed.

Estimation of the Valve Area

The gradient can be accurately measured with the modified Bernoulli equation, but we have described both technical and physiologic factors which can compromise the results of these measurements, such as low gradients in the setting of low cardiac output and severe stenosis, or high gradients in the setting of moderately severe stenosis and an increased stroke volume.

Several investigators have attempted to measure the stenotic valve area by a modified Gorlin formula, using the Doppler-derived gradient, and various methods of calculating the cardiac output [6,7,8,9,10,11,12,13]. While these investigations have demonstrated that it is possible to measure the valve area with acceptable accuracy, the necessity of measuring the cardiac output is time consuming. In addition, the cardiac output determination introduces the possible errors associated with flow volume calculations. Another approach for the calculation of the valve area implements the equation for the conservation of mass, or the continuity equation. Simply stated, in a closed flow circuit the flow volume measured at one site must equal the volume measured at another site. The circuit's cross-sectional area and the flow velocity may change, but these changes are inversely related and the volume will remain constant. The heart may be considered a closed flow circuit, as changes in flow volume are generally negligible. Therefore in aortic stenosis if one measures the prestenotic flow velocity and the cross-sectional area in the left ventricular outflow tract, the stroke volume can be obtained. The stroke volume at the level of the stenotic valve must be the same, and as the velocity of flow across the obstruction can easily be obtained, it is then possible to rewrite the equation to solve for the stenotic valve area. This method is applicable for the determination of aortic valve area, pulmonary valve area and the mitral valve area in the setting of valvular stenosis. The author's experience with this technique has been primarily in the measurement of aortic valve area, and good correlations with invasive measurements have been obtained. Casales and coworkers performed hemodynamic (Gorlin) and Doppler (continuity equation) measurements simultaneously in a series of patients; their results suggested that the measurement of the aortic valve area by the Gorlin formula method is more flow dependent than the Doppler-derived method based upon the continuity equation. The main problem with the implementation of this technique is determining the prestenotic flow region, and the geometric assumptions made when calculating the prestenotic cross-sectional area.

The protocol that we use in the case of aortic stenosis is performed from an apical position; either the long axis, two, or four chamber view may be used. The pulsed Doppler sample volume is moved in discrete steps from the apical region towards the stenotic valve. At a point proximal to the obstruction, a rapid increase in flow velocity is noted, and usually causes aliasing of the spectral trace. This site is then used for the prestenotic area and velocity measurements. It can be useful to implement the high pulse repetition frequency mode to resolve the aliased signal while retaining some degree of range resolution. The continuous mode is then used to measure the peak velocity across the stenotic valve, and the stenotic valve area (Aa) is calculated:

$$Aa = \frac{A\ ps \times Vps}{Va}$$

Equation 5-6

where Aa= aortic valve area, Aps= prestenotic cross-sectional area, Vps= prestenotic flow peak velocity and Va= aortic stenosis peak flow velocity.

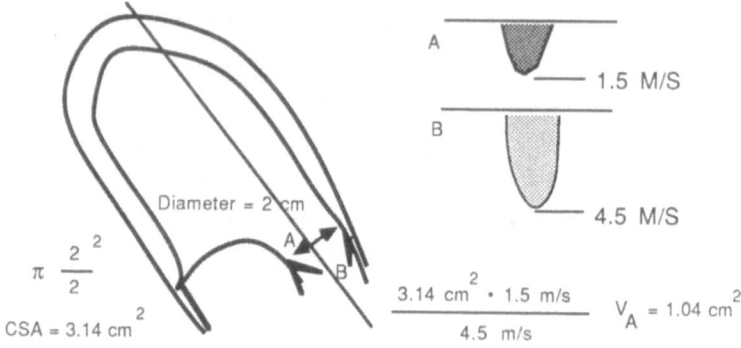

Fig. 5-12. This schematic demonstrates the method in which the continuity equation is used to calculate the orifice area in aortic stenosis. The prestenotic flow area and velocity are measured at the level of the left ventricular outflow tract (A), and the peak velocity is measured at the level of the obstruction (B) with CW Doppler.

Other methods of measuring the aortic valve area include the bioimpedance method described by Goli and associates [13]. With this method, continuous mode is used to measure the peak transvalvular flow velocity (and to derive the gradient), pulsed mode is used to measure the mean velocity and the two-dimensional image is employed to measure the cross-sectional area of the left ventricle at the level of the outflow tract. The cardiac output is measured by tetrapolar electrical transthoracic bioimpedance, yielding all the information required for the application of the Gorlin formula. In Goli's study, the valve area derived by the bioimpedance method was more accurate than the more conventional continuity equation method.

A more recently described method of measuring the aortic valve area is the direct planimetry of the aortic valve image obtained during the transesophageal echocardiogram (TEE). To apply the transesophageal approach, the short axis view of the aortic valve is obtained and the cross-sectional area of the valve planimetered from the frozen two-dimensional image. The experience of Kasper and coworkers demonstrated a close agreement in the value of the valve areas obtained by the Doppler continuity equation method and the TEE method. While the Doppler method is perhaps a more accurate predictor of the valve area, the TEE method yields more information regarding the morphology of the valve lesion.

Valvular Aortic Stenosis

Among the forms of aortic obstruction, valvular stenosis most frequently gives rise to symptoms in infancy. The malformed aortic valve may be unicuspid, bicuspid or myxomatous. Usually the unicuspid type will be encountered in cases of critical aortic stenosis. The application of two dimensional echocardiography has been widely used in the setting of left ventricular outflow obstruction to evaluate the anatomic parameters associated with this pathologic condition. The site of the obstruction can be localized by pulsed mode or color flow imaging. The presence of subvalvular or supravalvular narrowing or coarctation can be determined, and the nature of the obstruction characterized as fixed or dynamic. One can study the valves and observe if the leaflets are thickened or fused, and determine whether the motion of the leaflets in systole and diastole are abnormal. One can also observe the pathophysiology indirectly by evaluating the degree of ventricular hypertrophy if present. The application of imaging techniques in left ventricular outflow tract obstructions is generally more useful in the pediatric patient than in the adult patient because high quality images are easier to obtain in children, which is important as the location of the obstruction is more variable. However, it is not possible to directly evaluate the hemodynamic effects of the obstruction with imaging techniques, and this is where the implementation of pulsed and continuous wave Doppler is very useful. (Fig. 5-13, 5-14).

Aortic stenosis in children is often a progressive disease and the ability to reliably follow these patients is extremely important. To interrogate the transvalvular flow with the Doppler echocardiographic method the suprasternal, right parasternal and apical windows are most commonly used. The jet in congenital aortic stenosis can frequently be intercepted from the suprasternal position, and jet eccentricity is generally not so great a problem with children as it is in adult aortic stenosis. However, the right parasternal window is also useful in many pediatric patients when the suprasternal notch cannot be accessed. The continuous wave beam can usually be aligned with the stenotic jet by listening to the audio signal, and looking for a narrow band spectral trace. When the beam-to-flow angle is small, the audio signal has a characteristic high pitch and the spectral envelope is well delineated.

Once an adequate recording of aortic flow has been obtained, the peak velocity may be used to estimate the peak instantaneous pressure gradient by applying the modified Bernoulli equation. Since the peak velocity is sustained in a significant obstruction, the mean Doppler gradient should also be calculated. The Doppler-derived peak gradient represents an instantaneous pressure gradient, while the catheterization peak gradient represents a peak to peak pressure difference. The value of the Doppler-derived peak and mean gradients may vary significantly with the condition of the patient during the ultrasound examination. Also, if the patient is agitated, the calculated gradients can be much higher than those obtained when the patient is sedated.

Patients with bicuspid aortic valves have a slightly increased aortic flow velocity, or the value of the peak flow velocity may be within the normal limits during childhood (Fig. 5-15). Fibrotic thickening or calcification of the aortic valve cusps may gradually cause an increase in the transvalvular gradient with the development of left ventricular outflow obstruction. Increasingly higher aortic flow velocities will be recorded as the valve becomes obstructed. The application of the Bernoulli equation to calculate the pressure drop across the obstructed aortic valve in children has been verified by several investigators. Lima and coworkers demonstrated a very good correlation between invasive and Doppler derived measurements of the pressure drop across the stenotic aortic valve several years ago. They further suggested at this time that this could be an interesting method for both the initial diagnosis and quantitation of aortic stenosis, and the serial management of such patients. In recent years this statement on the potential usefulness of the technique has become generally accepted. In many institutions preoperative catheterization in the setting of aortic stenosis is frequently bypassed, based on the Doppler derived measurement of the pressure drop.

Robinson and coworkers evaluated this method in the setting of congenital aortic stenosis in the neonate. They demonstrated a good correlation between the invasive and noninvasive results, suggesting that the need for preoperative catheterization in the neonate could be obviated. This is of clinical interest as there are associated risks with catheterizing the sick neonate, and Doppler echocardiography permits the physician to follow the infant postoperatively. An alternative means of evaluating the severity of the valvular stenosis is to calculate the stenotic valve orifice with the continuity equation, as previously discussed. In the setting of valvular aortic stenosis, the prestenotic flow velocity and cross-sectional area are measured in the left ventricular outflow tract. High pulse repetition frequency mode may be useful, as this velocity frequently exceeds the conventional pulsed Doppler Nyquist limit. Continuous mode is then used to measure the peak transvalvular velocity and the calculation is performed as we have outlined.

Doppler techniques may also be used to estimate the aortic valve area and the residual gradient following valvulotomy, and to assess the degree of insufficiency created by the procedure. The Doppler-derived pressure gradient can be compared to the pre-operative value and that obtained at catheterization. Serial Doppler examinations of post-valvulotomy patients are a reliable means of detecting the development of significant outflow obstruction. This topic is discussed more rigorously in the section on valvuloplasty.

Subvalvular Aortic Stenosis

Obstruction of the left ventricular outflow tract can occur at various levels of the outflow tract, and be either fixed or dynamic. Two dimensional echocardiography is a useful tool in diagnosing these lesions, and in evaluation of the location and type of obstruction. However, attempts to quantify these lesions with imaging techniques h ve proven to be of limited practical value. The application of Doppler ultrasound provides valuable information, both qualitative and quantitative (Fig. 5-17, 5-18, 5-19)[15,16].

The location of the obstruction is usually quite easily established with color flow mapping techniques. Color wraparound, or aliasing, is noted just proximal to the obstruction, with a high degree of variance noted at the level of the narrowing. This flow may remain turbulent into the aorta, or it may become more organized distal to obstruction. In a serial obstruction with subvalvular and valvular stenosis, the flow becomes turbulent at the level of the subvalvular obstruction, reorganizes distal to the obstruction, and then becomes turbulent again at the level of the valvular stenosis. In a subvalvular aortic stenosis with coexisting mitral regurgitation, color flow mapping can be useful for finding the proper alignment with the stenotic jet, and separating it from the regurgitant jet. This is especially helpful in children, because there is little temporal or spatial separation of these abnormal flow patterns. In fact, to demonstrate the temporal sequence of these flows it is generally necessary to implement the color M-mode or the conventional pulsed Doppler, which can also be used to localize the obstruction and measure the velocity. The sample volume is positioned along the outflow tract until aliasing is noted. A sample volume length of 3-4 mm yields the best trade-off between sensitivity and axial resolution. But for the localization of the obstruction, color flow imaging does offer distinct advantages in terms of spatial resolution, resulting in a more rapid examination time (a point which should be appreciated by the pediatric echocardiographer) and a higher degree of confidence when interpreting the results.

Once the obstruction has been localized with pulsed Doppler or color flow imaging, the high pulse repetition frequency (high prf) mode or continuous mode is implemented to measure the peak blood flow velocity. In both pediatric and adult applications a highly sensitive continuous mode is of primary importance. In adult applications high prf is of limited value, but there are some advantages to having high prf capabilities available for pediatric applications. The biggest drawback of high pulse repetititon frequency Doppler in the adult patient is that the capability of detecting very weak, high velocity signals from flows at greater depths is much less than with CW Doppler. However, this is generally not a problem at the shallower interrogation depths encountered in children. The advantage is that some degree of range resolution is retained. If serial obstructions are present, it is often easier to separate the various velocity contributions of the multiple obstructions. The important issue is that the true peak velocity across the obstruction must be measured, regardless of which mode is selected. When the peak velocity has been obtained it is used to calculate the gradient, as in valvular stenosis. The Doppler derived pressure gradient has been demonstrated to correspond well with invasive measurements. As in the case of valvular stenosis, this offers a convenient, safe and accurate means of serially following the patient post -operatively.

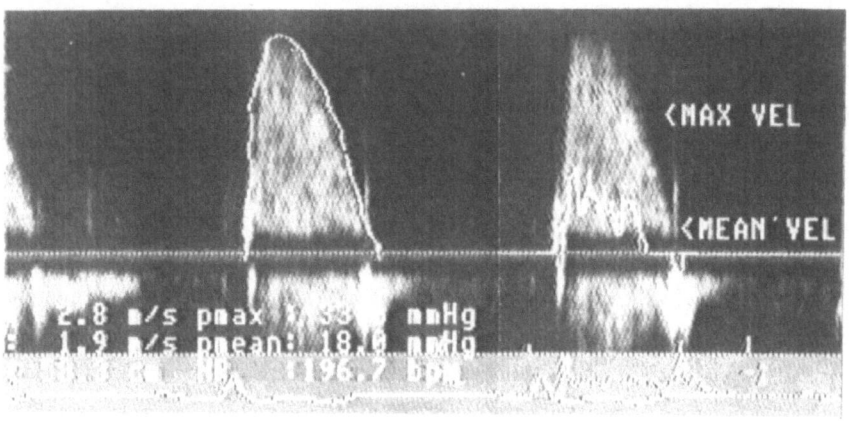

Fig. 5-13. The peak velocity can be much greater than the mean velocity in stenotic jets. In this example from a patient with a bicuspid aortic valve and mild stenosis, the peak flow velocity is 2.8 m/s (first complex), and the mean velocity is 1.9 m/s (second complex). The peak left ventricular-aortic pressure gradient is 33 mm Hg.

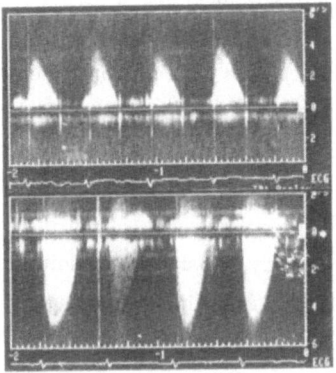

Fig. 5-14. The examination window from which the jet is interrogated can have profound impact on the accuracy of the gradient measurement. The top tracing of the jet in aortic stenosis obtained from the suprasternal notch yields a peak gradient of approximately 50 mm Hg. The bottom tracing from the apex of the same patient yields a gradient of more than 100 mm Hg.

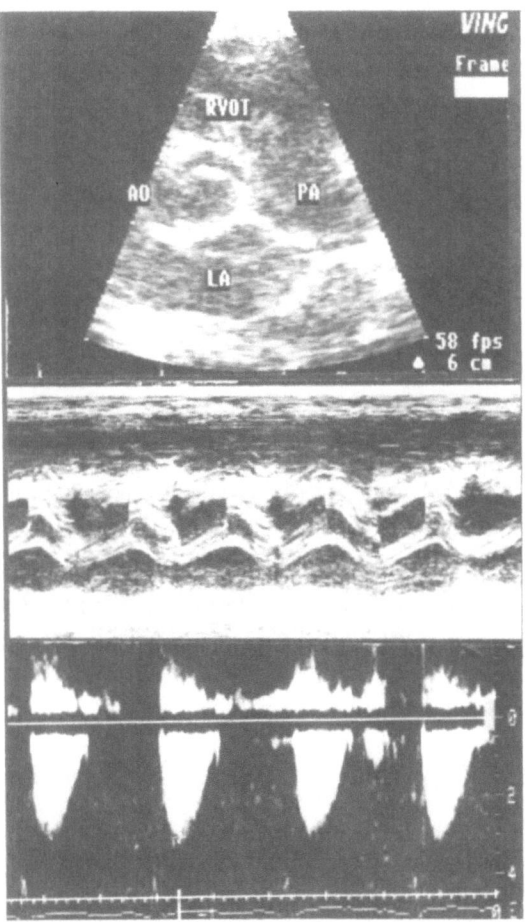

Fig. 5-15. A bicuspid aortic valve is demonstrated on the two-dimensional (top) and M-mode (center) examination. Note the thickened valve cusps on the two-dimensional image and the cusp eccentricity on the M-mode. The peak velocity (bottom) measured with continuous mode slightly exceeds 3.0 m/s with a corresponding peak gradient of 38 mm Hg, indicating the presence of a mild outflow obstruction. Right ventricular outflow tract (RVOT), aorta (AO), pulmonary artery (PA), left atrium (LA).

Coarctation of the Aorta

Coarctation of the aorta is a congenital anomaly in which there is an obstruction or narrowing of the distal aortic arch or the descending aorta. Juxtaductal coarctation occurs most frequently; a localized constriction of the aortic lumen can be found at the level of the ductus arteriosus. It may be difficult to define the coarctation site or to assess the degree of narrowing with imaging technique alone due to the presence of limitations in lateral resolution, artifacts, and echo dropout. Using continuous wave Doppler ultrasound, a characteristic flow pattern will be recorded from the suprasternal window in coarctation [17,18,19]. The distinctive spectral envelope has been described as sawtooth in appearance, and the audio signal has a characteristic grainy sound.

With increasing severity of the obstruction, the systolic volume of blood flowing in the descending aorta distal to the coarctation is significantly reduced. At the same time, the peak flow velocity increases and declines more slowly so that a relatively high velocity may be recorded in diastole as well. When there is a significant degree of narrowing, the diastolic flow velocities may exceed 2.0 m/s. The reduced volume of flow distal to the coarctation results in a high velocity but low intensity Doppler signal. Consequently, the peak flow velocity may be faintly recorded on the flow velocity curve. Since the coarctation creates a bending or kinking of the descending limb of the aorta, the jet may be eccentric and hard to track. Occasionally the peak flow velocities in the jet may be more clearly recorded by moving the transducer slightly to the left of the standard suprasternal position.

To calculate the pressure gradient across the coarctation, the peak velocity in the descending aorta must be included in the Bernoulli equation when it exceeds 1.0 m/s (Fig. 5-20). If the velocity proximal to the coarctation (V1) is neglected, the gradient (ΔP) will be overestimated. The gradient is calculated as:

$$\Delta P = 4\,(V2^2 - V1^2)$$

Equation 5-7

where V2 is the peak flow velocity distal to the coarctation. A parallel or nearly parallel alignment of the continuous wave beam to the jet is essential for accurate prediction of the pressure gradient.

Because the jet trajectory is unpredictable in coarctation, the jet may bend so acutely that a parallel position to flow cannot be achieved even with the use of an independent Doppler transducer. Stevenson et al have demonstrated that the jet angulation is probably responsible for the underestimation of the actual pressure gradient in coarctation. Although the potential for gradient underestimation exists, the Bernoulli equation still allows one to assess the relative severity of the outflow obstruction in patients with coarctation.

Color flow mapping can be used to localize the position of the coarctation and to roughly estimate the severity of the lesion. Simpson and associates have measured the ratio between the flow in the prestenotic range to the percent narrowing at the coarctation. In their experience, this measurement correlates well with the angiographically determined percent narrowing of the coarctation, even when the image of the descending aorta was not well visualized. In our limited experience of evaluating coarctation with transesophageal echocardiography, (TEE), we have found that the obstruction site can easily be demonstrated and the collateral runoff evaluated with color flow mapping during TEE. In one patient, we have been able to localize the coarctation and estimate the peak gradient with continuous mode during TEE while we could not address either issue with conventional transthoracic echocardiography.

The pulsed Doppler examination of flow in the descending aorta indicates the presence of high velocity flow at the level of, and downstream from, the coarctation site. Pulsed mode should be utilized to obtain V1, the peak flow velocity in the descending aorta proximal to the coarctation. When flow in the ascending aorta is interrogated, a normal aortic flow pattern is usually recorded in the absence of aortic stenosis. The peak flow velocity in the ascending aorta may be lower than normal due to left ventricular failure.

Aortic isthmus narrowing or infantile coarctation is another form of coarctation characterized by a region of luminal narrowing which frequently may extend from the left subclavian artery to the ductal level. A localized constriction may also exist near the ductus arteriosus. The Doppler examination is performed in the same manner as previously described, and the peak flow velocity may be used to predict the peak pressure gradient existing in the descending aorta. A patent ductus arteriosus is normally associated with infantile coarctation, while it may not be patent in juxtaductal coarctation. In coarctation syndrome the ductus is in direct continuity with the descending aorta, maintaining a fetal pattern of lower limb circulation. When the ductus constricts, the hemodynamic effects of the narrowed isthmus lumen become apparent and higher velocities are recorded in the isthmus. Ventricular septal defect is commonly associated with infantile coarctation, and the existence of this lesion should be established or ruled out during the Doppler examination.

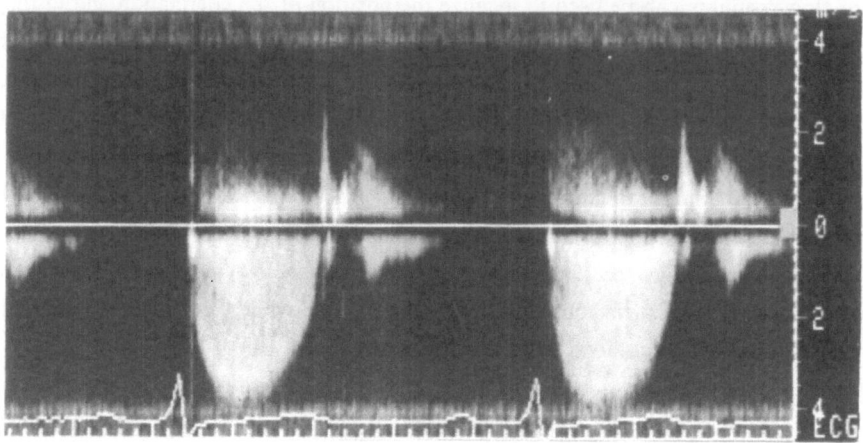

Fig. 5-16. This study is from a child with a fixed obstruction of the left ventricular outflow tract caused by a subvalvular membrane. The peak gradient measured was 64 mm Hg, and corresponded closely with the invasively measured gradient. Note the prolonged rise to the peak velocity and the slow decline of the peak flow velocity , resulting in a rounded spectral trace. This generally indicates that a severe obstruction is present. The strong spectral signal seen in the second trace of 1.0 m/s represents the flow in the ventricle proximal to the obstruction. In this case the term for P1 (4 mm Hg) is negligible. The strong vertical signals at the beginning and end of flow are generated by the aortic valve cusps passing through the continuous wave beam during valve opening and closure.

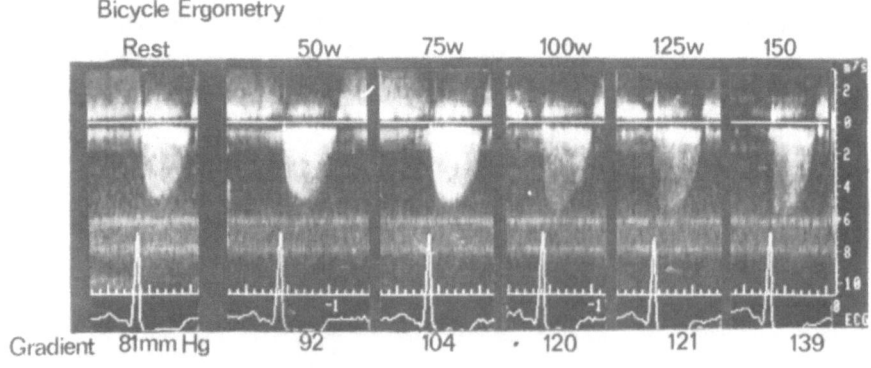

SUB AORTIC MEMBRANE

Fig. 5-17. The left ventricular outflow gradient increases from ≈ 80 mm Hg to ≈ 140 mm Hg under increasing workloads in a patient with a sub-valvular membrane.

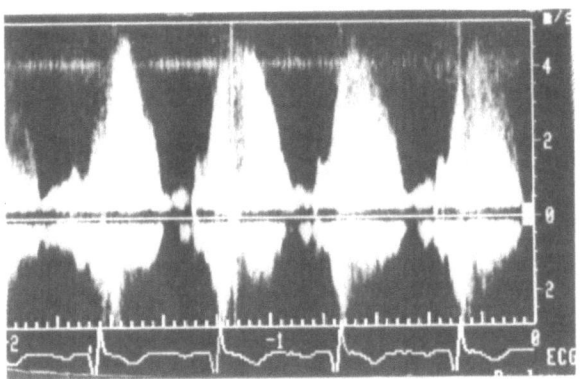

Fig. 5-18. The right parasternal window is used to interrogate the left ventricular outflow tract in an adolescent patient with a discrete subvalvular membrane and an associated severe dynamic outflow obstruction. The peak velocity is 4.8 m/s, yielding a gradient of 92 mm Hg. Note the late systolic peaking of the velocity trace. In the second trace, the strong vertical line appearing in mid-systole represents the motion of the membrane as it passes through the continuous wave beam.

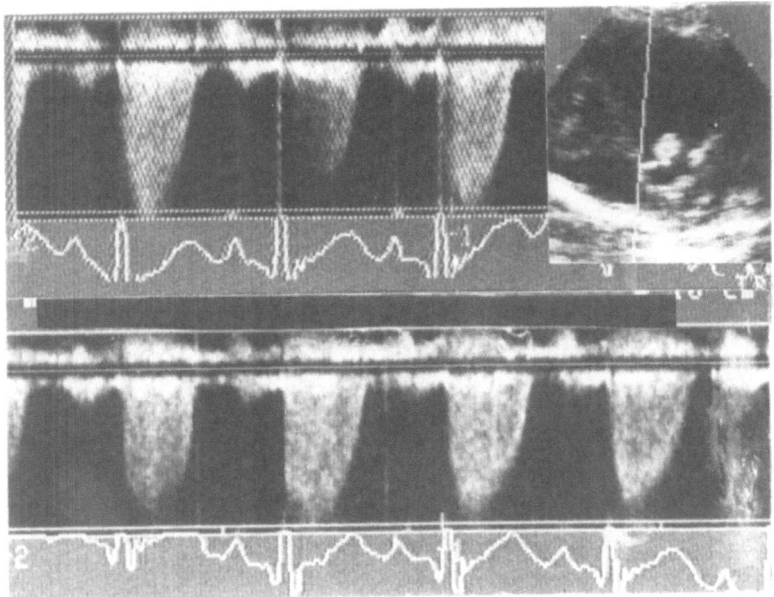

Fig. 5-19. This recording is from a patient with a pedunculated tumor in the left ventricular outflow tract, which causes an outflow obstruction with a gradient of 144 mm Hg.

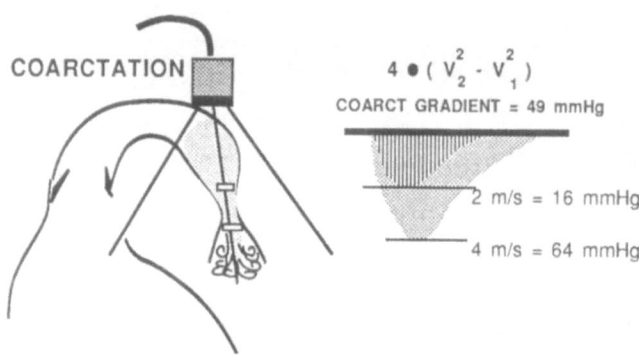

$$4 \bullet (V_2^2 - V_1^2)$$

COARCT GRADIENT = 49 mmHg

2 m/s = 16 mmHg

4 m/s = 64 mmHg

Fig. 5-20. To correctly estimate the gradient across a coarctation, it is necessary to measure both the prestenotic and stenotic flow velocity and to include both terms in the Bernoulli equation.

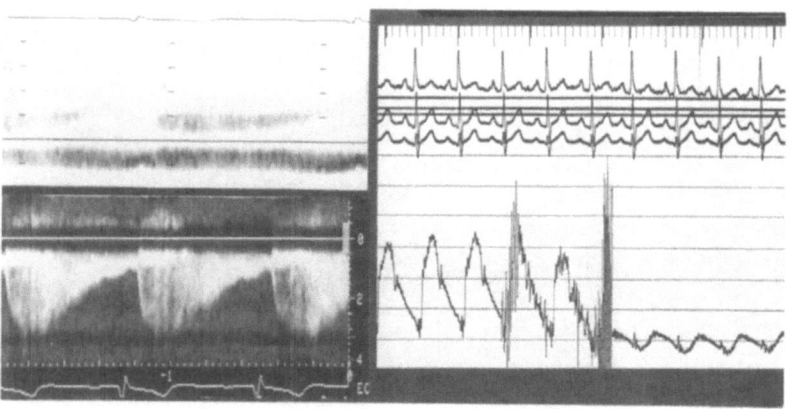

Fig. 5-21. In trace A, pulsed Doppler has been used to localize the site of a coarctation, and severe aliasing has occurred. The CW Doppler can resolve the true peak velocity (B) which corresponds quite well to the invasively derived gradient. The pressure recordings were obtained during pullback across the obstruction.

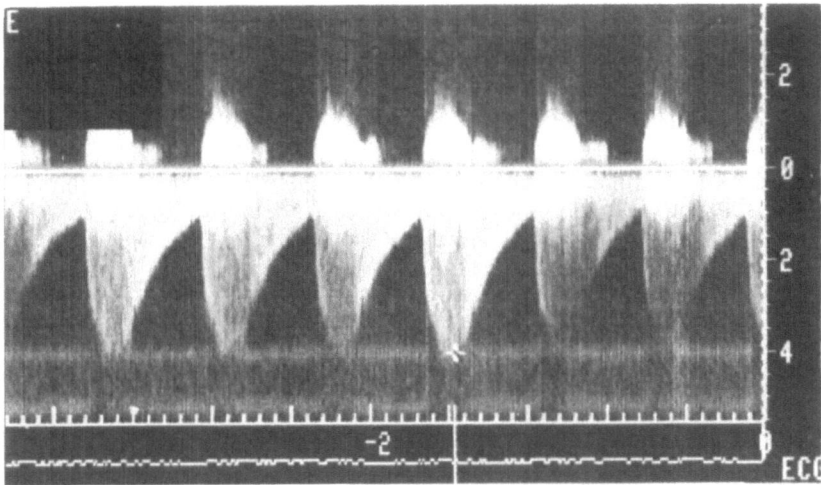

Fig. 5-22. This continuous mode tracing was obtained from the descending aorta of a patient with a coarctation. In this example the obstruction is severe, the peak velocity of 4.01 m/s yielded a gradient of 66 mmHg. There is continuous systolic and diastolic flow resulting in a flow velocity curve which has been described as having a saw-tooth appearance. This exponential deceleration of the velocity is almost always noted in severe coarctation. The positive flow originates from the left subclavian artery which has also been sampled by the CW Doppler beam.

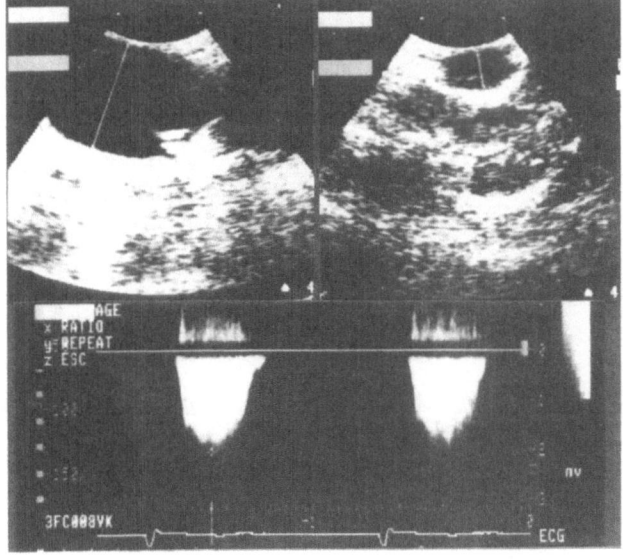

Fig. 5-23. Preceeding Page: This study was performed during a balloon dilatation of a recoarctation by transesophageal Doppler. A 7.5 MHz imaging frequency and 6.0 MHz probe with CW Doppler were used to measure the residual gradient. During the procedure, TEE monitoring permits the pressure gradients to be measured, the left ventricular function to be assessed, and global monitoring of cardiac hemodynamics to be correlated to morphology without compromising the surgical field.

Doppler techniques are also helpful in the evaluation of patients with coarctation after surgery. Using pulsed mode, flow in the ascending and descending aorta should be carefully interrogated (Color Plate 5-1). In a successful repair, the peak flow velocity in the descending aorta is still generally higher than normal. This finding may reflect the hyperdynamic state of the left ventricle which is frequently found in such patients. The peak flow velocity in the ascending aorta will also be higher than normal in these cases. When a localized significant increase in flow velocity is recorded in the descending aorta, re-coarctation should be suspected. To accurately assess the pressure gradient across the residual obstruction in the descending aorta, it is sometimes necessary to include the term for V1 in the Bernoulli equation, as explained earlier in this section.

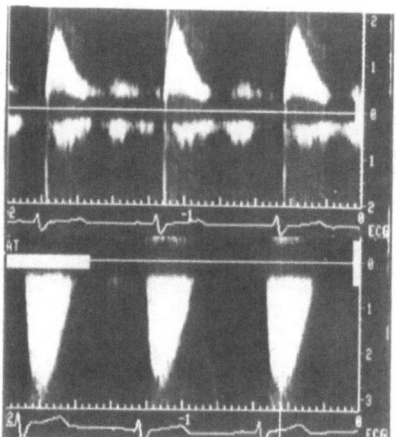

Fig. 5-24. Residual narrowing of the descending aorta in a patient with a corrected coarctation followed up several months post-operatively. The top trace was obtained from the ascending aorta, and the bottom trace from the descending aorta. The difference between the flow velocities in the ascending and descending aorta is quite small, indicating that the pressure drop across the residual narrowing is insignificant.

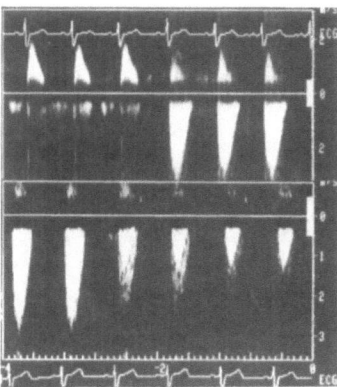

Fig. 5-25. Residual narrowing of the aorta. The first trace (top) was obtained by sweeping the continuous wave beam from the ascending to the descending aorta. The bottom trace was obtained by moving the high PRF sample volume back from the narrowing of the descending aorta into the proximal portion of the descending aorta.

Obstructive Cardiomyopathy

Conventional Doppler techniques allow one to assess the severity of the intraventricular obstruction present in patients with hypertrophic cardiomyopathy [20]. One of the principal roles of Doppler ultrasound is in the area of gradient determination. The peak systolic velocity in Figure 5-26 is used to calculate the pressure gradient using the modified Bernoulli equation. The gradient can also be obtained in the setting of dynamic obstructions (Fig. 5-27, 5-28) using continuous wave Doppler. This ability to evaluate hemodynamics is very valuable, and is an important adjunct to imaging. In Figure 5-29, an example of a patient with asymmetric septal hypertrophy, systolic anterior motion of the chordae tendinae, and absolutely no obstruction to left ventricular outflow is shown. This case emphasizes the need to monitor hemodynamics as well as performing tissue imaging. Besides allowing one to make quantitative measurements, the Doppler technique can be used to localize the site of obstruction. From the apical window, the left ventricular outflow can be examined with pulsed mode. By moving the sample volume further into the outflow tract, the level at which the increased velocity originates can be determined. The pulsed mode recording of left ventricular outflow will be heavily aliased at the level of the narrowest flow trajectory. Continuous mode should then be utilized to measure the peak flow velocity through the narrowed outflow tract. It may be difficult to record the low intensity but high velocity signals from the blood passing through this obstruction. An independent Doppler transducer is sometimes required to adequately record the peak velocities in the outflow tract.

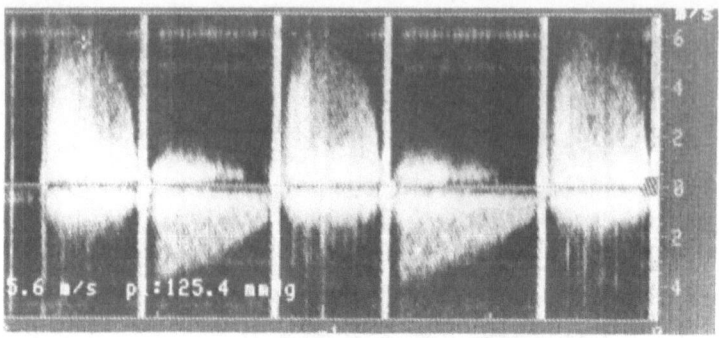

Fig. 5-26. A high velocity jet was recorded across the left ventricular outflow tract in a four year old boy with an obstructive cardiomyopathy and associated stenosis across a bicuspid aortic valve. The flow was measured from the right parasternal position and a peak outflow gradient of 125 mmHg was detected. In the aortic regurgitation (graded 2 + by the JET/LVOT area method), notes a very rapid pressure fall off. This reflects poor LV compliance rather than severe regurgitation. LVOT = left ventricular outflow tract.

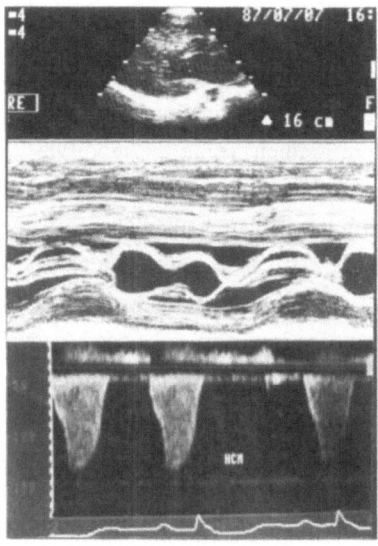

Fig. 5-27. The TM study (top) from a patient with a hypertrophic subaortic cardiomyopathy demonstrates the systolic anterior motion (SAM) of the mitral valve chordae. The continuous wave Doppler interrogation (bottom) yielded a peak gradient of 100 mmHg. Note the late systolic peak, a typical finding encountered in the setting of a dynamic outflow tract obstruction.

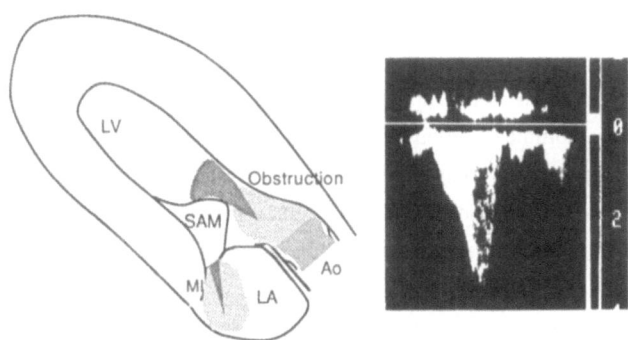

Fig. 5-28. The orientation of the left ventricular outflow obstruction and the mitral regurgitation are such that it is possible to align the continuous wave beam with both simultaneously. The peak velocity of the outflow curve occurs later in systole than the peak velocity of the mitral regurgitation, and is a characteristic finding in the setting of a dynamic obstruction.

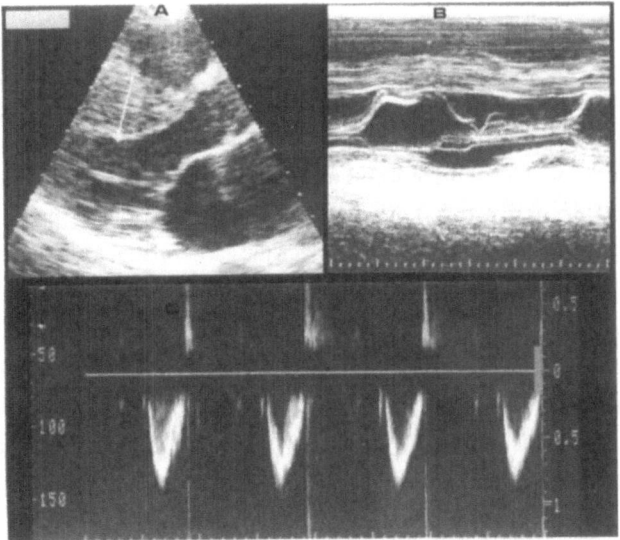

Fig. 5-29. A patient with significant septal hypertrophy (A), systolic anterior motion of the mitral valve chordae (B), but no outflow tract gradient recorded with continuous mode (C).

The continuous mode recording in left ventricular outflow obstruction has a late systolic peak which is characteristic of a dynamic obstruction to flow. The systolic anterior motion of the mitral leaflets serves to further narrow the outflow tract, causing the development of high flow velocities in late systole. The faded appearance of the spectral flow pattern in late systole is caused by the reduced volume of blood which has passed through the obstructed outflow tract. A high pass filter setting greater than 800 Hz should be selected when attempting to record the low intensity but high velocity outflow signal. Once the peak velocity has been optimally recorded, the peak intraventricular pressure gradient can be estimated by application of the modified Bernoulli equation.

Mitral regurgitation can often be detected in patients with hypertrophic cardiomyopathy. The outflow jet is more superiorly directed than the regurgitant jet, and the two flows can usually be differentiated. In addition, the morphology of the spectral flow patterns are different. The regurgitant flow peaks in mid-systole, whereas the outflow peaks in late systole. The regurgitant flow signal can usually be detected throughout systole, in agreement with reports that the regurgitation is not initiated by the systolic anterior movement of the mitral valve leaflets.

The peak velocities recorded in the aorta from the apical window may be within normal limits, indicating that the outflow jet has dissipated by the time the left ventricular outflow reaches the aortic annulus. When recording flow in the ascending aorta from the suprasternal window, a high degree of variability may be noted in the spectral flow pattern.

Pulmonic Stenosis

Valvular pulmonary stenosis is the most common obstructive lesion seen in congenital heart disease (10 % of all congenital heart disease). It may occur as an isolated lesion (15-20 percent of right ventricular outflow obstructions) or in conjunction with various complex lesions (Fig. 5-30). In valvular pulmonary stenosis, which is by far the larger patient population with right ventricular outflow obstruction, the thickened pulmonary cusps can be interrogated by various ultrasonic techniques.

The continuous wave Doppler is used to measure the peak transvalvular flow velocity. One must be certain that the true peak velocity has been obtained, and should therefore be selective in the signal choosen for measurement (Fig. 5-31). The two-dimensional and M-mode examinations yield structural information (Fig. 5-32, 5-33) such as the presence of thickened valves, chamber dilatation and hypertrophy, and doming of the valve cusp (Fig. 5-34). However, it is the Doppler modalities which permit the measurement of hemodynamic events, and transvalvular pressure gradients. The pulmonary cusps are often thickened and are highly reflective. Selection of a high pass filter setting near 1200 Hz will generally prevent saturation of the receivers when performing the Doppler examination.

The criteria established based on invasive pressure measurements can be applied in evaluating pulmonary stenosis by Doppler techniques, as the instantaneous peak and mean pressure gradients obtained by both methods are essentially equivalent. A peak pressure drop less than 30 mm Hg is considered to be mild in severity, while a peak pressure gradient of 30 to 60 mm Hg is considered to be a moderate obstruction. In severe cases, the peak gradient may exceed 160 mm Hg. The left parasternal transducer position from the second or third intercostal space is usually the best window for interrogating pulmonary flow (Fig. 5-35). Pulmonary regurgitation is seen in a large percentage of normal subjects, and is almost invariably found in patients with pulmonary stenosis.

The flow morphology reflects the severity of the lesion. In a more severe stenosis the peak pressure is sustained for a longer period, resulting in a higher mean pressure than would be seen in a less severe stenosis with the same peak gradient (Fig. 5-36). The comparison of a mild, moderate, and severe pulmonic stenosis in Figure 5-37 demonstrates how the systolic velocity trace becomes more rounded in the more severe lesion. The deceleration of an associated pulmonary regurgitation velocity tracing reflects the pulmonary artery pressure (Fig. 3-38). The flow at the level of the stenosis is organized, and the flow profile is flat. If one uses high pulse repetition frequency Doppler and places a small sample volume in the stenotic orifice, a relatively narrow band signal is obtained (Fig. 5-39). When interrogating the pulmonary artery with continuous wave Doppler, flow disturbances from other sites, such as a patent ductus arteriosus (Fig. 5-40) can be encountered. In complex lesions the ability to implement continuous wave Doppler with the imaging probe is quite useful. Color flow mapping can be used for the localization of the obstruction and to determine the presence of associated lesions, especially in the setting of complex anomalies. In the setting of tetralogy of Fallot for instance, patent ductus is not an uncommon finding (Fig. 5-41).

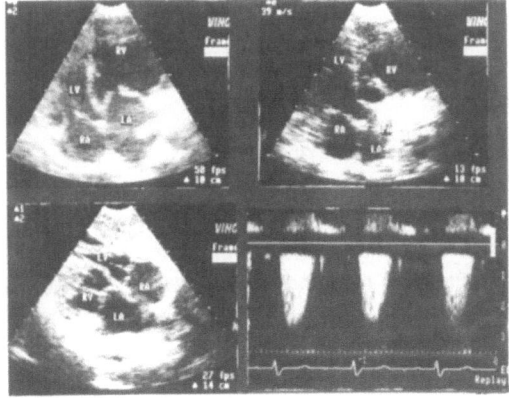

Fig. 5-30. A subcostal four chamber view in a child with an L transposition of the great arteries. A small gradient was measured across the pulmonic valve by continuous wave Doppler (lower). Left ventricle=LV, right ventricle=RV, left atrium= LA, right atrium=RA.

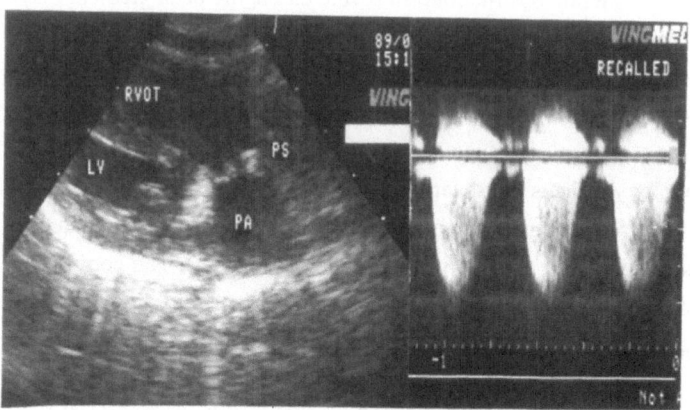

Fig. 5-31. The thickened PV opening motion is greatly reduced, as noted on the 2D image (left). The CW Doppler measurement of PV flow yielded a gradient of ~ 60 mmHg (right).

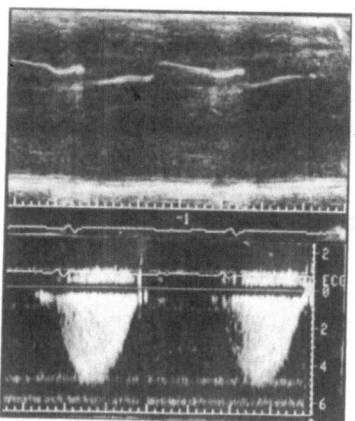

Fig. 5-32. The M-mode demonstrates a thickened pulmonary valve cusp (arrow). The peak velocity measured by CW Doppler was 5 m/s yielding a pressure of ≈100 mm Hg. The strong vertical spikes represent valve opening and closure.

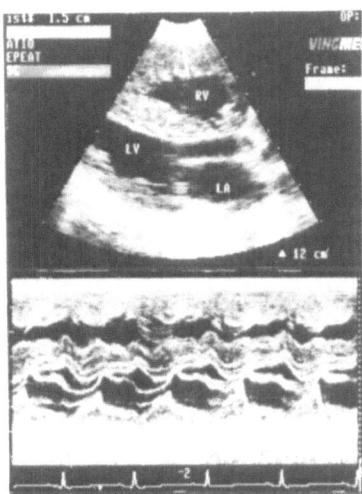

Fig. 5-33. Pulmonary stenosis. The two dimensional image (top) of the parasternal long axis demonstrates marked right ventricular hypertrophy. The TM mode (bottom) findings from the same transducer position. Right ventricle (RV), left ventricle (LV), left atrium (LA).

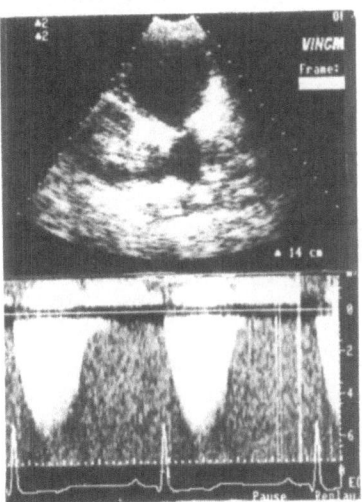

Fig. 5-34. The two dimensional image of the right ventricular outflow tract demonstrates the systolic doming of the pulmonic valve (top). The continuous wave Doppler was implemented to measure a flow velocity of 5.25 m/s (110 mmHg).

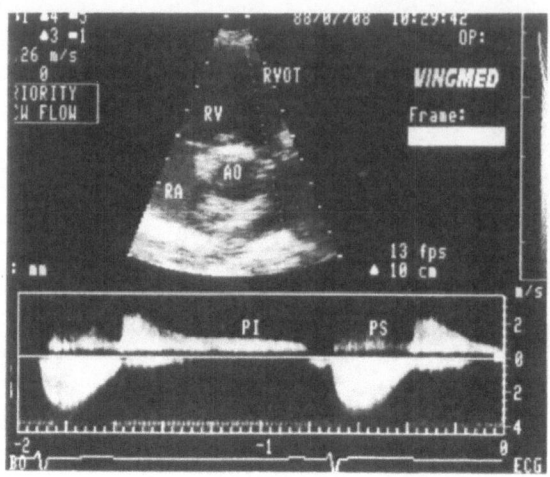

Fig. 5-35. A mild residual gradient and regurgitation recorded in a patient after pulmonary valvulotomy using continuous mode. The peak velocity is 3.2 m/s, and the mean velocity is approximately 2.0 m/s; the corrected gradient is approximately 20 mmHg. This study was obtained from the left parasternal position in the second intercostal space. This is frequently the best window for interrogating the pulmonary valve. Right ventricle=RV, right atrium=RA, Ao=aorta, PS = pulmonary stenosis, PI = pulmonary insufficiency.

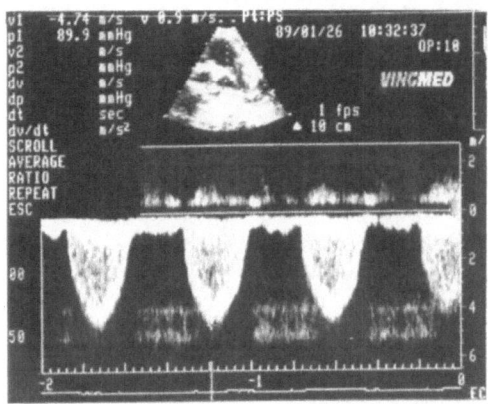

Fig. 5-36. A gradient of 90 mmHg was measured by CW Doppler in this patient with valvular pulmonic stenosis. If one compares the tracing of severe pulmonary stenosis in this figure to that of the moderate stenosis in the preceeding figure, a later peak velocity is noted with the more severe stenosis.

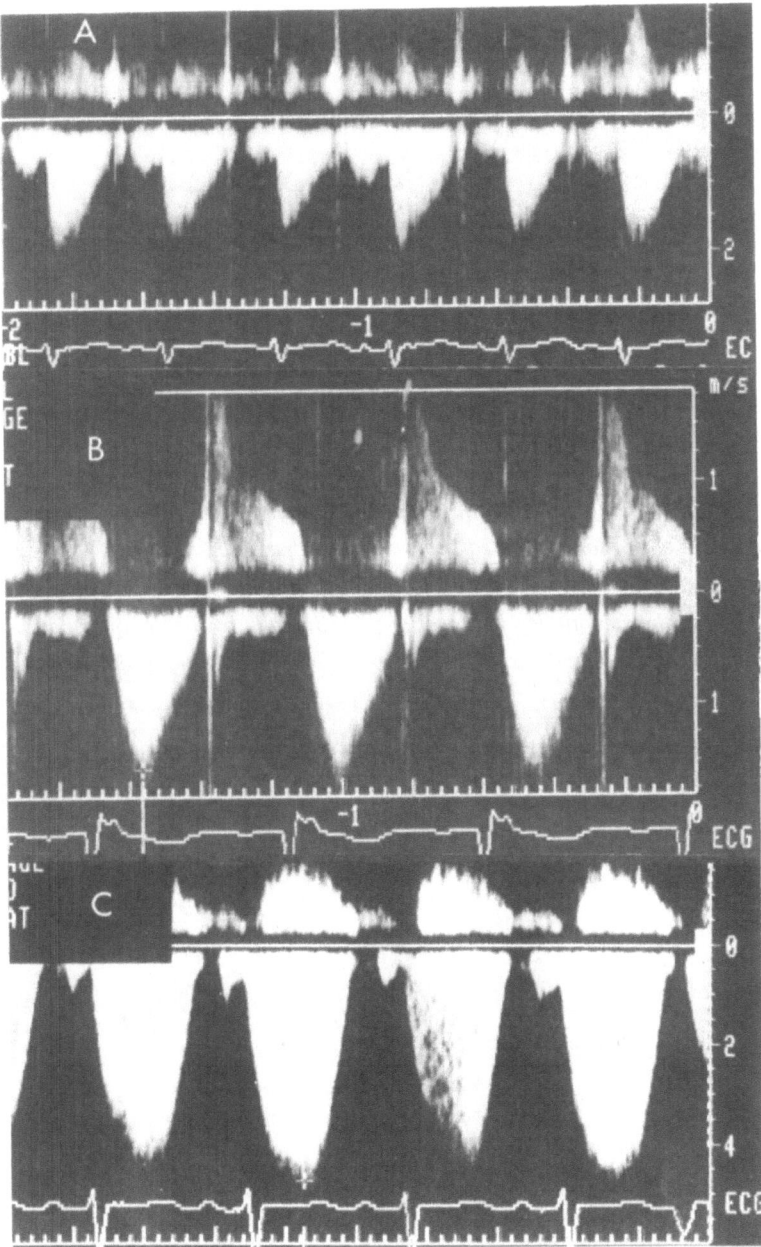

Fig. 5-37. This series of traces was obtained from three subjects with (A) mild infundibular narrowing, (B) mild stenosis following pulmonary valvotomy, and (C) severe valvular pulmonic stenosis. The time from onset of flow to peak is very rapid in A and B, but is delayed in C. This sustained high pressure is one reason that the mean gradient measurement is more representative of the lesion's severity than the peak gradient.

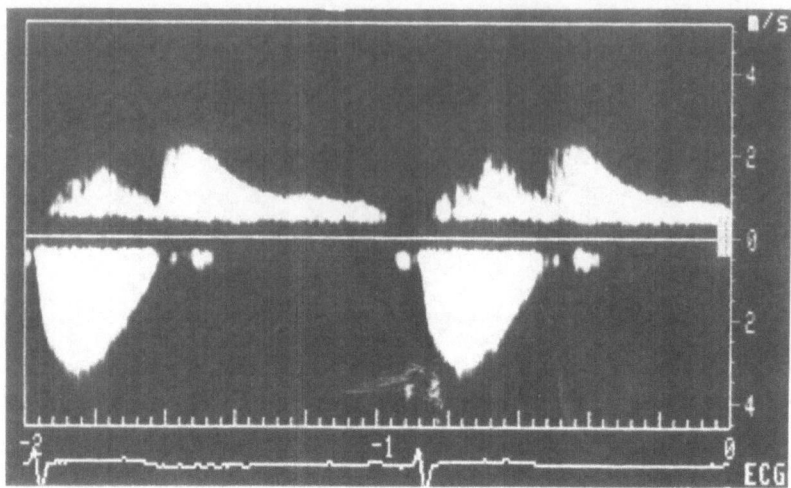

Fig. 5-38. As with aortic stenosis, the high pass filters should be set as high as possible to permit the optimal delineation of the peak flow envelope in pulmonic stenosis. When continuous wave Doppler is used the beam crosses various structures and flows which generate Doppler shifts not related to the stenotic jet. Removal of this clinically irrelevant information prevents saturation of the receivers and yields good envelope definition, as in this pulmonary stenosis and regurgitation tracing.

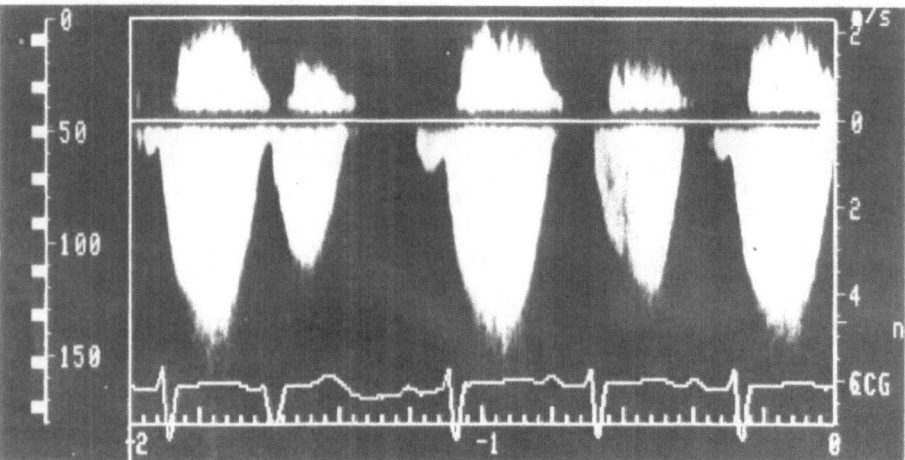

Fig. 5-39. High pulse repetition frequency Doppler can also be used to measure the peak velocity in certain situations, such as this severe pulmonary stenosis. A graphic representation of the multiple sample volume positions along the beam direction is displayed to the left of the spectral curve. Because the sample volumes are measuring flow in discrete areas, a very well defined envelope is usually obtained. Note the reduced peak/flow velocity with the occurrence of ectopic beats.

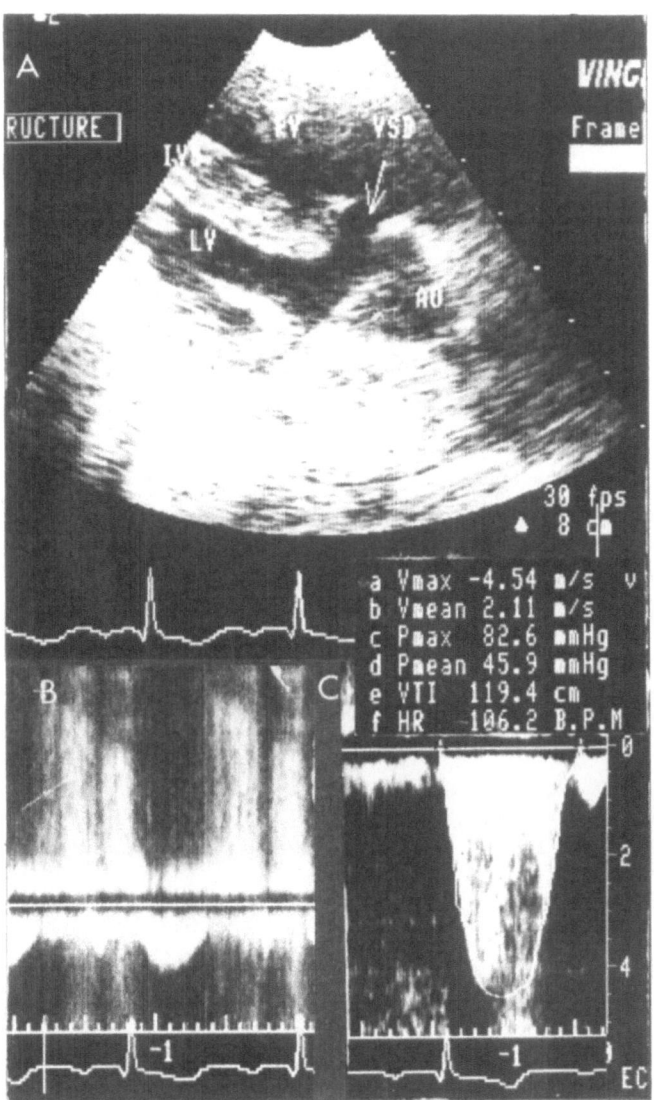

Fig. 5-40. This study was obtained from a child with an uncorrected tetralogy of Fallot. The two-dimensional image (A) demonstrates a large ventricular septal defect with overriding aorta. Pulsed Doppler interrogation of the main pulmonary artery demonstrates the presence of a patent ductus arteriosus (B). Continuous wave Doppler (C) is then used to quantify the gradient across the stenotic pulmonic valve. Both the peak and mean gradients (82 mmHg and 46 mmHg respectively) are displayed. Note that these values can be quite different, and that the same measurements should be used when comparing the values to those derived from catheterization data. Right ventricle (RV), ventricular septal defect (VSD), interventricular septum (IVS), left ventricular (LV), aorta (Ao).

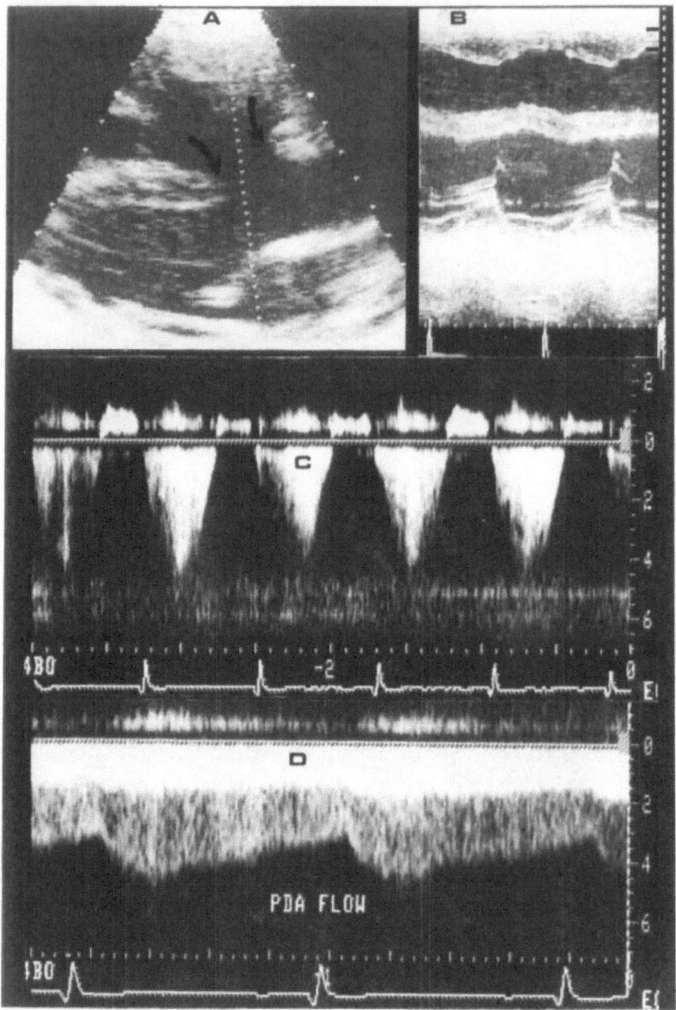

Fig. 5-41. This patient with a tetralogy of Fallot is seen to have a large ventricular septal defect with overriding aorta root in the parasternal long axis view (A). There is marked right ventricular hypertrophy (B) and a moderately high pulmonary flow velocity of approximately 4 m/s yielding a gradient of 64 mmHg (C). Two flows are detected in the proximity of the descending aorta (D). The flow velocity of 1.75 m/s originates from the ductus, and is interrogated at an oblique angle. A less intense high velocity signal of 4.25 m/s arises from flow through a Waterston shunt.

While in general there is no shunting associated with isolated valvular pulmonic stenosis, if the right ventricular systolic pressure is greatly elevated, one may detect flow across a patent foramen ovale.

The evaluation of pulmonary stenosis by Doppler techniques includes localization of the obstruction by pulsed Doppler mapping methods and the measurement of the pressure gradient by continuous wave Doppler . In infants and small children, it is often easier to obtain a good quality continuous mode recording of pulmonary flow from the subcostal window. The peak velocity measured from the subcostal window may actually be greater than that measured from the parasternal window. The jet direction in pulmonary stenosis tends to be more variable than the jet direction in congenital aortic stenois, and oblique jets may be encountered. Color flow analysis can be used at the beginning of the examination to determine the jet orientation and the optimal transducer position for the continuous mode scan. The localization, quantitation and evaluation of coexisting lesions can be carried out with a high degree of accuracy by Doppler ultrasound techniques. The peak instantaneous pressure gradient and the mean pressure gradient are calculated by applying the modified Bernoulli equation (Fig. 5-42 through 5-45).

In a study performed at the pediatric clinic of the CHU Geneva, we compared the results obtained by invasive and noninvasive methods, and there was a close correlation between both the mean and instantaneous peak pressure gradient measurements made by catheterization and Doppler. As in aortic stenosis, the peak instantaneous gradient measured by Doppler consistently exceeds the peak-to-peak gradient measured at catheterization.

Infundibular Pulmonic Stenosis

When infundibular and valvular obstruction coexist, the flow through the infundibulum will be superimposed upon the continuous wave recording of pulmonary artery flow. The infundibular obstruction represents a dynamic obstruction to flow, and has a late systolic peak velocity. The peak flow velocity through the infundibulum is increased, and should be included in the calculation of the peak transvalvular gradient (Fig.5-47, 5-48). Houston and coworkers studied the measurement of the pressure drop across the right ventricular outflow tract in patients with infundibular pulmonary stenosis by continuous wave Doppler and invasive methods.

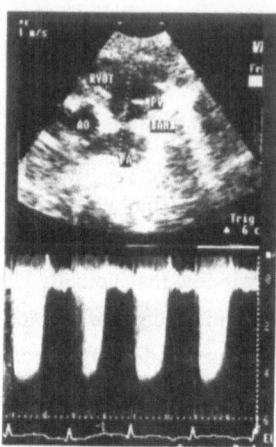

Fig. 5-42. The parasternal short axis image clearly demonstrates the pulmonary artery band. The pulmonary valve (PV) is noted proximally, and the right ventricular outflow tract is dilated. The continuous wave cursor is aligned with the pulmonary artery flow and a high velocity jet (4.25 m/s) is sampled (Color Plate 5-2).

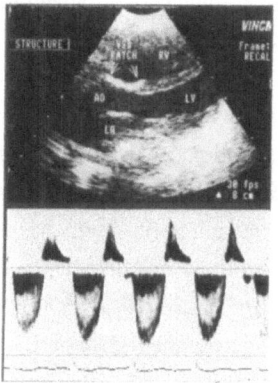

Fig. 5-43. This study is from a patient in a follow-up study of postoperative repair of tetralogy of Fallot. The two-dimensional view (A) demonstrates the septal defect repair. Either color flow mapping or conventional Doppler can be used to detect any residual leakage. The spectral trace from the pulmonary valve (bottom) demonstrates a peak systolic velocity of 2.8 m/s, and a relatively strong diastolic signal from a significant pulmonary regurgitation. Conventional Doppler and color flow mapping Doppler techniques offer a reproducible and accurate means of following these patients post-operatively.

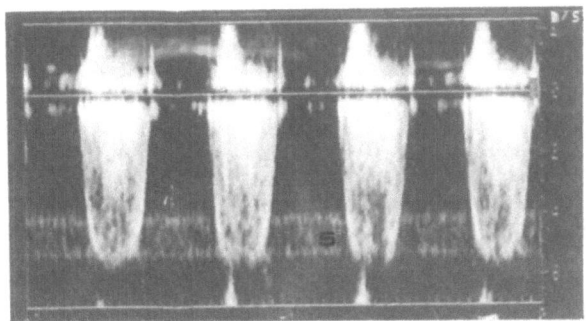

Fig. 5-44. This recording from a patient with a pulmonary artery band demonstrates the characteristic flow curve. The pulmonary outflow was interrogated with continuous wave Doppler and peak velocity of 5.25 m/s measured. Note the opening and closing movements of the valve at the beginning and end of flow.

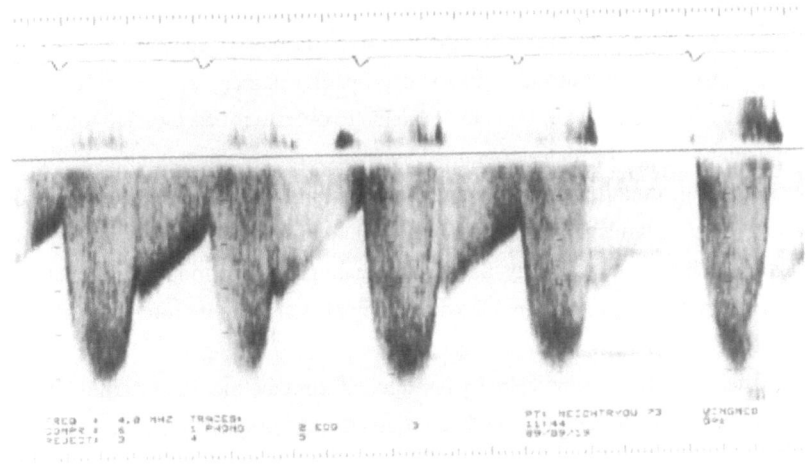

Fig. 5-45. This study was obtained in a child with a pulmonary artery band, which had shifted in position impinging on the right pulmonary artery branch. Using CW Doppler a gradient of 64 mmHg was measured across the band. With a slightly medial change in angulation a higher velocity systolic flow with a diastolic flow component was also sampled, though the origin of this jet could not be determined.

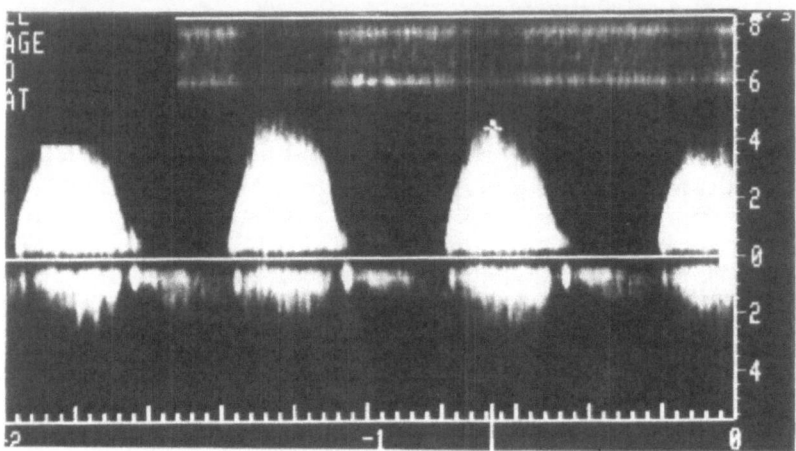

Fig. 5-46. A moderately severe pulmonic stenosis recorded from the right supraclavicular position in a patient with transposition of the great vessels. The peak velocity is approximately 4 m/s yielding a gradient of 64 mmHg.

They found that the simplified Bernoulli equation was an accurate means of measuring the total outflow tract gradient, and that the term for friction can be neglected, even in cases of long segment stenosis. They pointed out that the decision to operate is based on the total outflow tract gradient and anatomical information obtained by echocardiographic techniques. Moreover, the pathophysiologic information regarding the contribution of multiple obstructions to the total gradient is not of great clinical importance. We would add that the implementation of color flow imaging is helpful in that the pathophysiologic and anatomic information is demonstrated together in a real time format, and that continuous wave Doppler is still required for quantitative analysis of the severity of the gradient.

If the increased subvalvular flow velocity is excluded from the modified Bernoulli equation in a serial obstruction, overestimation of the peak transvalvular gradient will occur, but this error is generally not important. The pressure drop across the entire outflow tract can be calculated by substitution of the maximum pulmonary flow velocity into the modified Bernoulli equation.

Pulmonary Branch Narrowing

When examining the pulmonary artery with pulsed Doppler, the flow velocity is frequently seen to increase in the region of the bifurcation . The increased flow velocity is a physiologic occurrence in the neonate which normalizes within the first few months of life. The peak velocity can be two to three times higher at the bifurcation than at the level of the valve, but is still generally less than 2.5 m/s. In Fig. 5-49 the peak velocity recorded at the pulmonary valve level was approximately 0.80 m/s, and at the right pulmonary artery branch the velocity was over 2.0 m/s. In Fig. 5-50 the sample sites and velocity recordings in a two week old baby demonstrate the increased flow velocity as the sample volume is positioned closer to the right branch of the pulmonary artery . A continuous sweep of the pulmonary artery flow from the level of the valve to the level of the right pulmonary artery is demonstrated. The right pulmonary branch flow velocity exceeds 3.0 m/s.

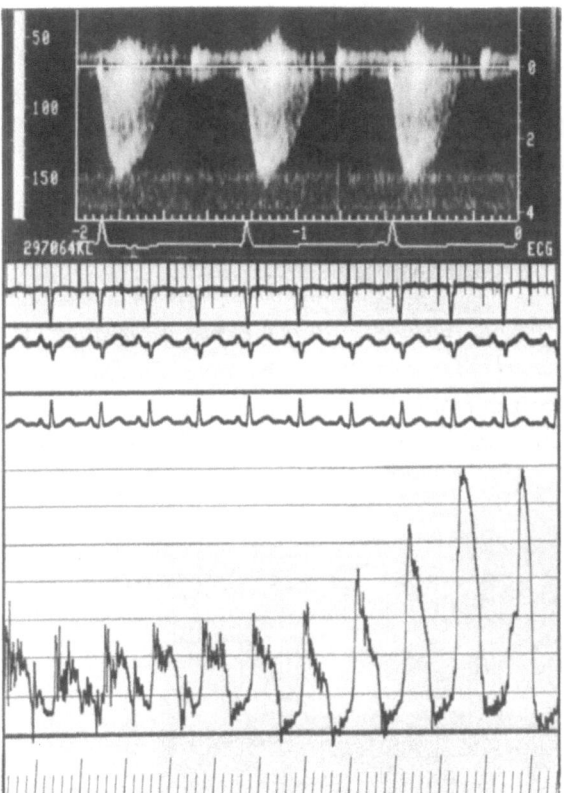

Fig. 5-47. The continuous wave Doppler tracing (upper panel) was obtained in the right ventricular outflow tract of a child with a subvalvular stenosis. The peak velocity measured (3.2 m/s) yielded a gradient of 41 mmHg which correlates well with the invasively measured gradient. The level of the obstruction can be localized using either conventional pulsed Doppler, or with color flow mapping Doppler. In this case, the level of the obstruction was confirmed at catheterization. The lower panel demonstrates the catheter pullback from main pulmonary artery to the right ventricle.

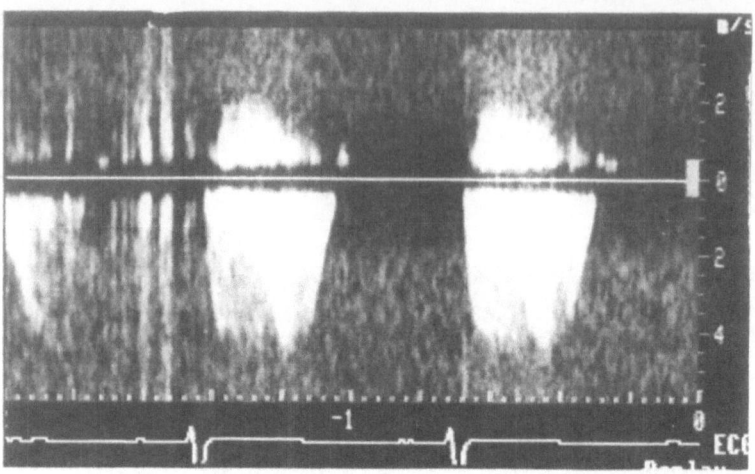

Fig. 5-48. Combined infundibular and valvular stenosis. The early systolic peak velocity is less intense than the bright white area on the spectrum with the exponential acceleration curve, which represents the infundibular stenosis. A peak velocity of 4.15 m/s was measured with continuous wave Doppler yielding a gradient of 69 mm Hg. In the setting of a dynamic obstruction it is necessary to filter the strong signals from the wall motion by setting a high threshold high pass filter. Note the beat-to-beat variation in trace quality; only well delineated curves should be measured.

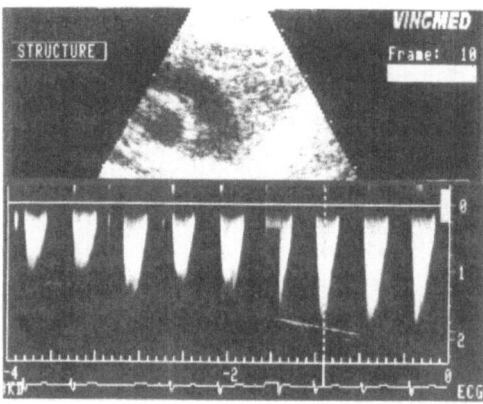

Fig. 5-49. The flow velocity at the valve level (left) is often two to three times lower than the velocity at the level of the pulmonary artery branch (right) in the neonatal patient. The peak velocity at the level of the branches does not usually exceed 2.5 m/s. This phenomenon probably explains the high degree of variance observed at the pulmonary bifurcation when implementing the color flow Doppler to study right ventricular outflow.

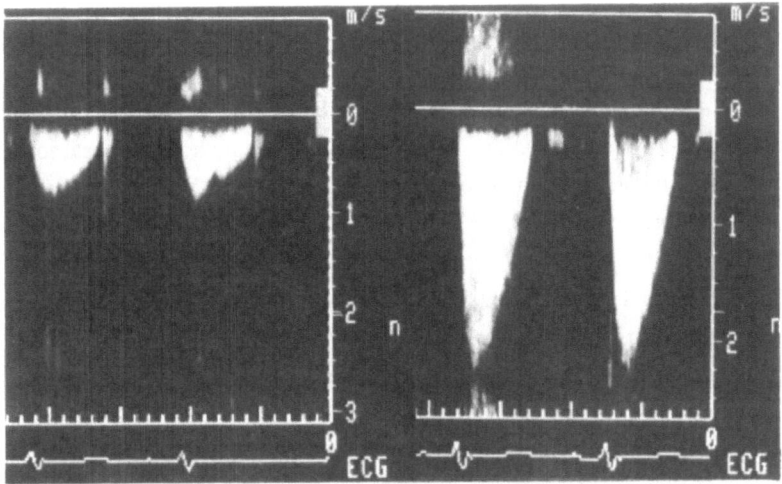

Fig. 5-50. An increase in the flow velocity at the level of both the left and right pulmonary artery branches is a frequent finding in the neonate. This "physiologic" branch stenosis is usually resolved within the first two to three months of life. The trace in this figure demonstrates the increase in flow velocity as the pulsed Doppler sample volume is positioned along several points from the right ventricular outflow tract to the left pulmonary artery branch in a 5 week old infant.

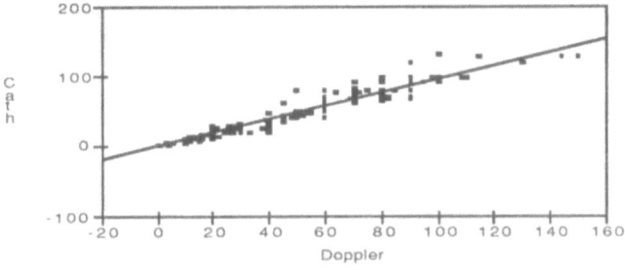

Data File: RV

Source	Sum of Squares	Deg. of Freedom	Mean Squares	F-Ratio	Prob>F
Model	150091.453	1	150091.453	1913.554	0.000
Error	10981.033	140	78.436		
Total	161072.486	141			

Coefficient of Determination (R^2)	0.932
Adjusted Coefficient (R^2)	0.931
Coefficient of Correlation (R)	0.965
Standard Error of Estimate	8.856
Durbin-Watson Statistic	1.817

Fig. 5-51. In this series of 141 consecutive patients with right ventricular outflow obstructions a close correlation between catheterization and Doppler derived gradients was noted.

Mitral Stenosis

Mitral stenosis is a disease in which the anterior and posterior leaflets of the mitral valve are fused together, resulting in a reduction of the effective cross-sectional flow area and an increased transvalvular pressure gradient. The fused leaflets can be clearly demonstrated during the two-dimensional and M-mode examination. Anterior diastolic motion of the posterior mitral leaflet is a common finding on the M-mode recording (Fig. 5-53). The M-mode study will also demonstrate a prolonged E to F slope of the mitral valve and increased left atrial dimensions. The left atrial diameter may be greatly increased in the setting of either pure stenosis or a coexistent mitral stenosis and regurgitation. When a severe stenosis is present one will usually find a greater degree of left atrial dilitation.

Rheumatic heart disease is rarely seen in pediatric clinics in the United States and Europe, although it is not uncommon in developing regions of the world. We have seen patients with severe rheumatic mitral stenosis as young as 5 or 6 years. The disease progresses in the pediatric patient much as in the adult, but at a much more rapid rate. The stenotic valve orifice does tend to be more concentric with the jet more centrally oriented than in adult patients (Fig. 5-54, 5-55). The young patient is quite often in sinus rhythm and a biphasic mitral flow pattern is recorded. The initial peak represents the passive filling component of mitral flow, and the second peak represents the atrial contribution to left ventricular filling. The peak velocity of the passive filling components usually lies in the 2.0 to 3.0 m/s range.

Congenital mitral stenosis is a rarely seen lesion in which the chordae tendinae as well as the rest of the mitral apparatus may be abnormal . The chordae may insert into two normal papillary muscles or a single fused papillary muscle, as in the case of a parachute mitral valve. The valve leaflets are often thickened and do not open as fully as the mitral valve; the presence of anomalous chordal attachment further restricts leaflet excursion.

These various causes of left ventricular inflow obstruction can be identified, localized, and quantified using a combination of color flow mapping, pulsed, and continuous wave Doppler techniques in conjunction with bidimensional and M-mode imaging [21,22]. The pulsed Doppler sample volume is positioned below the mitral valve in the left ventrical and moved in steps toward the left atrial side of the flow circuit. At the level of the obstruction, a strong aliasing is observed and high pulse repetition frequency mode or continuous mode can be used to resolve the peak velocity.

The continuous mode evaluation of congenital mitral stenosis is usually performed from the apical transducer position. Continuous mode should initially be utilized to obtain a parallel alignment to the jet. The atrial flow component often has the same velocity, or an even higher amplitude than the rapid filling component in congenital mitral stenosis. High pulse repetition frequency mode usually yields an acceptable flow pattern in these cases because the flow velocities are generally not very high (<3 m/s). Calculation of the peak diastolic gradient and mean gradient is useful in assessing the severity of the inflow obstruction.

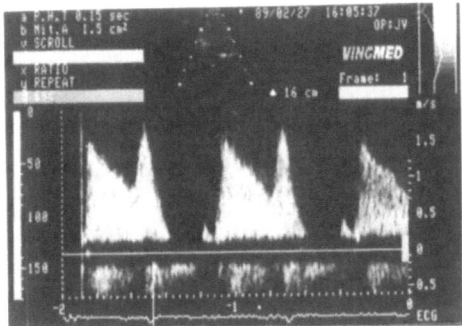

Fig. 5-52. In the pediatric patient with mitral stenosis the pressure halftime can be measured as in the adult patient. The proper slope for measurement of the pressure halftime can be difficult to define when an irregular contour of the velocity curve is present.

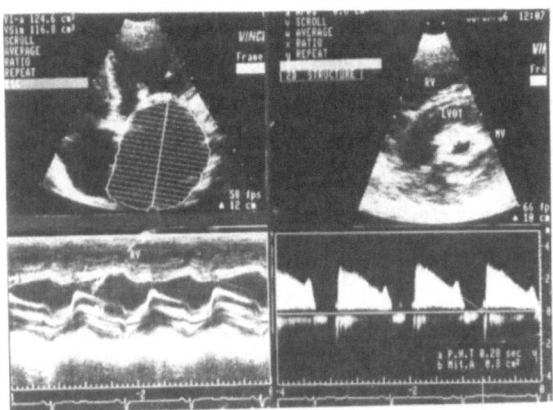

Fig. 5-53. Rheumatic mitral stenosis in the pediatric patient is similar to that in the adult patient, but progresses at a much more rapid rate. In this figure, the two-dimensional (A) and M-mode (B) images demonstrate the typical findings of thickened fused valve leaflets, left atrial enlargement, a dilated left atrium with an estimated left atrial volume of 116 cc (using a uniplaner Simpson algorithm) in an adolescent with rheumatic mitral stenosis and regurgitation. The mitral valve area is measured by planimetry of the valve from the parasternal short axis image (C) and by the Doppler-derived pressure halftime method (D). VSim =Simpson algorithm, Right ventricle = RV, mitral valve = MV, interventricular septum = IVS.

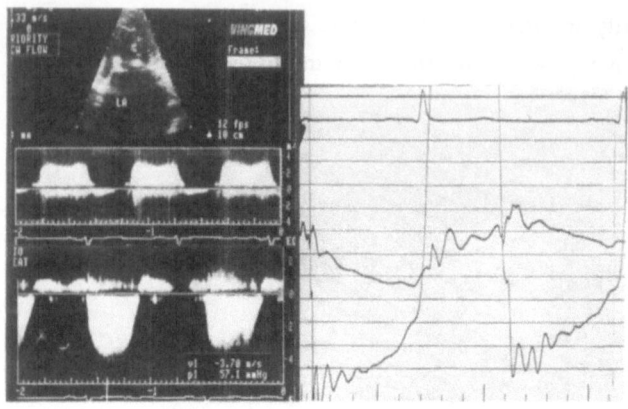

Fig. 5-54. *The mitral stenosis jet (A) is frequently interrogated from the apical transducer position using either a two-chamber or four-chamber view. Another important application of the continuous mode in mitral stenosis is to estimate the systolic right ventricular pressure (and by inference the pulmonary artery pressure) in those patients with tricuspid regurgitation (B). In this case, the peak regurgitant velocity of 3.7 m/s yielded an estimated systolic pulmonary artery pressure of 57 mm Hg, indicating the presence of pulmonary hypertension. The Doppler-derived measurement of the peak and mean gradient correlates quite well with the invasively measured pressure gradients (C). In this case, the Doppler peak gradient is 27 mm Hg, and the catheterization gradient is 28 mm Hg. In the pediatric patient, the diastolic flow is frequently biphasic, reflecting the presence of sinus rhythm.*

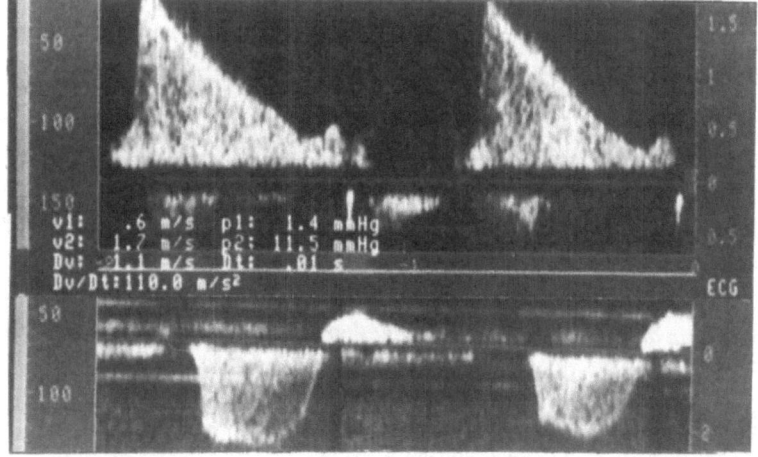

Fig. 5-55. This image was obtained in a patient with mitral stenosis and a tricuspid regurgitation. The CW Doppler trace of the mitral stenosis A) demonstrates a slightly prolonged pressure halftime. The tricuspid regurgitant flow signal strength is quite strong, indicating a relatively dense concentration of blood cells. The tricuspid regurgitation is used to estimate a pulmonary artery pressure of ≈ 18 mm Hg (B).

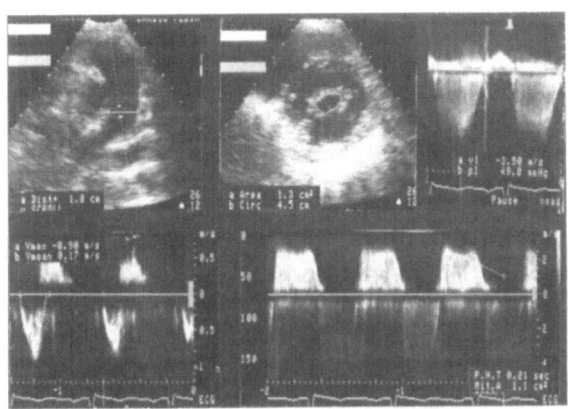

Fig. 5-56. The continuity equation was used to calculate the valve area in this 13 year old girl with rheumatic mitral stenosis. The pulmonary artery was measured and the cross-sectional area derived (A) and the pulmonary flow peak velocity measured (B). The peak mitral velocity (C) was measured and the mitral valve area calculated as A*B/C. The stenotic area measured by direct planemetry corresponded closely (D). The tricuspid regurgitation yielded a pulmonary artery pressure of ≈ 50 mm Hg.

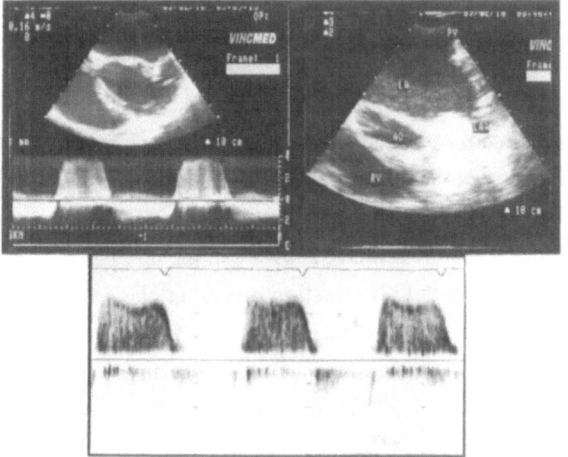

Fig. 5-57. Preceeding Page: Thickened fused leaflets can be seen in this same child with mitral stenosis and regurgitation by transesophageal echo / Doppler preoperatively in the operating theater. The continuous mode interrogation ot the mitral valve demonstrates a peak diastolic gradient of 25 mm Hg with a relatively long pressure halftime indicating a severe stenosis and a strong regurgitant signal (A). The transthoracic CW study is demonstrated for comparison (B). The left atrial appendage was then studied to detect the presence of thrombi (C).

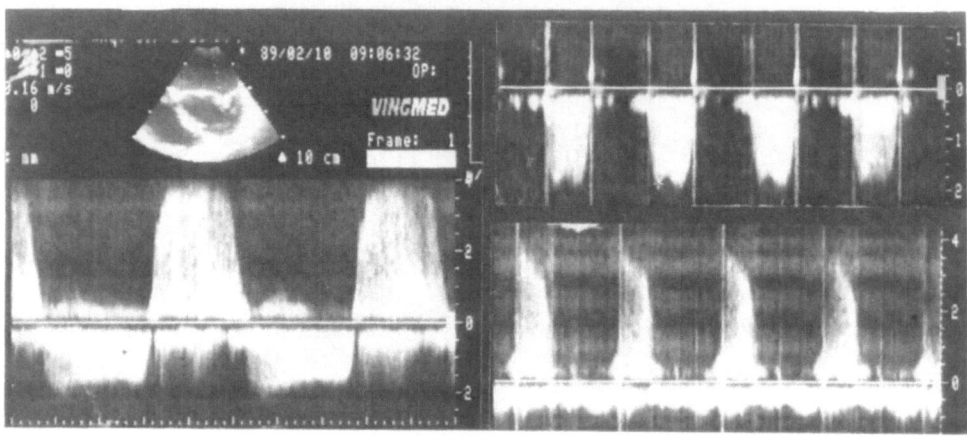

Fig. 5-58. In this series of images from the same patient, the baseline TEE study is demonstrated (A), and the post-operative trans-prosthetic flow (B) which is noted to have a significantly shorter pressure halftime and no insufficiency. The tricuspid regurgitation (C) yields a gradient consistent with that measured pre-operatively.

Another method of estimating the severity of the obstruction is to calculate the pressure halftime. This is the period of time required for the peak diastolic pressure to decrease to half its initial value. This parameter is not affected to the same degree as the pressure gradient by changes in heart rate or cardiac output . The pressure halftime velocity can be obtained by dividing the peak velocity by $\sqrt{2}$. The halftime is the interval between the peak velocity and the pressure half velocity . Hatle and coworkers have shown that the normal range for the pressure halftime is 20-60 ms in adults. When mild obstruction is present, the pressure halftime ranges from 100-200 ms. Moderate obstruction is indicated when the pressure halftime lies between 200-300 ms, and severe obstruction is indicated by a pressure halftime greater than 300 ms. Slightly prolonged pressure halftimes of 60-120 ms are frequently found in a nonobstructed valve when significant mitral regurgitation exists. The measurement of the pressure halftime is made on the passive filling component of the flow velocity curve regardless of the amplitude of the atrial component.

Hatle and coworkers have also described a method of calculating the mitral orifice area from the estimated pressure halftime using the following empirical formula:

$$MVA = 220/PHT$$

Equation 5-8

where MVA is the mitral valve area in sq cm and PHT is the pressure halftime. When the cardiac rhythm is irregular, at least five beats should be measured and the mean value of the pressure halftime used to estimate the orifice area. In our experience, the pressure halftime method of measuring the valve area is not as accurate for small children as in the adolescent and adult patient. This is probably due to the more rapid heart rates encountered in the pediatric patient group. An empirical constant should probably be derived for smaller valves and faster heart rates for application in the pediatric patient .

Nakatani and coworkers have applied the continuity equation to calculate the valve area in mitral stenosis. They suggest that this method is a more reliable predictor of stenotic mitral valve area than the pressure halftime. The method appears as accurate as the halftime in adults, but is somewhat more difficult to apply in routine clinical use. Considering the aforementioned limitations with the pressure halftime derived area in small children, it is not unreasonable to expect better results with the continuity equation .

To perform this measurement the cross-sectional area is measured in the main pulmonary artery and the pulmonic flow curve is sampled at the same site and planimetered to obtain the velocity time integral . The mitral flow peak velocity is then planimetered and the mitral valve area (MVA) is calculated :

$$\frac{PA\ csa \cdot PA\ vti}{MV\ vti} = MVA$$

Equation 5-9

where PA csa = pulmonary artery cross-sectional area, PA vti = pulmonary artery flow velocity integral, and MV vti = mitral valve flow velocity integral. The peak flow velocities can be substituted for the terms PA vti and MV vti, somewhat simplifying the measurement.

Valvuloplasty

The use of pulmonary valvuloplasty was first reported by Kan and coworkers in 1982. The application of this technique in the pediatric patient with aortic, pulmonary, and mitral stenosis was performed and the results published over the next few years. The application of the balloon valvuloplasty method in patients of various ages, and under various clinical circumstances, has yielded mixed results. There appear to be some limitations in the efficacy of balloon valvuloplasty in the older adult patient with a heavily calcified stenosis, however, long term follow up studies are unavailable at this time.

Doppler ultrasound offers a convenient way of selecting those patients with valvular stenosis who would benefit from valvuloplasty and to evaluate the efficacy of the procedure after it has been performed, and for the long term follow-up of these patients [23,24]. In the setting of pulmonary stenosis, aortic stenosis, or mitral stenosis, those lesions in which the valve leaflets are pliable respond the most favorably to valvuloplasty. Abascal and coworkers found that patients with thickened nonpliable leaflets undergoing mitral valvuloplasty experienced a greater degree of restenosis at the six month follow-up examination than those with pliable mitral leaflets [23]. Continuous mode permits one to estimate the peak and mean pressure gradients before and after the valvuloplasty. One should note that the peak post-operative gradient may be nearly as high as the pre-operative value if the ventricular function has improved in the adult, or due to an increased infundibular reaction in the pediatric patient. We therefore suggest that the mean gradient should always be calculated with inclusion of the term for the pre-stenotic flow velocity.

Measurement of the valve area is probably a better means of evaluating the effectiveness of the procedure, as this parameter is not affected by changes in flow to the same degree as the gradient measurement. A more recently described method of measuring the valve area in mitral and aortic stenosis is by direct transesophageal imaging. This allows the investigator to monitor the valve throughout the procedure, planimetering the valve directly. Color flow imaging during the transesophageal examination aids in the estimation of the severity of the valve insufficiency before and after the valvuloplasty. The site of the incompetence can readily be detected with color flow mapping yielding relevant hemodynamic and anatomic information.

The correlation between gradient measurements made by Doppler and catheterization is quite good, both pre- and post-operatively (Fig. 5-59). In Fig. 5-60, continuous mode has been used to measure the peak velocity across the pulmonic valve in a candidate for pulmonary balloon valvuloplasty . The peak velocity obtained was 5.1 m/s, corresponding to a peak pressure drop of 104 mm Hg. Based on the results of the Doppler examination, this patient underwent valvuloplasty with a significant reduction in the transvalvular gradient . Note the excellent definition of the peak flow envelope in this recording, which is an indication that a good angle to flow has been achieved. In Figure 5-63, a study from a patient in whom post-valvuloplasty M-mode and Doppler studies have been performed, the valve is noted to open well and no significant gradient is recorded.

In Fig. 5-65, recordings of both the Doppler gradient and the pressure tracings are demonstrated. The Doppler-derived gradient is slightly overestimated due to the difference between the instantaneous and peak-to-peak gradients measured by Doppler and catheterization respectively. There was some infundibular narrowing in this case, causing an increase in flow velocity proximal to the obstruction. Consequently, the flow velocity before the obstruction can be included in the Bernoulli equation to calculate the true gradient. As previously mentioned though, from a practical standpoint, the error caused by neglecting this term in post-valvulotomy cases is not usually clinically relevant.

The peak velocity can be measured at short intervals, plugged into the modified Bernoulli equation, and the results averaged to calculate the temporal mean gradient . It is of course more convenient to make this measurement with either an online or an offline analysis system . But it can also be performed manually by measuring the velocity every 20-40 milliseconds, calculating the peak pressure gradient and averaging the results.

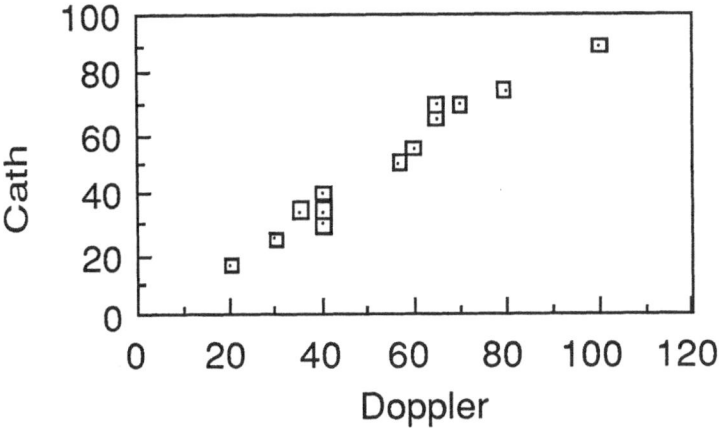

Fig. 5-59. The Doppler-derived gradient is a useful method of evaluating the effectiveness of the valvuloplasty procedure. In this graph, pre- and post-valvuloplasty Doppler and catheterization-derived gradients are compared. Both pre-and post-valvuloplasty gradients measured by Doppler techniques correspond well to those measured during catheterization.

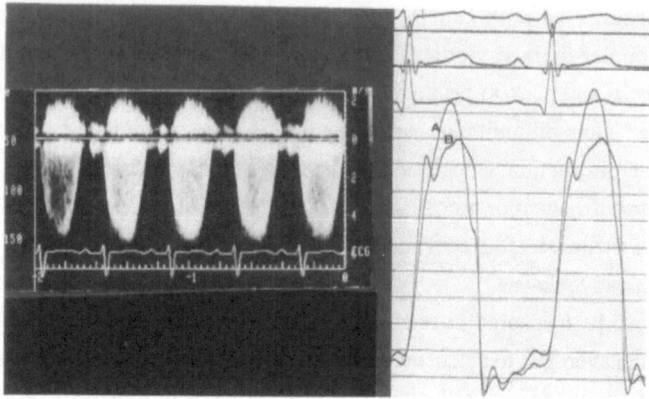

Fig. 5-60. Continuous mode recording of a high velocity flow (5.0 m/s) from a patient with pulmonary stenosis before valvuloplasty (left). Note the delay in the acceleration of flow across the obstruction. The right and left ventricular pressure can be of equal values in such patients (right).

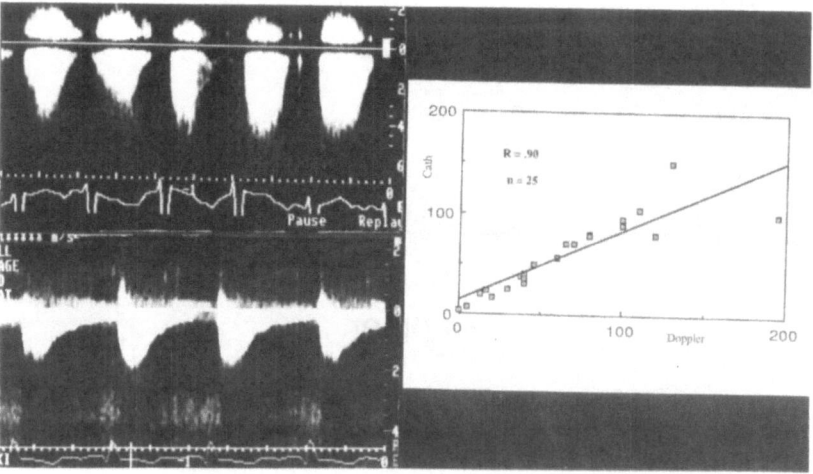

Fig. 5-61. Top. Continuous mode recording of pulmonary flow in a patient with pulmonary stenosis before valvuloplasty; a peak gradient of 65 mm Hg is measured. Bottom. Pulmonary flow in the same patient one day after valvuloplasty; the peak gradient is 16 mmHg. The comparison of pre and post pulmonic valvuloplasty gradients by Doppler and catheterization are demonstrated.

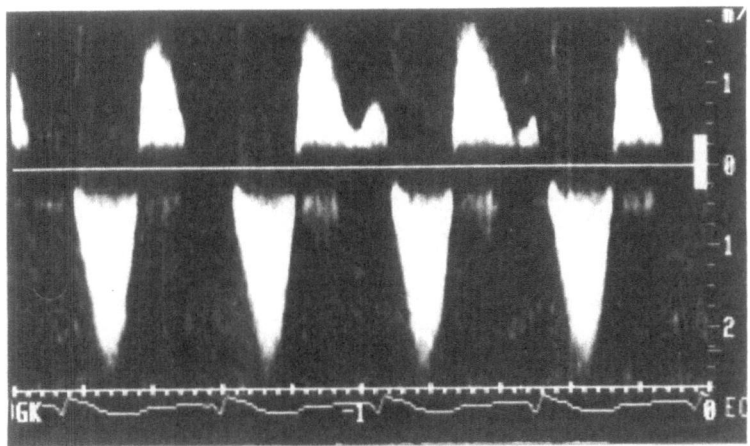

Fig. 5-62. *Doppler techniques can be used to detect the development of complications such as regurgitation and restenosis in the post-valvulotomy patient. In this example, an adequate reduction of the mean gradient was noted along with the presence of a moderately severe regurgitation. Pulmonary insufficiency = PI, pulmonary valve flow = PV.*

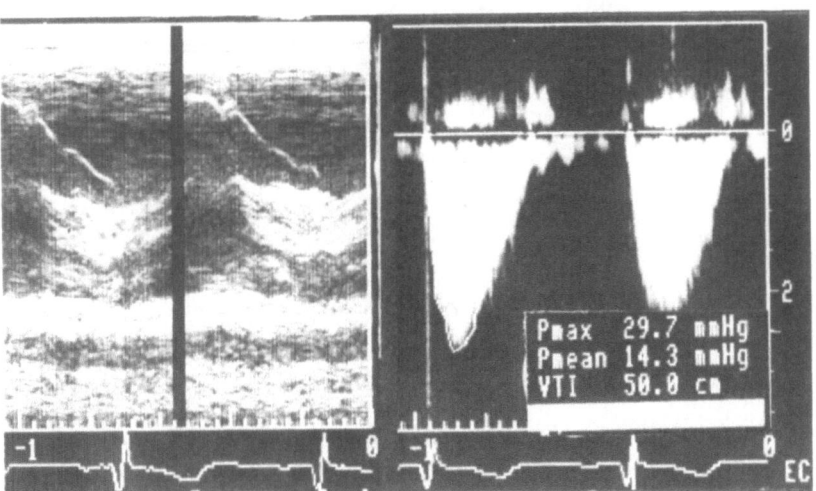

Fig. 5-63. *The M-mode study in this post-valvulotomy patient demonstrates a thin pliable cusp (left). A peak gradient of 30 mm Hg is estimated from the continuous mode recording (right). Valve opening and closure is recorded as vertical spikes on the spectral trace at the beginning and end of pulmonary flow.*

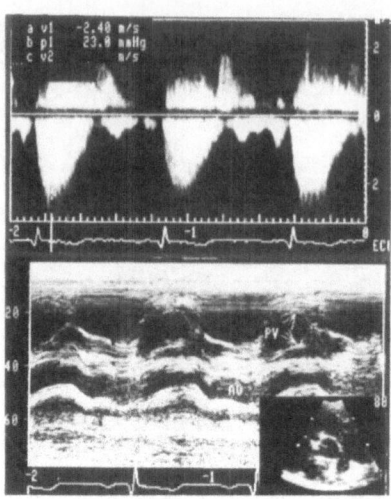

Fig. 5-64. Continuous mode has been used to measure a peak velocity of 2.4 m/s with a calculated gradient of 23 mm Hg in this example (top). The M-mode study of the pulmonary valve demonstrates good excursion of the pulmonary cusp (bottom). Pulmonary valve = PV, aorta = AO.

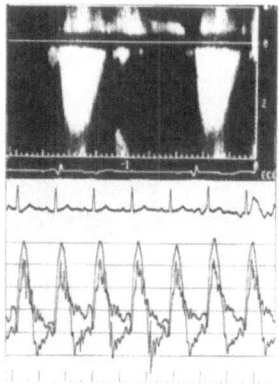

Fig. 4-65. Continuous mode recording in a patient after valvulotomy demonstrates a peak residual gradient of 34 mm Hg (top). The infundibular flow velocity is 2.0 m/s; inclusion of this term in the gradient calculation yields a corrected peak transvalvular gradient of 18 mm Hg. The pressure recording obtained on the same day as the Doppler examination demonstrates a peak systolic gradient of 14 mm Hg (bottom).

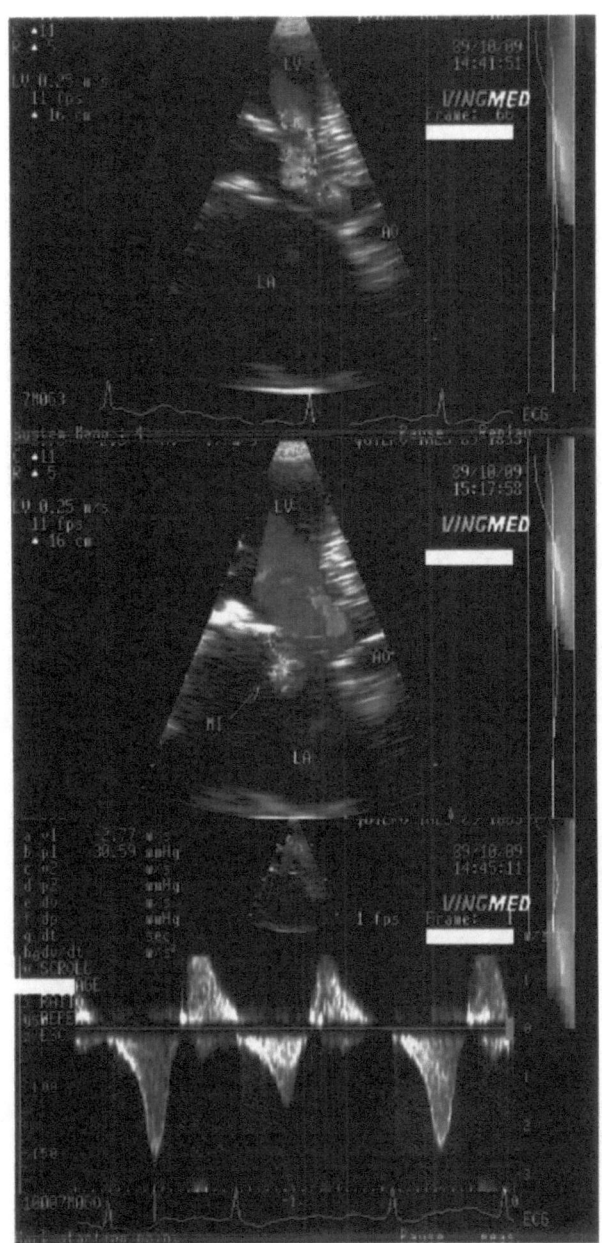

Color Plate 5-1. This series of images is from a patient with a dynamic obstruction to LV outflow. One notes a flow disturbance 3-4 cm below the aortic valve in systole encoded in bright green (A). Mitral regurgitation is also present, the timing and alignment of the obstruction and the mitral insufficiency is such that, both flows may be sampled simultaneously (B), continuous wave Doppler permits measurement of the left ventricular outflow gradient, 30 mmHg in this case (C). The mitral insufficiency flow is superimposed on the left ventricular outflow tracing in the second and third complex.

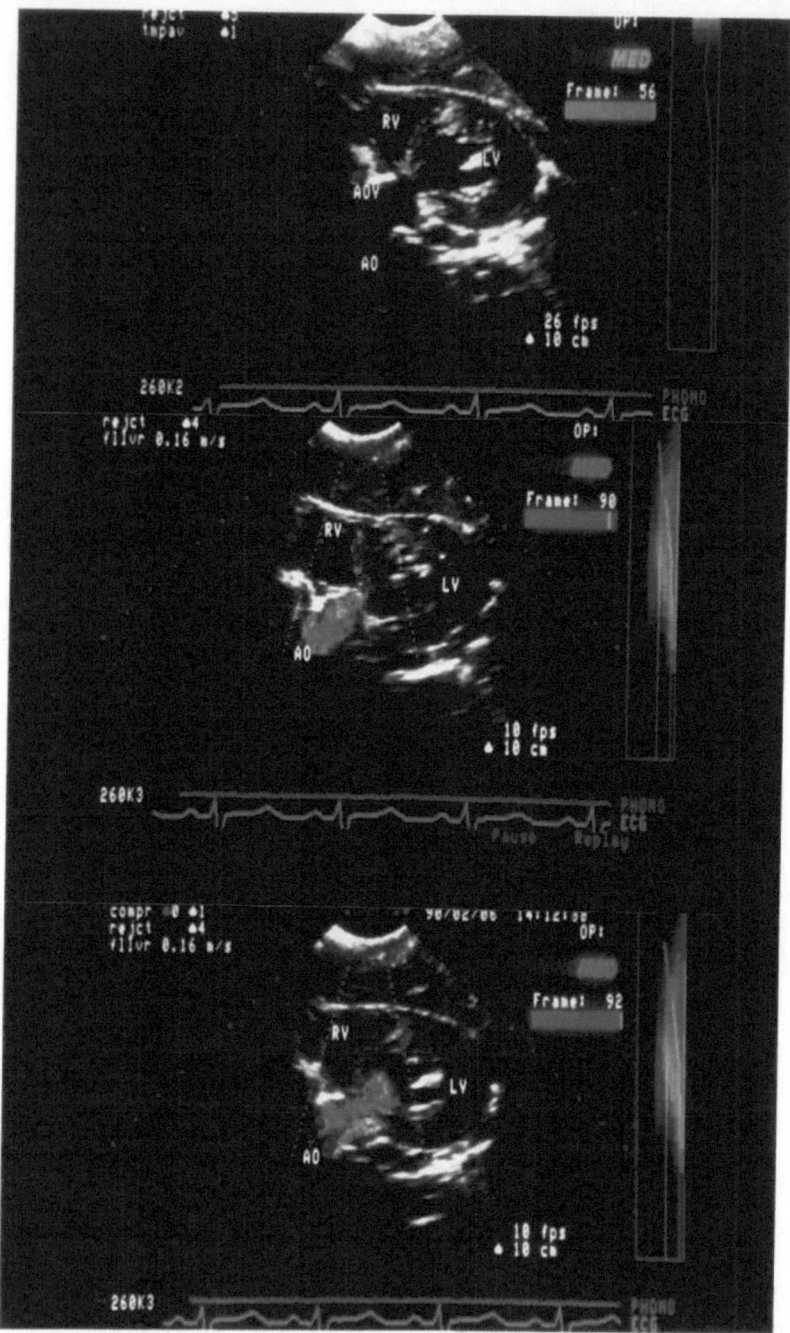

Color Plate 5-2. This study was performed in a patient with a subvalvular left ventricular outflow tract obstruction. The 2D image is used to demonstrate the subvalvular ring (top), which has caused a severe outflow tract obstruction. The highly aliased CFM signal demonstrated in the middle and lower frames is quite useful in determining the exact location of the obstruction.

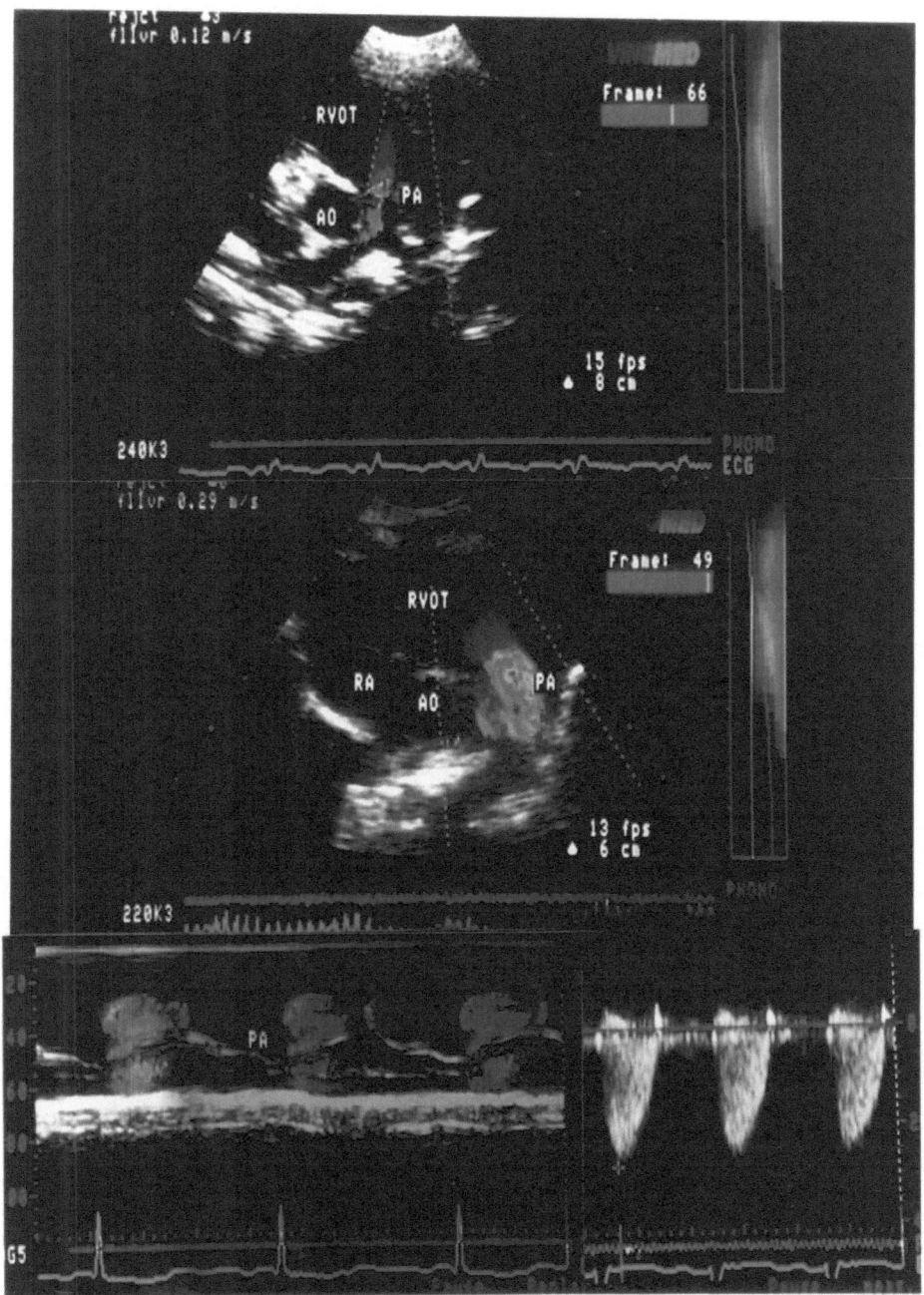

Color Plate 5-3. The neonatal patient in the first frame with severe pulmonic stenosis is studied by CFM Doppler. Note the very narrow jet width across the valve, with an intense aliasing of the flow map. The jet in the pulmonic stenosis in the second frame is from a patient with a moderately severe lesion. The jet width is much wider than that noted in the first case, and the aliasing less pronounced. The temporal resolution of the flow is better with the color TM, but for quantitative measurements CW is required (lower frames).

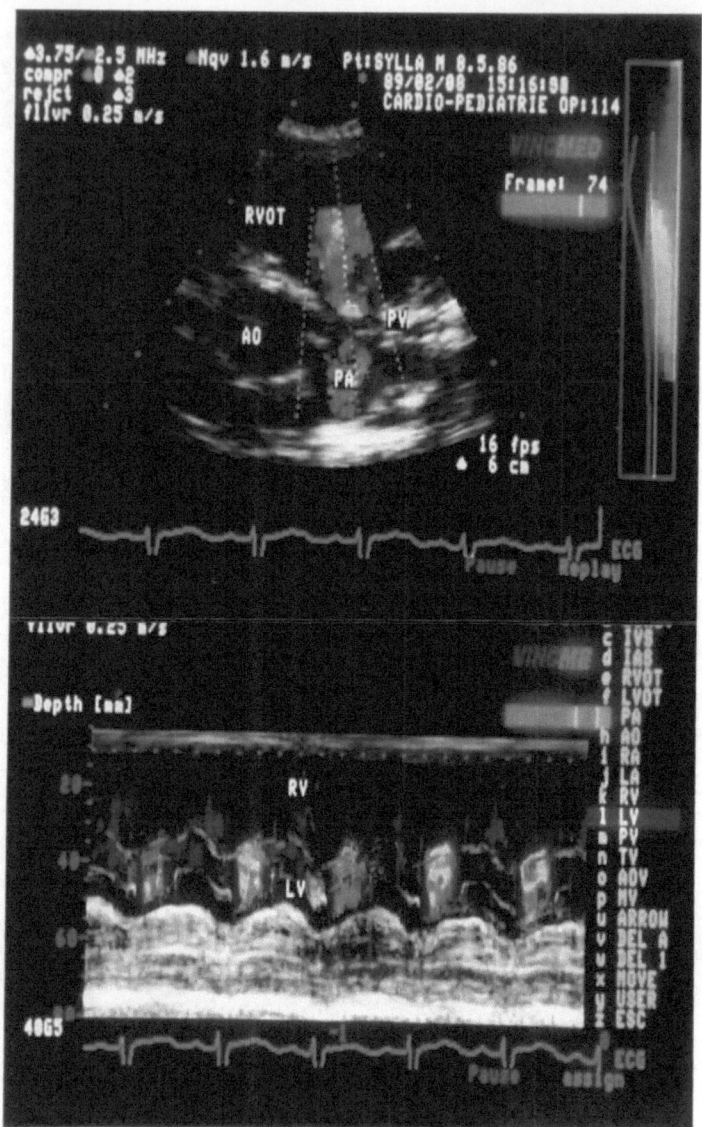

Color Plate 5-4. These images were obtained in a patient with a combined infundibular (IS) and valvular pulmonic stenosis (PV). The flow is noted to become quite disturbed far below the valvular level (top). This is also demonstrated by the color TM mode image (middle). The peak velocity measured by continuous wave Doppler was 4.8 m/s yielding a gradient of 91 mm Hg.

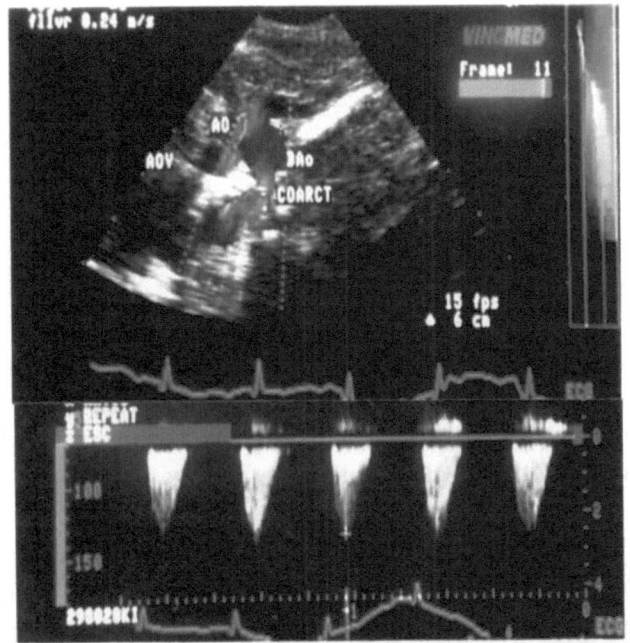

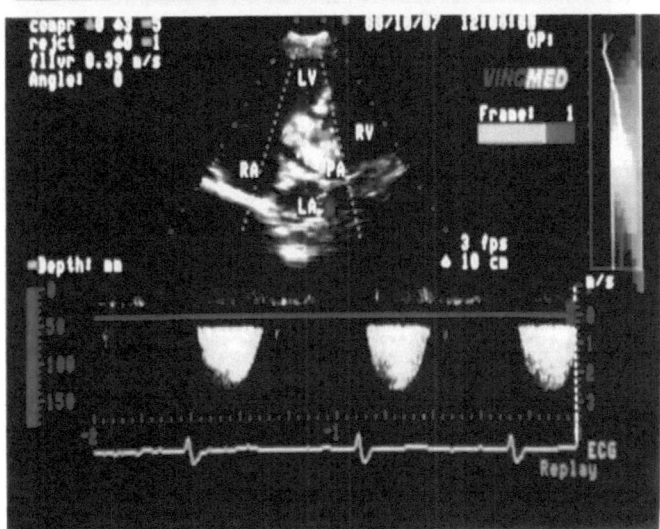

Color Pate 5-5. (A) Suprasternal long-axis view of the descending aorta in an infant several days after correction of severe coarctation (top). Residual narrowing of the descending aorta results in increased flow velocities. This is demonstrated by the presence of brighter shades of blue in the color flow interrogation. Shades of red indicate approaching flow; shades of blue receding flow. Continuous mode is used to measure the residual gradient which is 25 mm Hg .

Color Plate 5-5. (B) These images were obtained in the same patient as fig. 5-30 with transposition of the great vessels. The subcostal 2D image of the four-chamber view is demonstrated. The standard apical four-chamber view is used for the implementation of CFM to localize the stenotic valve, the continuous wave Doppler is then used to measure the peak velocity .Aorta = AO, Aortic valve = AOV, descending aorta = Dao, coarctation site = COARCT.

Summary

In this chapter, we have reviewed the various applications of Doppler techniques in the setting of obstructive lesions. Several important parameters used to assess the severity of an obstruction can be derived by Doppler methods; without the use of Doppler ultrasound these parameters can only be obtained by cardiac catheterization. Doppler-derived pressure gradient measurements are extremely accurate if performed with care and precision. Calculation of the valve area by means of the continuity equation is reliable, cost effective and safe for the patient. The fact that Doppler echocardiography is safe, reproducible and reliable in experienced hands makes it an important tool not only in the initial evaluation of obstructive lesions, but in their follow-up as well.

In general, continuous mode is the most useful modality in evaluating obstruction, although high pulse repetition frequency mode can also be used to measure high velocity flows. Measurements derived from the spectral trace include the peak gradient and the temporal mean gradient. The examiner must be aware of the potential limitations of the methods which were discussed in this chapter. These include high pass filter settings, Doppler gain settings, patient size, and the interrogation angle, among other factors. The hemodynamic information obtained by Doppler techniques complements the anatomic information obtained from the two-dimensional examination, and enables a more accurate noninvasive assessment of the obstructive lesion to be made.

As valvuloplasty and other nonsurgical means of correcting valvular lesions become more widely used, the role of Doppler echocardiography in the evaluation and follow-up of patients undergoing these procedures will also expand.

References

1. Holen J, Aaslid R, Landmark K, Simonsen S. Determination of the pressure gradient in mitral stenosis with a noninvasive Doppler technique. Acta Med Scand 1976; 199: 455-60.
2. Houston AB, Sheldon CD, Simpson IA. Assessment of the value of continuous wave Doppler echocardiography in 121 infants and children with congenital heart disease (abstr). Sixth Symp on Echocardiology, Rotterdam, June 1985.
3. Stam BR, Martin RP. Quantification of pressure gradients across stenotic lesions by Doppler ultrasound. J Am Coll Cardiol 1984, 2;707-718.
4. Horowitz S, Lima CO, Valdes-Cruz LM, et al. Validation of an echo-Doppler method for calculating severity of discrete stenotic obstructions in a canine model with a pulmonary artery band. Pediat. Res 1983, 17:114A.

5. Stevenson JG, Kawabori, French JW. Critical importance of sedation when measuring pressure gradients by Doppler (abstr). Circulation 1984 (supp II), 70:363.

6. Hatle L, Angelsen BA, Tromsdal A. Noninvasive asessment of atrioventricular pressure halftime by Doppler ultrasound. Circulation 1979, 60: 1096-1104.

7. Kosturakis D, Allen HD, Goldberg SJ, Sahn DJ. Noninvasive quantification of stenotic semilunar valve area by Doppler echocardiography. J Am Coll Cardiol 1984; 3: 1256-62.

8. Thomas JD, Weyman AE. Doppler mitral half-time: A clinical tool in search of theoretical justification. J Am Coll Cardiol 1987; 10: 923-9.

9. Skjearpe T, Hegrenaes L, Hatle L. Noninvasive estimation of valve area in patients with aortic stenosis by Doppler ultrasound and two-dimensional echocardiography. Circulation 1985, 12: 810-8.

10. Teirstein P, Yeager M, Yock P, Popp RL. Doppler echocardiographic measurement of aortic valve area in aortic stenosis: A noninvasive application of the Gorlin formula. J Am Coll Cardiol 1986; 8: 1059-65.

11. Ohlsson J, Wranne B. Noninvasive assessment of valve area in patients with aortic stenosis. J Am Coll Cardiol 1986; 7: 502-8.

12. Richards KL, Cannon Sr, Miller JF. Calculation of aortic valve area by Doppler echocardiography: A direct application of the continuity equation. Circulation 1986; 76:964-9.

13. Goli VD, Teague SM, Prasad, et al. A Doppler-bioimpedance hybrid for aortic stenotic area: Better than continuity (abstr) Circulation 1987, 76;IV-354.

14. Berger M, Bergdoff RL, Callerstein PE, Goldberg E. Evaluation of aortic stenosis by continuous wave Doppler ultrasound. J Am Coll Cardiol 1984; 3: 150-6.

15. Lima CO, Valdes-Cruz LM, Sahn DJ, et al. An echo-Doppler method for prediction of the severity of left ventricular outflow obstruction. Pediatr. Res. 1983, 17:180.

16. Simpson IA, Yoganathan A, Valdes-Cruz, et al. Flow Velocity acceleration and turbulence in serial subvalve tunnel and valvular obstructions: An in vitro study using color Dopler flow mapping (abstr). Circulation 1987, 76; IV-355.

17. Stevenson JG, French JW, Kawabori I. Doppler estimation of the pressure drop in coarctation of the aorta (abstr). Int Symp on Doppler Echocard. 1986;36.

18. Sahn DJ, Simpson IA, Powell JB, Swensson RE. Color Doppler flow mapping observations in coarctation of the aorta (abstr). Circulation 1987, 76, supp IV:174.

19. Morrow WR, Vick GW, Nihill MR, et al. Balloon dilatation of unoperated coarctation of the aorta: Short and intermediate-term effects. J Am Coll Cardiol 1988, 11: 133-8.

20. Henry WL, Clark CE, Glancy DL, Epstein SE. Echocardiographic measurement of left ventricular outflow gradient in idiopathic hypertrophic subaortic stenosis. N Engl J Med 1973; 288: 989-93.

21. Henry WL, Griffith JM, Michaelis LI, et al. Measurements of mitral orifice area in patients with mitral valve disease by real time two dimensional echocardiography. Circulation 1975; 51: 827-31.

22. Hatle L, Brubakk A. Tromsdal A, Angelsen BA. Noninvasive assessment of the pressure drop in mitral

stenosis by Doppler ultrasound. Br Heart J 1979,40: 131-140.

23. Abascal VM, Wilkins GT, Choong CY, et al. Echocardiographic evaluation of mitral valve structur and function in patients followed for at least 6 months after percutaneous balloon mitral valvuloplasty. J Am Coll Cardiol 1988, 12;3:606-615.

24. Wilkins GT, Abascal VM, Thomas JD, etal. The mitral valve pressure halftime: Accuracy at six months after valvuloplasty (abstr). J Am Coll Cardiol 1988, 11;2:21A.

CHAPTER VI

REGURGITANT LESIONS IN CONGENITAL HEART DISEASE

James V. Chapman

Introduction

The methods of evaluating regurgitant lesions in congenital heart disease are similar to methods used for acquired heart disease. Of course, the abnormal structure of the heart often noted in these cases requires the application techniques to be somewhat modified. In this chapter, we will present a general review of the application techniques used to evaluate the severity of regurgitant lesions rather than discuss specific issues (such as mitral regurgitation in atrio ventricular canal defect). The discussion of specific disease entities will be presented in the appropriate chapters.

The primary methods discussed in the evaluation of valvular regurgitations include flow mapping (using both pulsed Doppler and CFM Doppler modes), mapping the area of the incompetences (using CFM Doppler), and monitoring intracardiac pressures (using CW Doppler). These methods form the foundation on which the evaluation of aortic, mitral, and right sided regurgitations are based.

The evaluation of regurgitation in pediatric patients is affected by the rapid heart rates and small chamber sizes. The high heart rates are the source of artifacts originating from the rapid valve and wall motion, this problem is further exacerbated by the high frequency probes which are usually applied in pediatric echocardiography. The jet structure also undergoes rapid temporal changes, complicating the measurement. The small chamber size is important because even small regurgitations can persist further into the retrograde chamber than one might expect to find in an adult patient with the same severity of insufficiency. Also, in the setting of congenital abnormalities one may note several coexistent lesions with little spatial or temporal separation. Following is a discussion of the Doppler derived evaluation of valvular regurgitations.

Aortic Insufficiency

Aortic insufficiency as an isolated congenital lesion, except in the setting of congenital bicuspid aortic valve, is unusual. Small regurgitations are often noted in the setting of bicuspid aortic valve, though the hemodynamic importance of these leaks is generally minimal. In addition, aortic regurgitation is sometimes noted in the setting of complex congenital lesions such as tetrology of fallot, double outlet right ventricle, etc., but once again these are usually small insufficiencies. The various Doppler methods for evaluating aortic regurgitation in the pediatric patient are much the same as the methods used in adult Doppler echocardiography. These include pulsed Doppler and color flow mapping, calculation of the regurgitant fraction, evaluation of the left ventricular end diastolic pressure, and various methods of measuring the incompetence area. Each of these applications techniques will be discussed in this chapter and both the theoretical basis and practical application considerations discussed. The questions which would ideally be resolved by the Doppler examination are ; 1) the etiology of the lesion 2) the hemodynamic significance of the lesion 3) the timing of surgical intervention and 4) follow-up of postoperative patients. There are several limitations to consider when using the Doppler methods, but if the information from various techniques is considered together , a useful picture regarding the regurgitation and its hemodynamic consequences can be obtained.

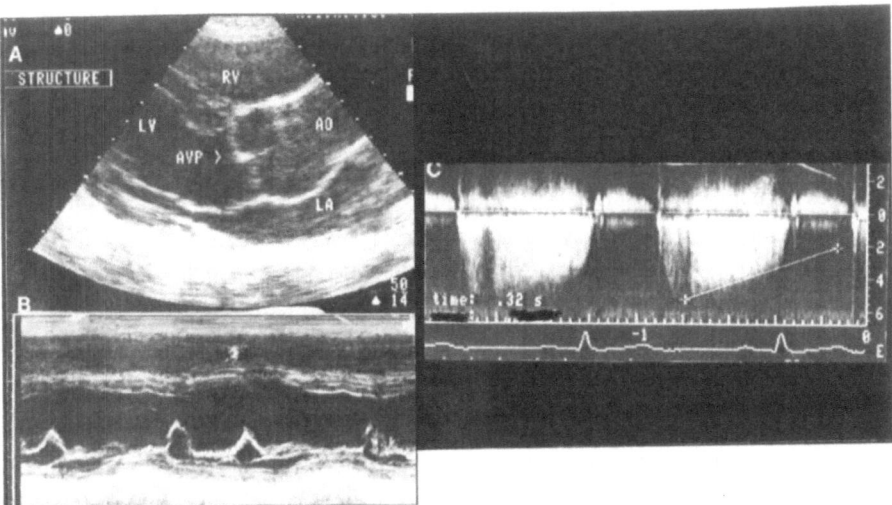

Fig. 6-1. This study demonstrates the 2D image (A), the TM mode study (B), and the continuous wave Doppler study (C) in a young adult patient with aortic valve prolapse and moderately severe aortic regurgitation.

Bidimensional and TM Imaging in Aortic Regurgitation

The 2D and M-mode echocardiographic examinations can yield a great deal of information pertaining to cardiac structure and function in the presence of aortic regurgitation. The findings in hemodynamically significant aortic insufficiency include left ventricular dilatation and hypertrophy, and ultrasonic imaging is an ideal way to evaluate and follow these changes. While no direct hemodynamic observation is possible in these modes, the effect of the regurgitant jet can be visualized. Fluttering of the anterior mitral valve leaflet or the ventricular septum may be recorded on TM mode if the regurgitant jet is oriented towards the mitral leaflets or the septum. While the echocardiographic findings of left ventricular dilatation and hypertrophy are indicative of a significant incompetence, such findings are detected at a late stage in the course of the disease. The presence of a diastolic septal or mitral valve flutter is related more to the direction of the jet than the severity of regurgitation.

Pulsed Doppler Techniques in Aortic Insufficiency

Flow mapping was one of the first applications of pulsed Doppler in cardiology. The development of color flow mapping was greatly enhanced by the intuitive acceptance of the applicability of a real time flow imaging system for an angiographic type mapping.

Doppler echocardiography allows one to semi-quantify the severity of the aortic insufficiency with a high degree of accuracy. With conventional pulsed mode or color flow mapping, the regurgitant flow can be mapped in the left ventricle simular to angiography. However, one must realize that Doppler and angiographic methods are quite different. While the angiographic methods rely on a mixing of the contrast medium with the regurgitant volume of blood to permit visualization of the regurgitation, color flow mapping methods observe motion, which not only originates with the regurgitant jet, but also from the displaced volume of blood in the outflow tract, eddies from both the regurgitant jet and the left ventricular inflow. The regurgitant jet is a complex flow structure and the ability to evaluate the jet is very much dependent on the ability to accurately analyze and encode the Doppler shifted blood signals. Mapping the intrusion of the aortic insufficiency jet into the left ventricle by conventional pulsed Doppler is performed by positioning the sample volume at various points in the left ventricular outflow tract and to ascertain the presence of diastolic aortic insufficiency flow. This study is usually best performed from an apical four-chamber or an apical two-chamber view with the transducer angled to permit a good alignment to the LVOT. The sample volume is positioned at the level slightly beneath the aortic cusp, then tracked in steps back into the LVOT and LV. These samples are interpolated to form a map of the regurgitant flow in the left ventricle. In the grading system we use, an aortic insufficiency signal localized to the area of the valve is considered grade 1, to the tips of the open mitral valve is grade 2, to the papillary muscles is grade 3, and to the ventricular apex grade 4.

In a conventional pulsed Doppler system one must be aware of the possible effect of range ambiguity (see chapter I) when mapping the jet towards the apex. If the Doppler instrument has been preset by the manufacturer to increase the pulse repetition frequency as the sample volume depth is decreased, the possibilty of sampling the jet at the level of the valve instead of at the apex must be considered.

Some of the other limitations with the technique have been mentioned, however there are two other important factors which are applications related. The jet can vary spatially as a function of time, and other flows mix with the aortic insufficiency jet, making delineation of the jets boundaries difficult. We prefer to make measurements early in diastole before significant eddy formation occurs. This also allows the aortic insufficiency jet to be measured before mixing with mitral inflow. It has been demonstrated that when two jets converge, as in the setting of aortic insufficiency and mitral inflow, the jets merge into a single flow structure, they do not remain separated as one might expect. This uncertainty as to which flow is being sampled is probably *the* limiting factor in flow mapping techniques. Fig. 6-3 demonstrates the correlation between pulsed Doppler flow mapping and angiography. This data was collected in a series of 40 patients aged 2 years to 64 years presenting with aortic insufficiency in various disease settings. Graph (A) demonstrates the pulsed Doppler flow mapping results obtained, with an acceptable correlation, though an important overlap of adjacent grades occurs. In a small subgroup (B, C) the results of pulsed Doppler and color flow mapping methods were compared. The results suggested that the accuracy of both methods is roughly equivalent, but from a practical perspective it should be stated that color flow mapping could be performed much more rapidly and with less ambiguity than pulsed Doppler methods.

The width and extension of the regurgitant flow may be used to estimate the degree of incompetence. This measurement is performed by meticulously mapping the area of the incompetence using a small pulsed Doppler sample volume. One can reconstruct a fairly accurate idea of the area of the incompetence in many patients with this technique. However, it is quite time consuming (a major disadvantage in pediatric applications) to manually plot out the area, and the spatial resolution of conventional pulsed Doppler is far inferior to color flow mapping of the incompetent area. This is because the sample volume length is several times shorter in a color flow mapping system, and this of course is the limiting factor in the systems radial resolution.

After aortic valve replacement, the Doppler methods can be implemented to follow the patient post-operativly as well. Indeed the noninvasive nature of the technique makes this an ideal tool for post or follow up.

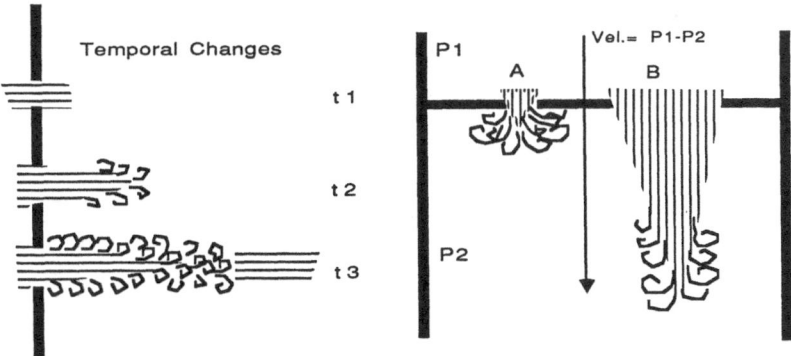

Fig. 6-2. The regurgitant jet structure changes with time. Early in the regurgitant cycle the jet is primarily organized (1), shortly after the onset of eddies are noted (2), and finally there is a mixing of eddies, displaced blood volume, and competing flows (3). If there is a large and a small flow circuit with the same pressure drop across them (P_1-P_2) the velocity of flow will be the same. The extension of flow will be greater in the large flow circuit.

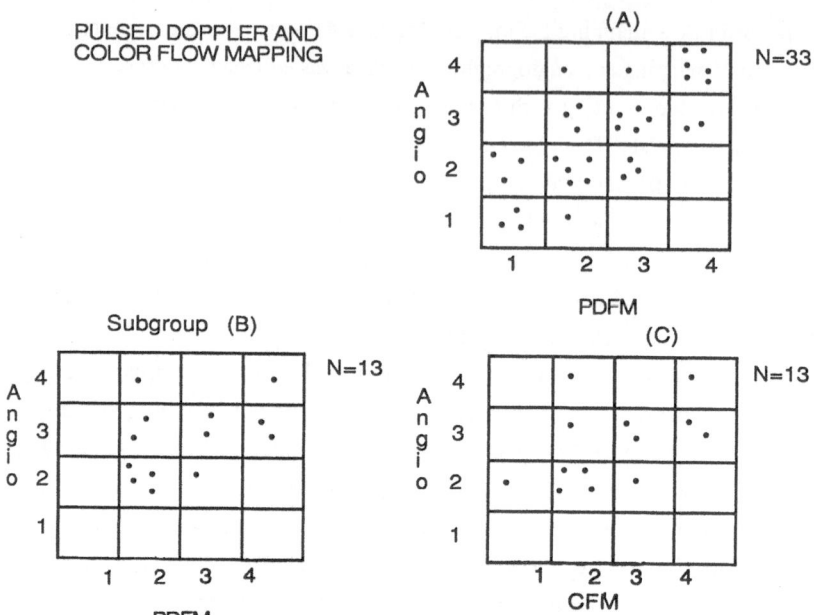

Fig. 6-3. *In this study we compared results from biplaner PD flow mapping to angiographic grades (A). While a correlation exists the significant overlap of grades is a limitation. In a subgroup of 20 patients we performed all the techniques previously described. In graph B we see that there is still considerable overlapping of grades, which is also noted in the CFM study in graph C .*

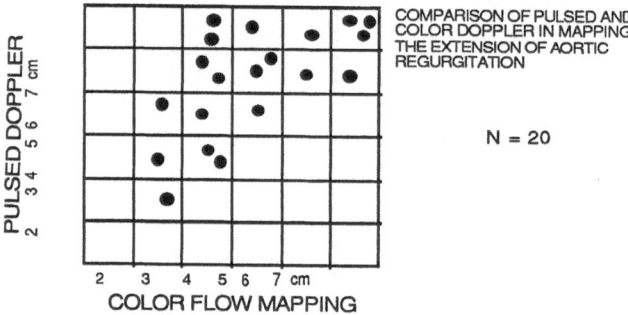

Fig. 6-4. *In this study the extension of flow measured by pulsed Doppler and color flow mapping methods were compared. The flow was tracked further into the retrograde left ventricular chamber by pulsed Doppler, but this was probably influenced by the left ventricular inflow tract contamination of the pulsed Doppler sample volume as much as by an inherently superior sensitivity.*

In conclusion, the pulsed Doppler flow mapping method permits one to evaluate the presence and severity (in a semi-quantitative manner) of aortic insufficiency. The technique is tedious and time consuming, but the results yield an acceptable means of classifying lesions which is quite helpful, especially in terms of patient follow-up. While the correlation to angiography is slightly better with color flow mapping, the main advantage is that the time of examination is much shorter. Whichever method is used, we found various technical and physiologic considerations which can affect the results of both. These include instrument set up, i.e. transducer frequency, prf, gain, reject, high pass filtering, etc., plus anatomical and physiologic considerations such as patient size, window access, jet direction, and left ventricular function.

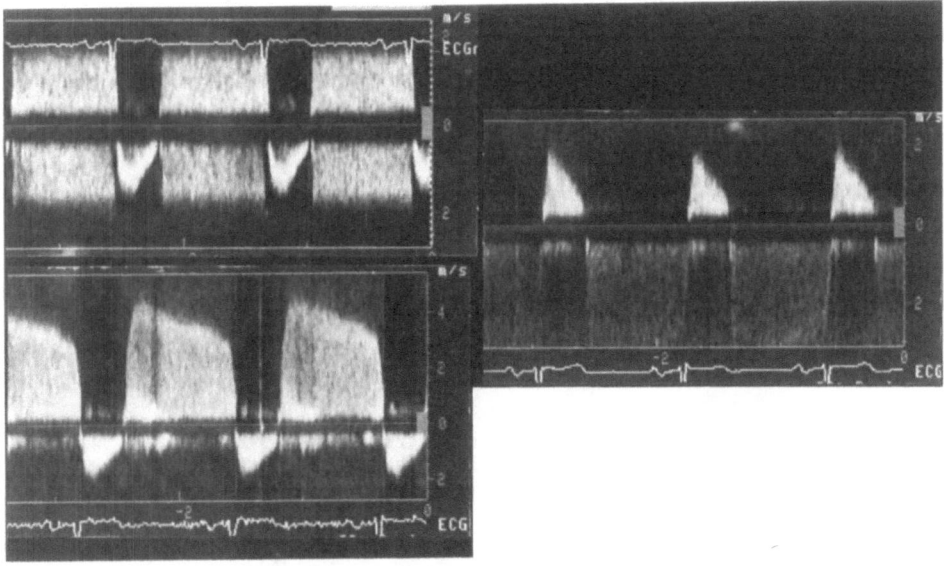

Fig. 6-5. This study demonstrates the pulsed Doppler recording from the apical window(A), the continuous wave Doppler recording from the same window (B), and the continuous wave Doppler study from the suprasternal notch in a 13 year old boy with pure aortic regurgitation.

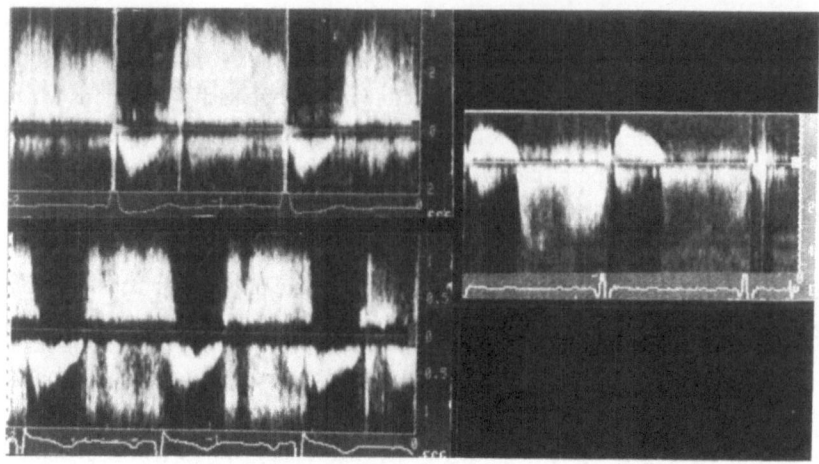

Fig. 6-6. *This study demonstrates the continuous wave Doppler recording from the apical window (A), the pulsed Doppler recording from the same window (B), and the continuous wave Doppler study from the right parasternal position aortic regurgitation. Note the strong "spikes" in the recordings obtained at the apical position.*

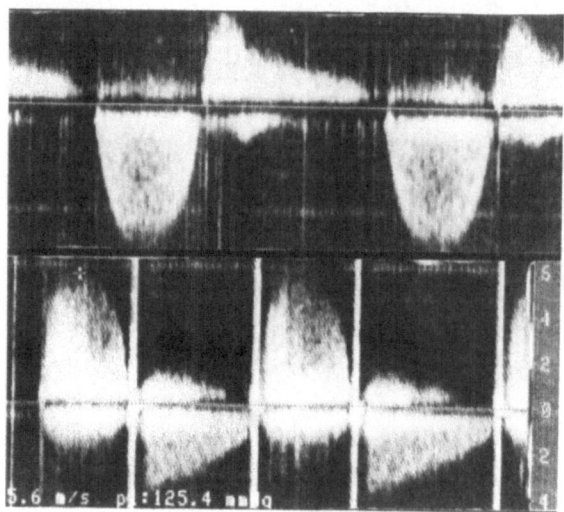

Fig. 6-7. *This figure demonstrates the timing differences in a patient with mitral stenosis and regurgitation (A), and aortic stenosis and regurgitation (B).*

Continuous Wave Applications in Aortic Insufficiency

The presure halftime is an accurate means of assessing the severity of mitral stenosis. More recently, this parameter has been applied in the evaluation of aortic insufficiency (Fig. 6-8) [1,2]. Continuous mode is used to record the high velocity regurgitant jets signal, most often from the apical window or right parasternal window. Parallel alignment with the regurgitant jet is essential in order to record the peak regurgitant flow velocities. The pressure halftime of the regurgitant flow signal is calculated in the same manner as in mitral stenosis. The peak regurgitant flow velocity is divided by $\sqrt{2}$, and the pressure halftime is the time interval required for the peak velocity to decrease to the pressure half velocity. If the maximum regurgitant velocity is not recorded, the pressure halftime measurement will not be accurate. The envelope of the aortic insufficiency signal can be difficult to obtain, due to both the orientation of the jet and the inherent problem of measuring high velocity jets with low signal intensity in the peak velocity range. An independent Doppler transducer is sometimes used to track these high velocity low intensity signals. The PHT cannot be used to measure valve area in aortic insufficiency, as it is in the setting of M.S.

It has been demonstrated that pressure halftimes tend to decrease with increasing severity of aortic incompetence. Several investigators have found that pressure halftimes less than 250 ms indicates the presence of severe insufficiency. One must be cautious when using this method as there are other factors which can result in a shortened halftime, such as reduced left ventricular compliance associated with various types of left ventricle dysfunction.

In a group of 32 patients (Fig.6-9) CW Doppler was used to measure the peak velocity of the aortic insufficiency jet. This, in turn, was used to measure the pressure halftime. As mentioned, the rational for this measurement is that the peak Flow velocity is related to the pressure difference between the Aorta and left ventricle in diastole. If the LVEDP is increased, the pressure difference, and so the velocity, are decreased. A) The pressure halftime parameter in these subjects corresponded quite well to semi-quantitative angiographic methods, though the correlation with absolute values of LVEDP was disappointing. B) The findings of this study demonstrated a good correlation with a slight degree of underestimation in the less severe lesions. In fact this was the most reliable Doppler based predictor of severity in our experience. When applying this technique it is important to obtain the peak regurgitant jet velocity. This may be difficult as the signal can be quite weak. We find that the apical and right parasternal window yields the best recordings. In addition one must be aware of the influence of non aortic insufficiency related changes in left ventricular compliance, which can cause a rapid decrease in the aortic insufficiency slope.

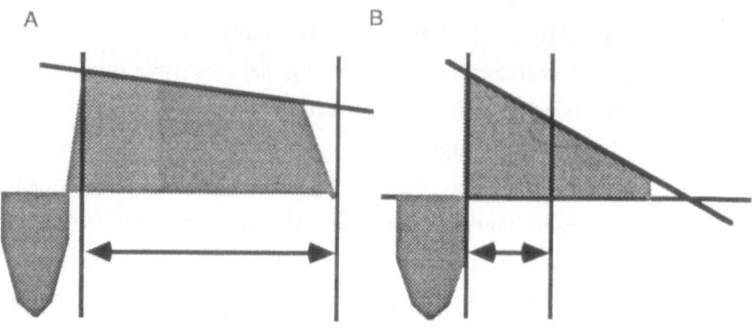

Fig. 6-8. *This schematic represents the aortic regurgitation wave forms which would be encountered in a mild (with the long pressure halftime), and severe (with the short pressure halftime) aortic regurgitation.*

PRESSURE HALFTIME METHOD

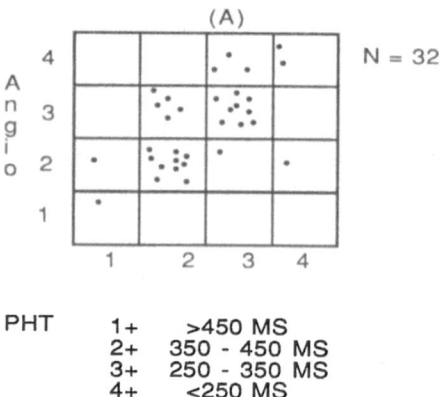

Fig. 6-9. *This graph demonstrates the correlation between angiographic measurement of the regurgitant grade and the Doppler derived grade of severity. The grading criteria used for the Doppler pressure halftime method (PHT) are demonstrated.*

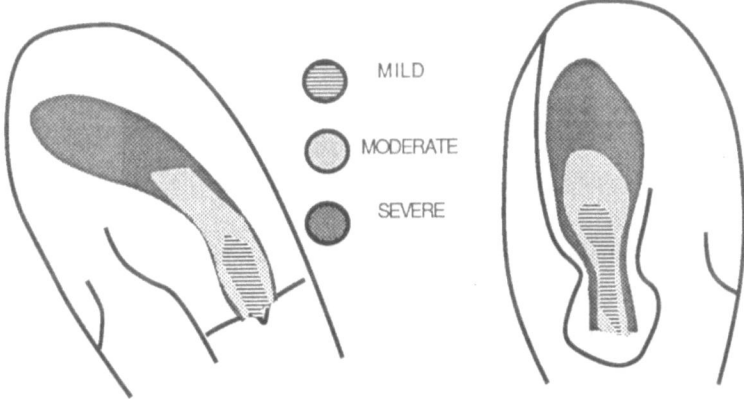

Fig. 6-10. This schematic demonstrates a color flow mapping biplaner grading system which can be implemented from an apical position. This is one means of addressing the problem of irregular jet geometry.

Color Flow Mapping in Aortic Insufficiency

Color flow analysis provides several posible methods of evaluating the severity of aortic insufficiency [4,5,6]. One may measure the regurgitant jets intrusion into the left ventricle along with multiplane flow mapping. Several color flow mapping methods of tracking the aortic insufficiency jet have been proposed. One may apply the criteria used for conventional pulsed Doppler flow mapping discussed earlier. The advantage is that the measurement can be made from a single frame with color flow mapping rather than requiring a systematic plotting of the regurgitant jet over several complexes. In Fig. 6-10 we demonstrate a schematic representation of the biplaner grading system we now routinely apply. The regurgitation is interrogated from both the apical long axis and four-chamber views, and graded as shown in the Figure. The examiner interpelates this biplaner information into a three dimensional map of the regurgitation. We feel that considering the significant overlap of grades in a four grade system, stratifying the patients into three grades is sufficient and less misleading.

The aortic insufficiency jet and left ventricular outflow width can also be measured, and a ratio of the jet's width to the outflow tract width calculated. This ratio increases with greater degrees of incompetence. Since the flow velocity in the regurgitation is not of interest in this application, a non-parallel transducer position is utilized. Either a parasternal long-axis or short-axis view of the left ventricle can be selected in order to measure the jet and outflow width (Fig. 6-11, 6-12).

Perry and coworkers have shown that the ratio of the jet area to the left ventricular outflow area is more sensitive in the prediction of severity than the width ratio. Short-axis views of the left ventricular ouflow and the regurgitant flow are used to determine the area. However, if the jet width or jet area is measured too far beneath the aortic valve, the severity of the regurgitation will be overestimated. The reason is that the jet appears to be larger in the color flow area at this level due to the presence of flow eddies. To avoid overestimation, the measurements should be made at a level immediately beneath or above the aortic valve. Another source of error can be sample contamination by flow in the elevational plane, however the use of a concentrically focused beam can help minimize such an error.

One must consider factors which can cause larger regurgitant areas to be measured than actually exist. As mentioned in the chapter on blood flow, if a very small incompetence is present, the jet tends to be spray-like. This results in an erroneously area of turbulent flow being noted in the short axis, relative to the outflow tract area. For this reason one should also look to the extension of the jet. While there are problems with using either width or extension measurement alone (i.e. gain depending, frequency depending, etc.) the findings of a large cross-sectional area of turbulent flow which is localized in extension to a region proximal to the valve indicates a small insuffciency.

Another factor to consider with this method is the influence of temporal changes in the regurgitant jet structure on the interpretation of the study (Fig. 6-2). Early in the regurgitant time phase the flow primarily represents the high velocity jet across the incompetence, but later in the regurgitant flows cycle eddies off the core flow occur. If the accuracy of the frequency analysis has been compromised in favor of high frame rate, or if the color maps implemented do not have good differentiation of the various flow components, these eddies can be erroneously included in the measurement of jet area. To circumvent these limitations, the instrument should be set up so that a) the pulse packet is as high as possible to optimize the accuracy of obtained frequency shifted signal measurements, b) the high pass filter is increased to remove the low velocity flow eddy components, c) the sample volume length reduced to improve the radial resolution and d) ECG gating or cineloop applied to capture the image to be measured early in the regurgitant flow cycle.

The reason the short axis of the jet is more accurate for this type of measurement is that the diameter measurements can vary greatly in an irregularly shaped orifice depending on the direction from which the jet is intersected. In one plane the diameter of the jet can be narrow, from another quite wide. We have also encountered very eccentric jets in which neither the area or diameter could be adequately studied (Fig. 6-11)

In an extension of a study reported earlier, we found a good correlation between the severity of aortic insufficiency graded by the Jet/Area method and angiography grading methods (Fig. 6-13). It is not unreasonable to assume that if the spatial and frequency resolution are optimized, the effective flow area at the level of the vena contracta can be measured with a clinically acceptable degree of accuracy.

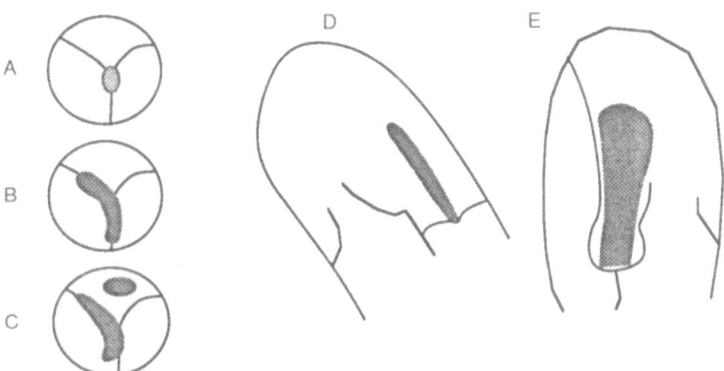

Fig. 6-11. Three different types of commonly seen incompetences. A central concentric
incompetence (A), a leak along a commisure (B), and multiple leaks (C). The application of a
biplaner mapping algorithm circumvents the problem of irregular jet geometry to some degree.

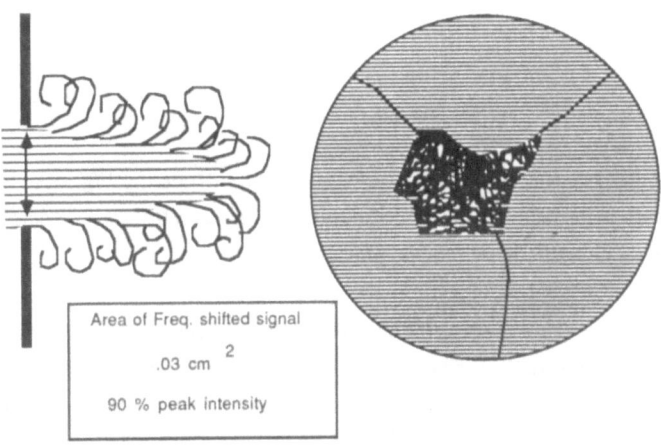

Area of Freq. shifted signal

.03 cm ^{2}

90 % peak intensity

Fig. 6-12. If the high pass filter is increased so that the low velocity eddies are removed, the
area of the high velocity core flow can be used to measure the area over which the incompetence
occurs.

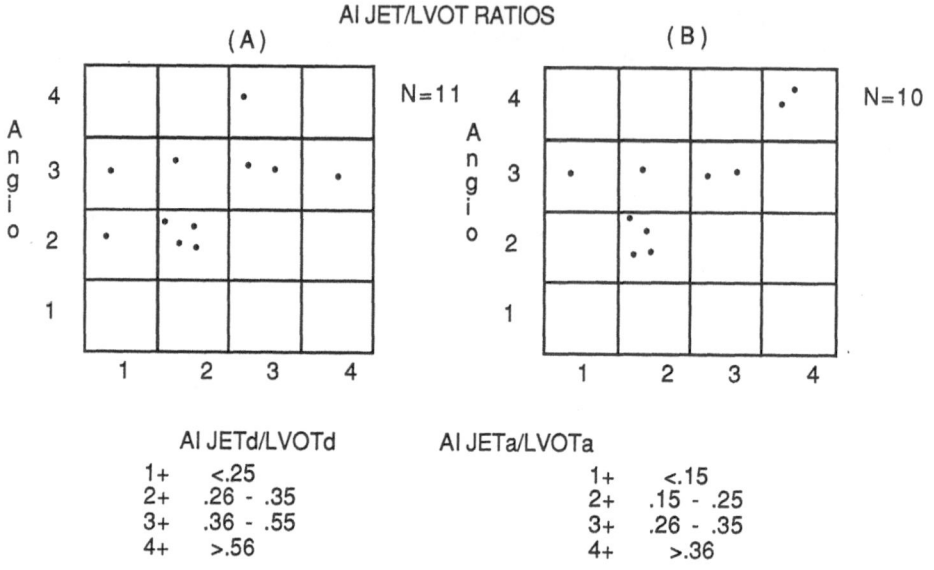

Fig. 6-13. *The comparison of the ratio between the aortic insufficiency jet and left ventricular outflow tract measurements to angiography. The area method is more accurate, but more difficult to apply.*

To optimize the the data used to perform both techniques demonstrated in Fig. 6-13, we set up the low velocity reject to remove low velocity components, reduced the sample cell length to improve radial resolution, and compressed the color scale so that the high amplitude signals were clearly delineated. Furthermore, we measured the earliest diastolic frame obtained, before significant eddy formation occurred. A) Of the 30 patients studied, adequate images were obtained on 25. The eccentric direction of the jet was responsible for two inadequate studies. While a separation of small from large regurgitations is possible, this study demonstrates that there is considerable overlap of grades, probably in part due to the non-uniform geometry of the incompetence. B) This is not so much a problem when the cross-sectional area is used, rather than the diameter. Though the angle of the Doppler plane must of necessity bisect the jet obliquely, an acceptable correlation to angiography was obtained, indicating that this factor is probably negligible. The table of criteria for both techniques are displayed in this Figure.

The Multi-modality Approach

As we have outlined, the possibilities for noninvasive evaluation of intracardiac hemodynamics have evolved at a rapid rate. The objective of this section has been to explain and compare Doppler derived grading systems for aortic regurgitation to angiographic methods. The Doppler methods presented include: A) Pulsed Doppler and color flow mapping from an apical four-chamber and long axis position. B) Ratios between aortic insufficiency jet to left ventricular outflow tract diameter or area and C) Measurement of the pressure halftime.

Whichever method is used, we have noted various technical and physiologic considerations which can affect the results. These include instrument set up, i.e. transducer frequency, prf, gain, reject, high pass filtering, etc., plus anatomical and physiologic considerations such as patient size, window access, jet direction, and left ventricular function.

In conclusion, we found the pressure halftime the most predictable indicator of severity but this was very much dependent on the ability to detect the peak flow velocity. One must also be cognizant of the fact that other non-aortic insufficiency related changes in left ventricular compliance can affect the pressure halftime as well.

The implementation of biplaner color flow mapping yields a rapid semi quantitative analysis of the severity of regurgitation, but is subject to the influence of several variables related to both the instrument and the patient. The aortic insufficiency jet to left ventricular outflow tract area ratio corresponds to angiography with acceptable accuracy when the examination can be performed, but the proper interrogation window cannot always be accessed. Our experience suggest that if one observes several of the relevant parameters outlined, and makes the interpretation on this increased information base, a higher diagnostic yield will result.

Mitral Insufficiency

Mitral regurgitation is noted in the setting of several congenital lesions and less frequently occurrs as an isolated lesion. As an isolated lesion it is noted with mitral valve prolapse, cleft mitral leaflet, and other structural abnormalities of the valve apparatus. In the setting of lesions such as atrioventricular septal defect, dilated cardiomyopathy, and Marfan's syndrome, mitral regurgitation is invariably present.

The application of conventional Doppler and color flow mapping methods can be used to evaluate the presence and severity of these mitral insufficiencies. As with aortic regurgitation, mitral regurgitation is usually evaluated by flow mapping techniques. In this section we will discuss the various methods implemented to evaluate mitral regurgitation.

Pulsed Doppler in Mitral Insufficiency

The pulsed mode technique of flow mapping can also be applied in the assessment of mitral insufficiency [7]. The apical transducer position usually permits a good alignment to flow to be achieved. The sample volume is placed in the left atrium behind the mitral annulus. When the systolic regurgitant flow signal is detected, an aliased signal will be recorded. The sample volume is then moved further back into the left atrium in an attempt to follow the regurgitant flow. When a severe incompetence is present, the regurgitant signal may be detected at the atrial wall near the entrance of or into, the pulmonary veins. The jet width is estimated by sweeping the sample volume laterally at various depths. In general, the greater the flow width and extension, the more severe the incompetence. Figure 6-14 demonstrates a mapping scheme which can be used to grade mitral regurgitation. The limitations of this method are the same as those of flow mapping in aortic insufficiency, i.e. gain and reject dependency, jet direction, and patient size.

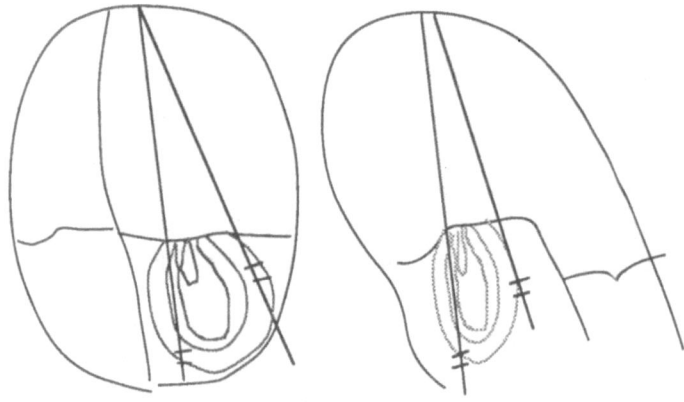

Fig. 6-14 . The pulsed Doppler can be used for flow mapping. This schematic demonstrates the way in which the regurgitation can be graded. The sample volume should be made as small as possible to optimize the radial resolution, this is especially true for pediatric patients due to the small heart size.

A standard apical transducer position may be used but often an intermediate position between the apex and the sternum offers a better window for the Doppler examination. The distance between the probe and the regurgitant flow is decreased, and the flow signal may be stronger than that recorded from the apex. The jet in mitral insufficiency is often eccentric, and is directed towards the left atrial wall. Due to the jet eccentricity, the intermediate transducer position provides a better alignment to the regurgitant flow. The parasternal window is often useful for mapping MI when the jet is eccentric, as a good alignment to the jet can be obtained. If the regurgitant signal is very intense, the regurgitation may generally be considered to be at least moderate in severity. There are of course exceptions, the signal intensity can be strong in a mild regurgitant lesion if the patient is particularly easy to examine, with acoustic windows permitting the transducers to be positioned close to the jet. The frequency of the transducer also has an impact on the signal intensity, lower frequencies tend to yield stronger signals. A narrow peak velocity envelope of the spectral trace usually indicates a more severe mitral insufficiency, but is quite angle dependent. A smaller sample volume can be used in flow mapping to improve the radial resolution. This permits a more precise definition of the regurgitant flow extension, although the signal-to-noise ratio of the signal is decreased.

The pulsed Doppler flow mapping technique represents a semi-quantitative approach to grading mitral regurgitation, but the technique is time -consuming. In the presence of left ventricular dilatation, the increased depth of interrogation can result in a reduced signal strength even when an intermediate transducer position is used. Patient movement may cause erroneous localization of flow. When reduced ventricular function coexists with mitral insufficiency, the flow mapping results may be equivocal.

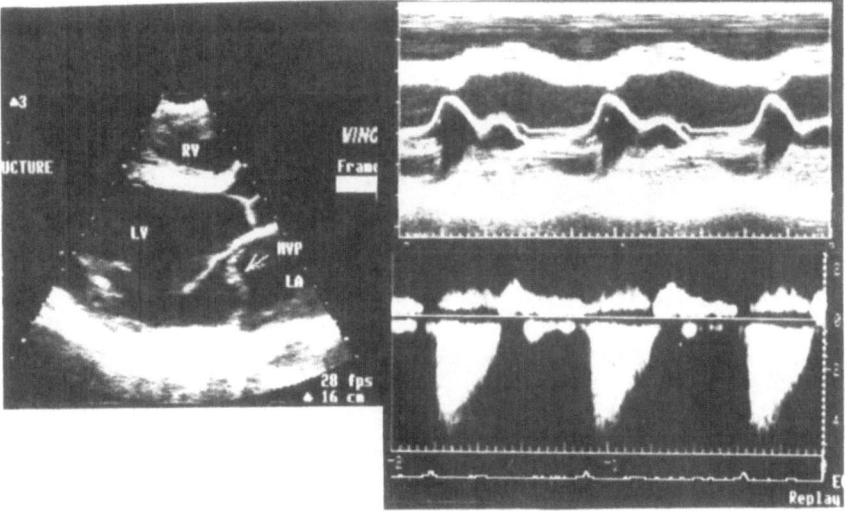

Fig. 6-15. In this adolescent patient with a mitral valve prolapse the 2D image permits visualization of the posterior leaflet into the left atrium (A), The TM study obtained from the same transducer position demonstrates that the prolapse is holosystolic (B). The continuous wave trace demonstrates a high velocity jet which rapidly decreases during systole indicating a severe regurgitation .

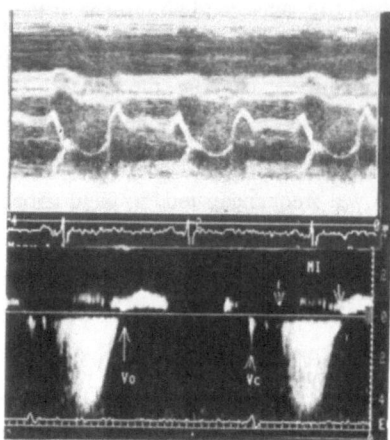

Fig. 6-16. In this adult patient with a mitral valve prolapse the 2D image permits visualization of the mitral leaflet into the left atrium (top). The continuous wave trace demonstrates a high velocity jet which commences ≈ 100 msec after mitral valve closure, demonstrating that this is a pansystolic prolapse.

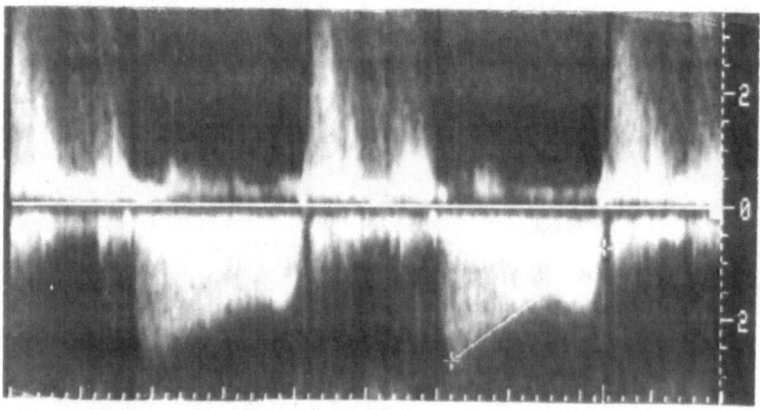

Fig. 6-17. This transesophageal tracings was recorded in a child with rheumatic mitral valve disease undergoing repair of the mitral valve. The stenosis was severe with mild to moderate regurgitation.

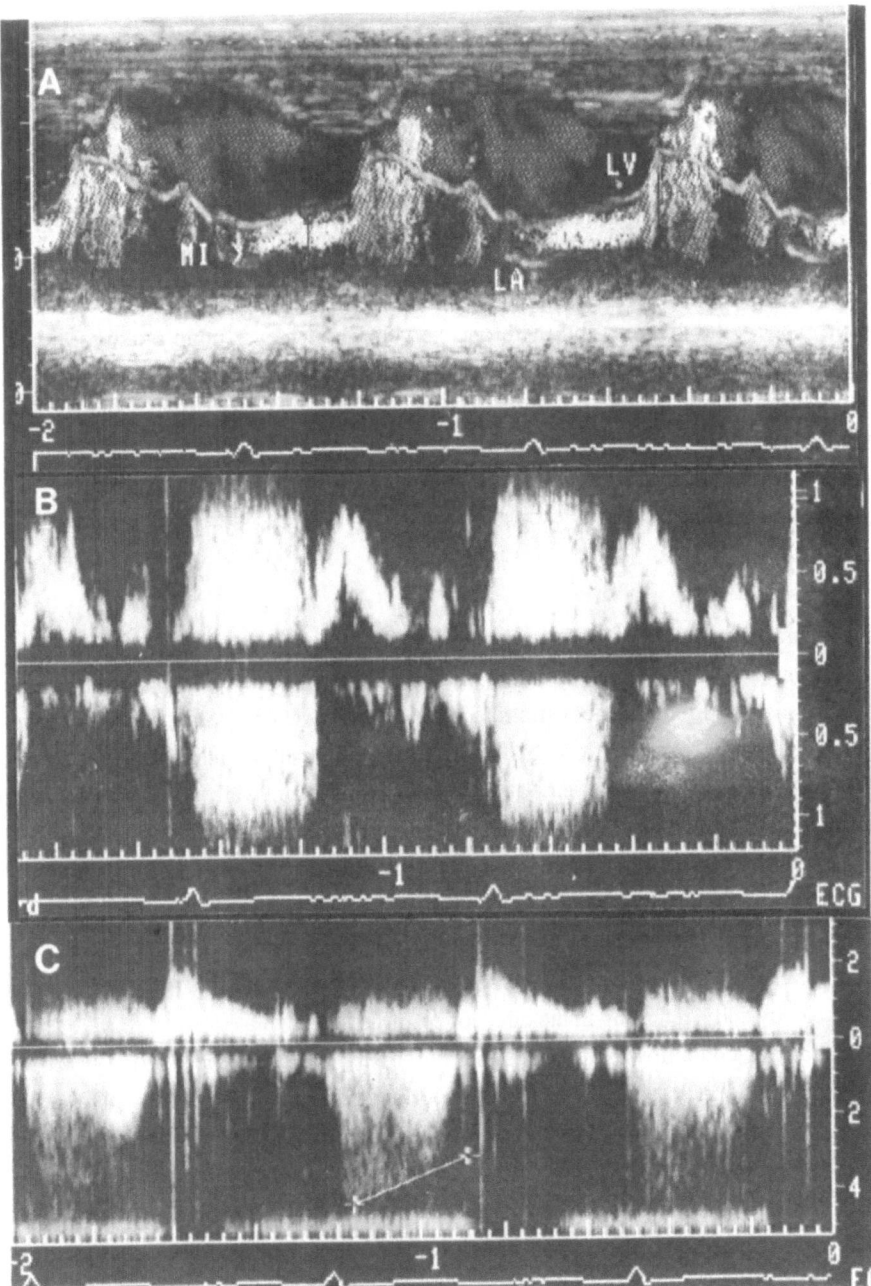

Fig. 6-18. This study was obtained from a patient with a mitral valve prolapse and severe regurgitation. The flow is localized using multigate TM mode (top), the extension of flow was mapped to the ceiling of the left atrium (middle), the continuous wave Doppler demonstrates a high velocity jet which rapidly decreases in velocity during late systole.

Continuous Wave Applications in Mitral Regurgitation

In order to supplement the pulsed Doppler flow mapping examination, continuous mode may be used to determine the orientation of the regurgitant jet. The relative intensity of the forward mitral flow and the regurgitant flow can be compared in the continuous wave recording. The Doppler derived pressure drop between the left ventricle and left atrium in systole correlates quite well to the invasive pressure measurements [8]. The CW Doppler can be used to measure the peak mitral insufficiency velocity and the rate of velocity deceleration, which is related to the reduced gradient between the left ventricle and left atrium. As the left atrium pressure increases in a severe mitral insufficiency, the gradient and therefore the velocity decrease quite rapidly. So in the presence of a rapidly decelerating mitral insufficiency jet velocity one should suspect a severe regurgitation. When moderate to severe incompetence is present, the forward flow velocity across the mitral valve will be increased. The increased velocity reflects the increased forward flow compensating for the regurgitant volume. The diastolic mitral flow peak velocity will be disproportionately increased when compared to the flow velocities across the non-diseased valves.

Color Flow Mapping in Mitral Regurgitation

Mitral regurgitation is one of the most difficult valvular lesions to quantify. This is due to variables such as jet direction, acoustic shadowing, distance from the probe, transducer frequency, the effect of competing flows on the jet, etc... Many methods have been described for implementing color flow mapping to semi-quantify these lesions, and while they are all limited in some way or another they are useful in the clinical setting when properly applied.

The most common method is to CFM map the flow into the left atrium as described for pulsed Doppler [3,9]. The regurgitant flow which is localized proximal to the valve is grade 1, grade 2 defines flow which extends less then a third of the left atrial length. In grade 3 the regurgitant jet extends to the left atrial ceiling, and in grade 4 a wide organized jet extends to the atrial ceiling with a high velocity eddy returning in the direction towards the valve.

The advantage of color flow mapping is that one obtains a global view of the heart with relatively good temporal resolution. The map is performed in a single frame with an image construction time of ≈ 50 ms, as opposed to a pulse Doppler flow map constructed over several cardiac cycles.

One of the most important factors when implementing a color flow mapping of the MI jet is knowing how the frequency shifted signals are analyzed and encoded. The area of interest is the jet core, but a larger area is obtained if the flow eddies of displaced blood and pulmonary venous flow are incorporated into the measured flow area. A color flow map should be selected which allows differentiation of these flow components.

The area of the jet and the area of the left atrium can be measured and the ratio between them used to evaluate the severity of the lesion. The jet and the left atrial chamber are planemetered, and the ratio between the two calculated. The apical four-chamber or the apical long axis are usually the best view for this application. The area of the jet measurement is affected by gain settings, reject settings, color maps, transducer frequency and patient size, and different instruments will yield different results. It is probably necessary for each lab to develop its own grading methods, taking these points into consideration for optimal results.

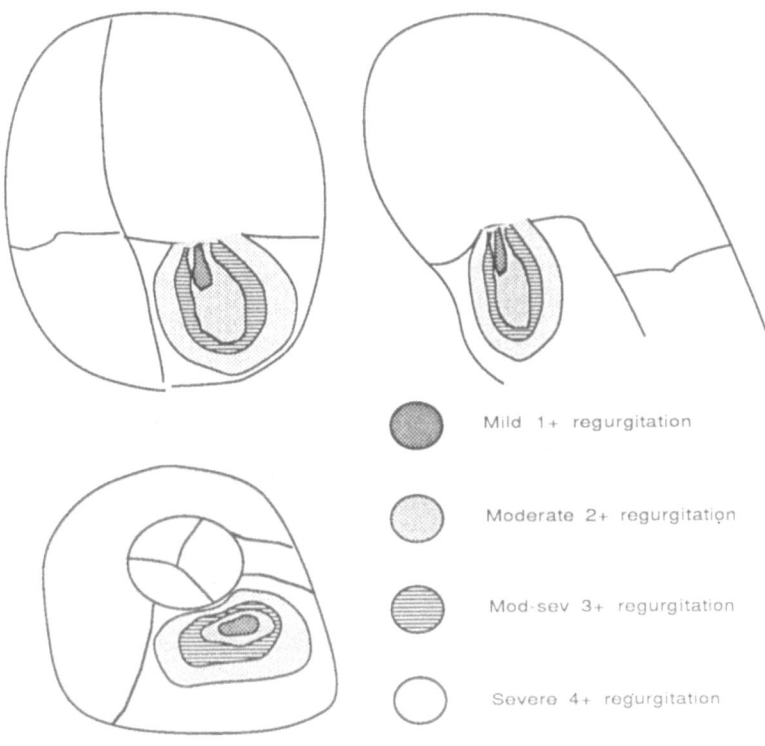

Fig. 6-19. A grading system for mitral regurgitation based on measurements from the apical four-chamber view, the apical two-chamber view, and the parasternal short axis view.

Pulmonary Regurgitation

Mild pulmonary regurgitation is a frequent finding in both adults and children [10]. As a pathologic entity this lesion is most often noted in children post pulmonic valve valvuloplasty or in the setting of pulmonary hypertension [11]. It may also occur in combination with complex congenital defects, as the result of endocarditis, or rarely, absent pulmonic valve. The right ventricular outflow tract can usually be well visualized in both pediatric and adult patients from the left parasternal transducer position. However, the subcostal position can be a good alternative window, especially in children. The regurgitant flow can be demonstrated using pulsed, continuous wave, and color flow mapping Doppler. Continuous wave applications are more useful in the measurement of the pulmonary artery diastolic pressure than in the evaluation of the regurgitation, and will be discussed in chapter VII.

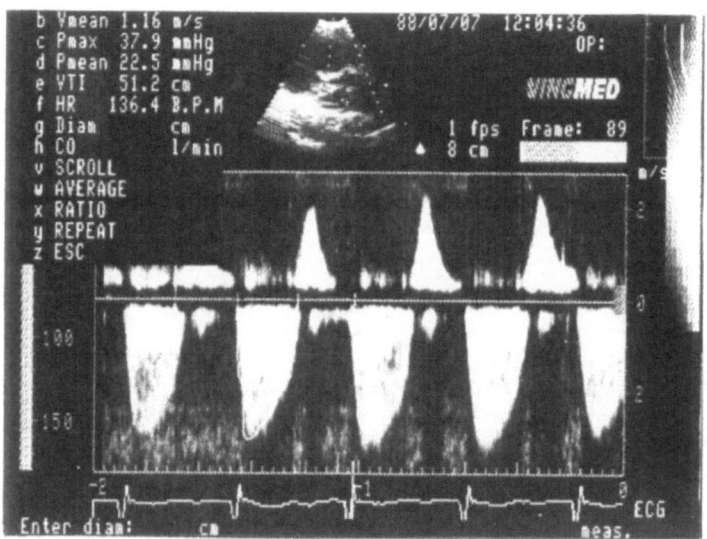

Fig. 6-20. This figure demonstrates the 2D parasternal view frequently used to measure pulmonary regurgitation flow (A), the pulsed Doppler recording of a mild insufficiency (B), a severe pulmonic stenosis with a mild regurgitation and a moderate residual stenosis with a small regurgitation (C), and a large regurgitation post valvuloplasty (D).

Pulsed Doppler Applications in Pulmonic Valve Regurgitation

The examination technique applying pulsed Doppler is performed by positioning the sample volume in the outflow tract proximal to the pulmonic valve, and searching for a diastolic flow towards the transducer. The velocity of this flow is related to the pressure gradient between the pulmonary artery and the right ventricle, and not the severity of the regurgitation. As the gradient is usually small, aliasing of the pulsed Doppler recording may or may not occur. It can be useful to initially increase the size of the sample volume dimension to search out the flow. Once the flow is located, the sample volume length can be reduced to improve the radial resolution and the regurgitant flow tracked into the right ventricular outflow tract. In our experience, it is possible to differentiate physiologic insufficiency from small and large insufficiencies, however quantitation of the degree of regurgitation is not possible. Figure 6-19 demonstrates the qualitative method used by the author. In addition, one may consider the strength of the regurgitant jet as larger regurgitations usually yield higher intensity signals. However, the interrogation site is close to the transducer and even small insufficiencies can yield relatively strong signals, especially in children.

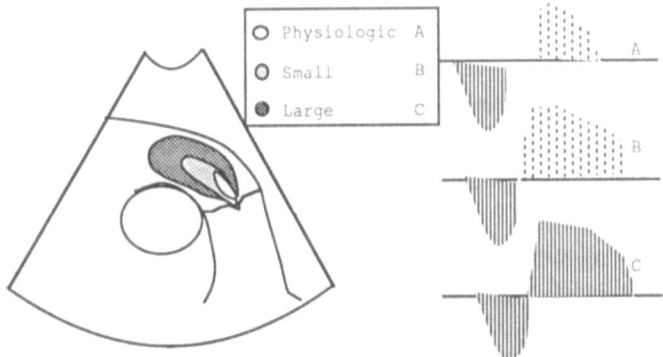

Fig. 6-21. This figure demonstrates a qualitative method for the evaluation of pulmonary regurgitation. Physiologic regurgitations are generally localized to the region of the valve and occur primarily in late diastole (A). Small regurgitations are localized to the area of the valve but tend to occur from valve closure to opening (B). Large regurgitations occur over a larger area, the signal is usually quite strong, and the regurgitation occurs from valve closure to opening (C).

Color Flow Mapping in Pulmonic Valve Regurgitation

The color flow mapping applications in the setting of pulmonary valve regurgitation are quite simular to those proposed for pulsed Doppler, and are subject to the same limitations. An advantage however, is that the color flow mapping method permits a much more rapid interrogation of the right ventricular outflow tract to be performed. While it is our opinion that the usefulness of flow mapping (by either pulsed Doppler or CFM) is of limited value, it is of interest to observe the acceleration of flow from the main pulmonary artery towards the pulmonic valve incompetence in diastole. The rational for this statement is that as the severity of the regurgitation increases, a larger volume of blood returns from the main pulmonary artery resulting in a retrograde flow being measured deeper in the artery. Figure 6-22 demonstrates a schematic representation of this method.

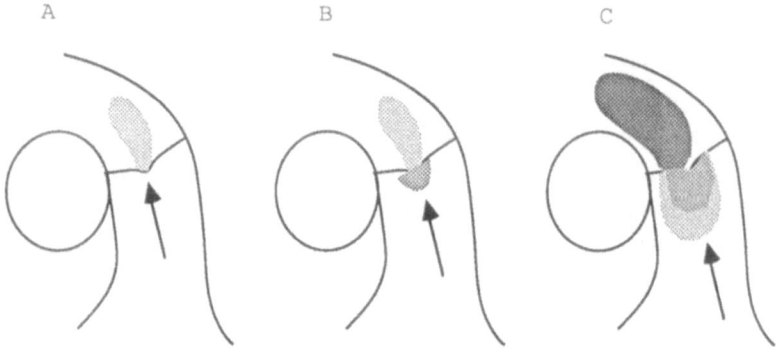

Fig. 6-22. As the severity of the regurgitation increases, a larger volume of blood returns from the main pulmonary artery resulting in a retrograde flow being measured deeper in the artery. This schematic represents a physiologic (A), moderate (B), and severe regurgitation (C).

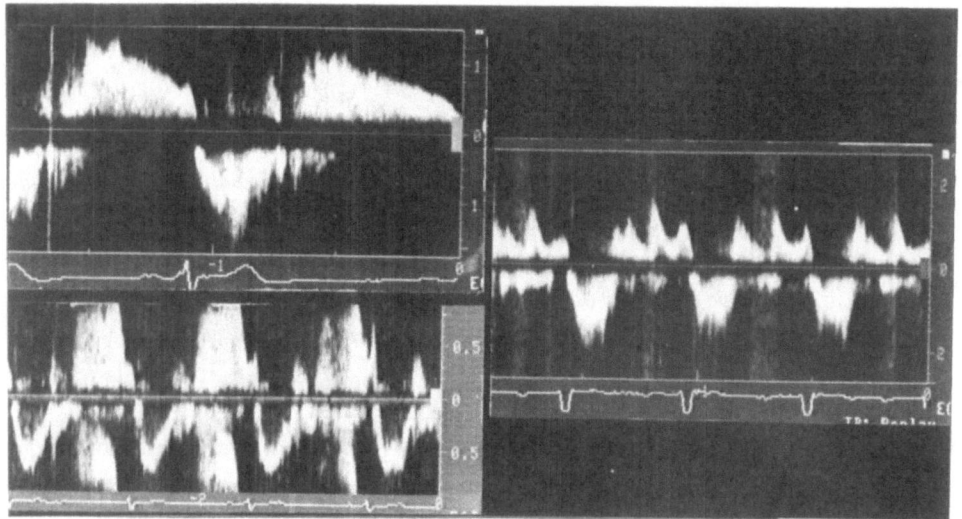

Fig. 6-23. Three examples of mild pulmonary regurgitation from patients post valvuloplasty (A), idiopathic dilatation of the pulmonary artery (B), and in a patient with an atrial septal defect (C).

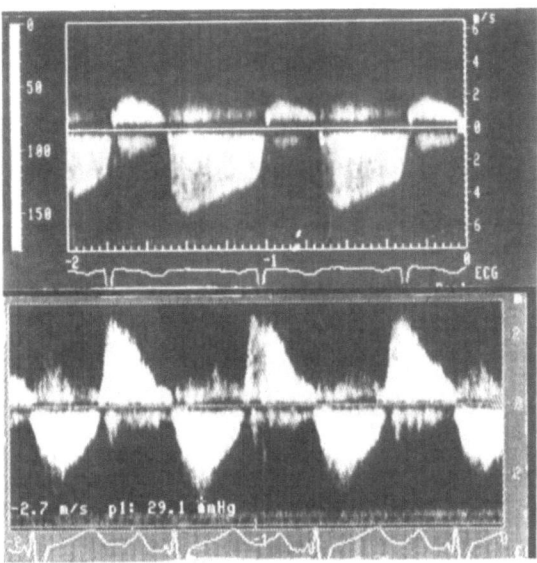

Fig. 6-24. The recordings of aortic regurgitation (top) and pulmonary regurgitation (lower) are compared in this figure. Unless a severe pulmonary hypertension exists, the velocity of the pulmonary regurgitation will be significantly lower than the velocity measured from an aortic regurgitation jet.

Tricuspid Regurgitation

As with pulmonary regurgitation, there is a high incidence of physiologic tricuspid regurgitation [10]. As a pathologic entity this lesion may be organic and is often found in the setting of complex lesions such as Ebstein's anamoly and atrioventricular canal defects. Or it can be functional, and is invariably noted when pulmonary pressure or right ventricular pressure is increased. Tricuspid regurgitation can be evaluated by pulsed Doppler, color flow mapping, or continuous wave Doppler [12,13]. However, continuous wave Doppler is more useful in determining the pulmonary artery and right ventricular systolic pressure than in the quantitation of severity, and will therefore be discussed in chapter VII.

Pulsed Doppler Applications

The most frequently used windows for examination of the tricuspid valve are the parasternal right ventricular inflow view, the standard short axis view, and the apical four-chamber view. The sample volume is positioned proximal to the valve and a systolic flow from the right ventricle to the right atrium is searched for. Increasing the sample volume length initially may help to localize the regurgitant jet. The flow is away from the transducer and the signal will typically be aliased.

The severity of the regurgitation can be measured semi-quantitatively by flow mapping, as with mitral regurgitation. The regurgitant jet is tracked into the right atrium step by step, flow localized to the immediate area of the valve is classified grade I, to the middle of the atrium grade II, to the ceiling of the atrium grade III, and into the hepatic veins grade IV. Fig. 6-24 demonstrates schematically the grading system applied by the author. The accuracy of this technique is determined by the ability to adequately sample the flow, the right atrial chamber size, the direction of the jet, and the effects of coexisting lesions.

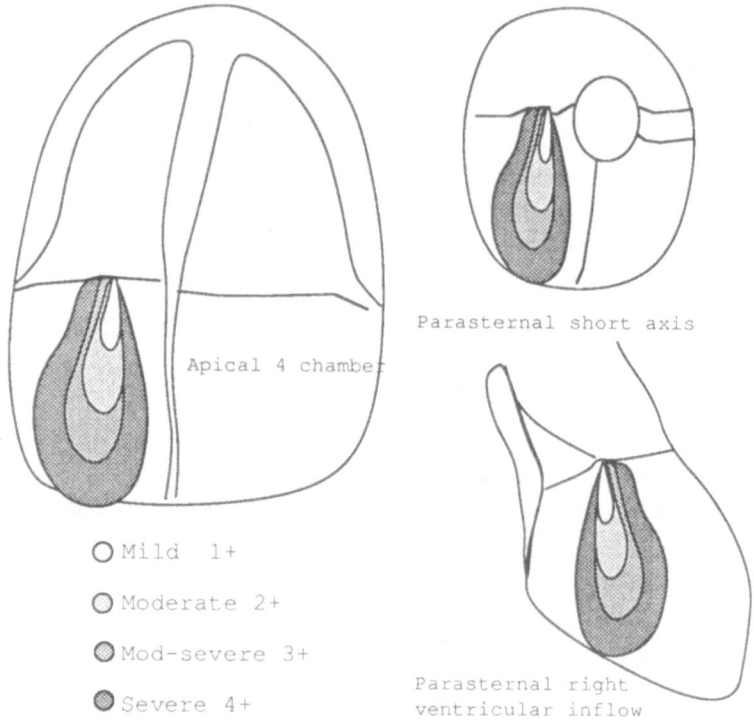

Fig. 6-25. This figure demonstrates a flow mapping method for the semi-quantitation of tricuspid regurgitation which can be applied from the apical four-chamber position, the parasternal short axis view, or the parasternal right ventricular inflow view. The same grading criteria are used for pulsed and color flow mapping modalities.

Color Flow Mapping Applications

The color flow mapping method is applied in essentially the same way as pulsed Doppler, i.e. the same imaging windows and same grading criteria are used. The advantage of using color flow mapping is that the study can be performed much more rapidly, temporal and spatial changes in the flow are more clearly defined, and one can localize and identify multiple leaks more clearly. On the debit side, the temporal resolution of the 2D color flow mapping mode is not as good as with spectral Doppler, but this problem is circumvented with the color TM mode which offers very good temporal resolution.

The color 2D mode is also quite useful for localizing retrograde flow into the inferior vena cava, the hepatic veins, and occasionally the superior vena cava. It is also used for positioning the pulsed Doppler sample volume so that quantitative measurement of flow velocities at these sites can be measured.

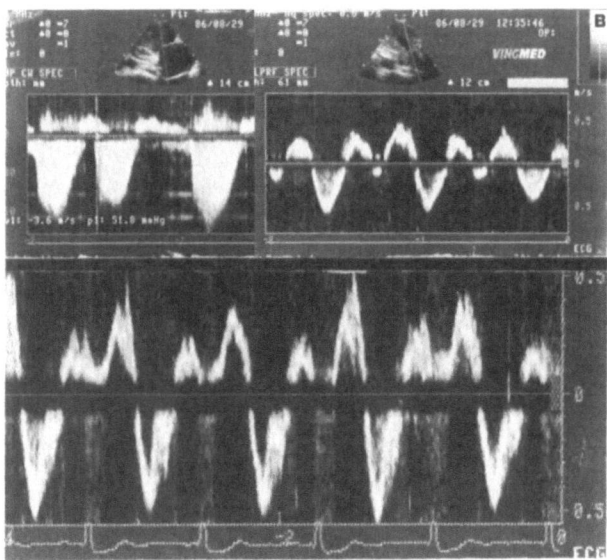

Fig. 6-26. In this patient with a severe tricuspid regurgitation the flow in the hepatic veins demonstrates a large systolic "V" wave. (B,C). The continuous wave Doppler was used to measure the high velocity regurgitant jet which indicates an increased pulmonary artery pressure but yields little relevant information regarding the lesion's severity.

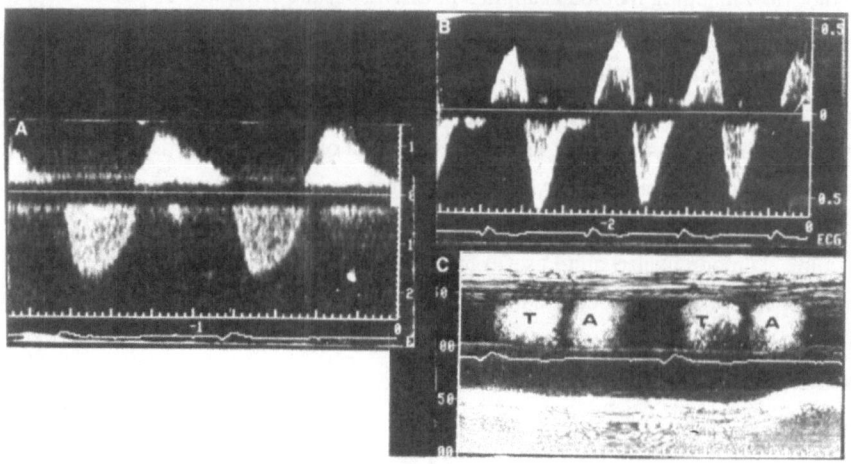

Fig. 6-27. The continuous wave Doppler was used to measure a low velocity regurgitant jet in this patient with a severe tricuspid regurgitation, the flow in the hepatic veins demonstrates a large systolic "V" wave by pulsed Doppler (B), and multigated TM mode Doppler interrogation.

References

1. Oh JK, Hatle LK, Sinak LJ, et al. Characteristic Doppler echocardiography pattern of mitral inflow velocity in severe aortic regurgitation. JACC Vol.14 No.7.1989; 1712-1717.

2. Labovitz AJ, Ferrara RP, Kern MJ, et al. Quantitative evaluation of aortic insufficiency by continuous wave Doppler echocardiography. JACC Vol.8 No.6 1986; 1341-1347.

3. Smith MD, Grayburn PA, Spain MG, et al. Observer variability in the quantitation of Doppler color flow jet areas for mitral and aortic regurgitation. JACC Vol.11 No.3 1988; 579-585.

4. Come PC, Riley MF, Carl LV, et al. Pulsed Doppler echocardiographic evaluation of valvular regurgitation in patients with valve prolapse. JACC Vol.8 No.6 1986; 1355-1364.

5. Pandis IP, Ross J, Munley B, et al. Diastolic mitral regurgitation in patients with atrioventricular conduction abnormalities. JACC Vol.7 No.4 1986;768-774.

6. Spain MG, Smith MD, Grayburn PA, et al. Quantitative assessment of mitral regurgitation by Doppler color flow imaging. JACC Vol. 13 No.3 1989; 554-564.

7. Come PC, Riley MF, Berman AD, et al. Serial assessment of mitral regurgitation by pulsed Doppler echocardiography in patients undergoing balloon aortic valvuloplasty. JACC Vol.14 No.3 1989; 677-682.

8. Nishimura RA, Tajik AJ. Determination of left-sided pressure gradients by utilizing Doppler aortic and mitral regurgitant signals. JACC Vol.11 No.2 1988; 317-321.

9. Sahn DJ. Instrumentation and physical factors related to visualization of stenotic and regurgitant jets by Doppler color flow mapping. JACC Vol.12 No.5 1988; 1354-1365.

10. Berger M, Hecht SR, van Tosh A, et al. Pulsed and continuous wave Doppler echocardiography assessment of valvular regurgitation in normal subjects. JACC Vol.13 No.7 1989; 1540-1545.

11. Marantz PM, Huhta JC, Mullins CE, et al. Results of balloon valvuloplasty in typical and diastolic pulmonary valve stenosis. JACC Vol.12 No.2 1988; 476-479.

12. Yoganathan AP, Cape EG, Sung HW, et al. Review of hydrodynamic principles for the cardiologist. JACC Vol.12 No.5 1988;1344-1353.

13. Simpson IA, Valdez-Cruz LM, Sahn DJ, et al. Doppler color flow mapping of simulated in vitro regurgitant jets. JACC Vol.13 No.5 1989; 1195-1207.

14. Schnittger I, Appleton CP, Hatle LK, et al. Diastolic mitral tricuspid regurgitation by Doppler echocardiography in patients with atrioventricular block. JACC Vol.11 No.1 1988; 83-88.

15. Berman AD, Weinstein JS, Safian RD, et al. Combined aortic and mitral balloon valvuloplasty in patients with critical aortic and mitral valve stenosis. JACC Vol.11 No.6 1988; 1213-1218.

16. Martin RP, Ettedgui JA, Quershi SA, et al. A quantitative evaluation of aortic regurgitation after anatomic correction of transposition of the great arteries. JACC Vol.12 No.5 1988; 1281-1284.

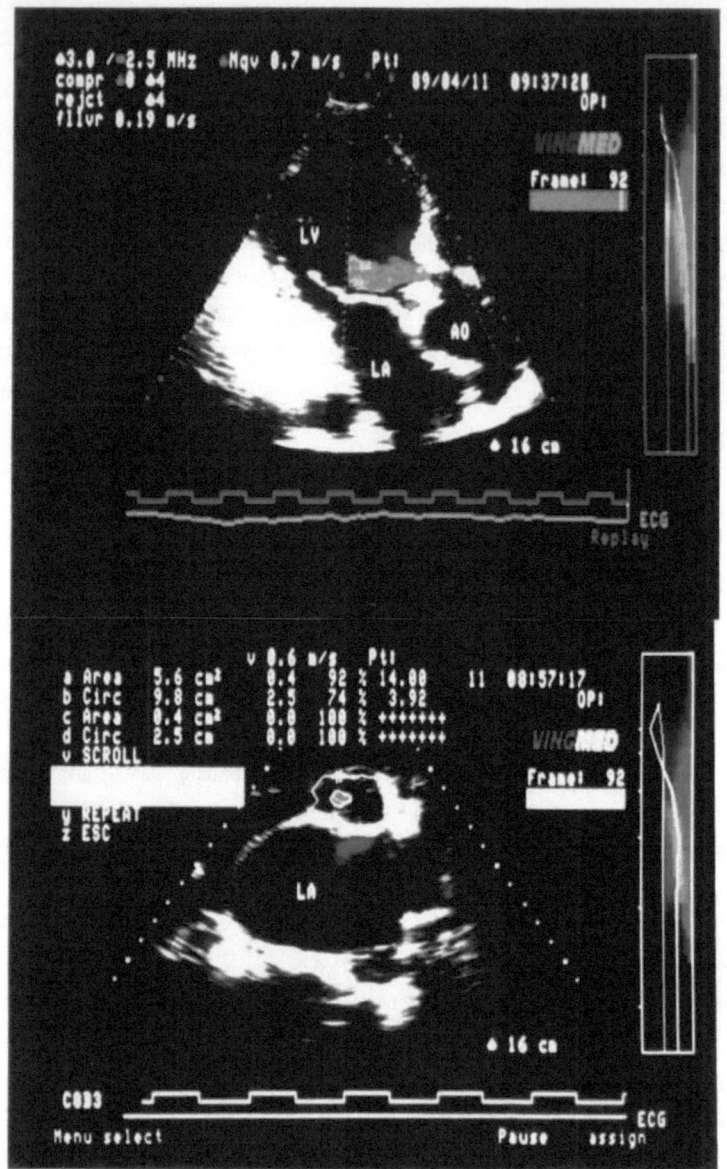

Color Plate 6-1. In this adult patient with a congenital bicuspid aortic valve, the presence of an outflow tract obstruction is denoted by the severely aliased flow signal at the level of the aortic valve (top). The continuous wave Doppler (not shown) yielded a systolic gradient of 40 mm Hg. The presence of a moderate aortic regurgitation (middle) is visualized. One also notes the left ventricular inflow and eddy formation mixing with the regurgitant jet as it follows the anterior mitral valve leaflet (lower).

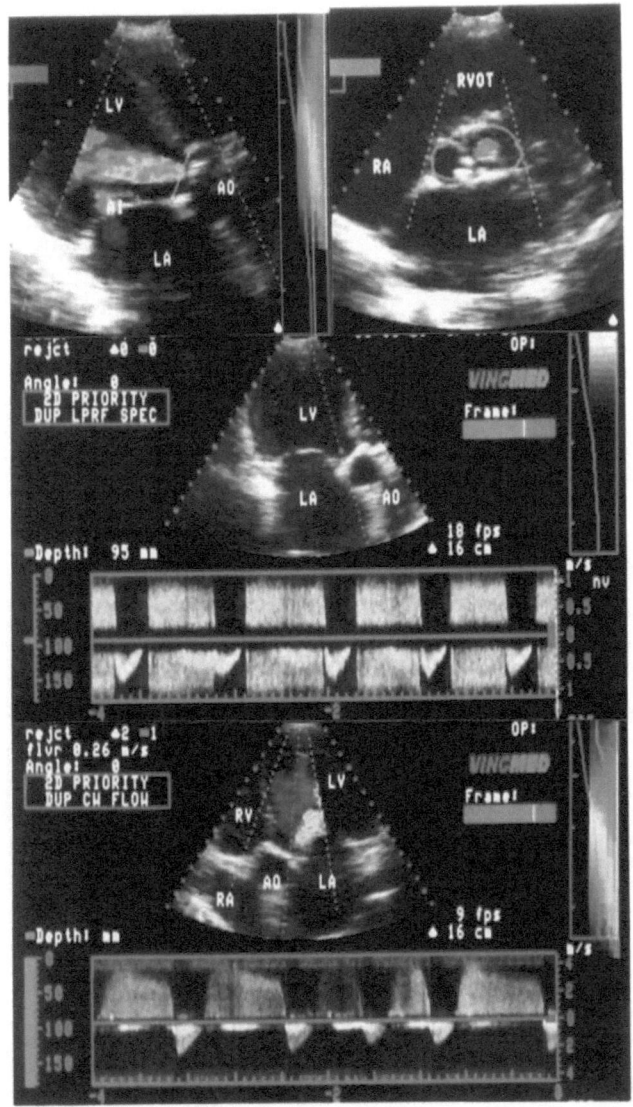

Color Plate 6-2. *In the setting of endocarditis the 2D image is used to localize the vegitation and measure the left ventricular dimensions, and the color flow mapping mode is used to assess the aortic regurgitation (top) In a patient with a bicuspid aortic valve and a small regurgitation the ratio between the regurgitation area and the aorta is measured (lower).*

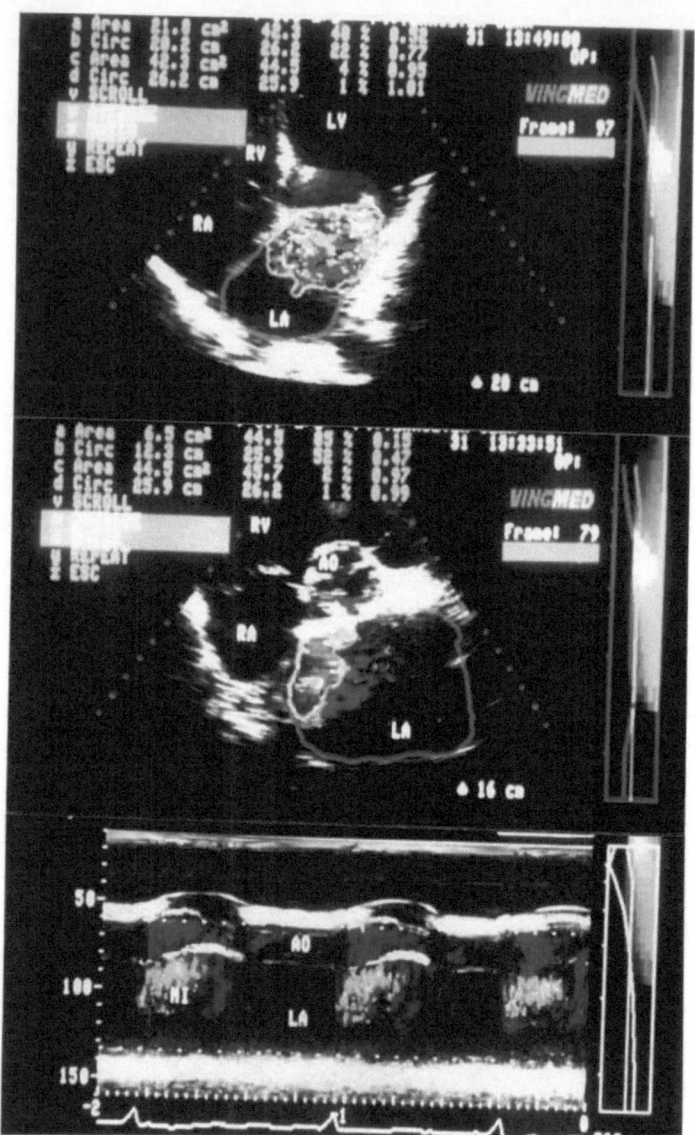

Color Plate 6-3. This series of images demonstrates the views used for the calculation of the ratio between mitral regurgitation jet area and left atrial area in the apical four-chamber view, and the parasternal short axis (middle). The color TM mode can be used to observe the timing of the regurgitant flow.

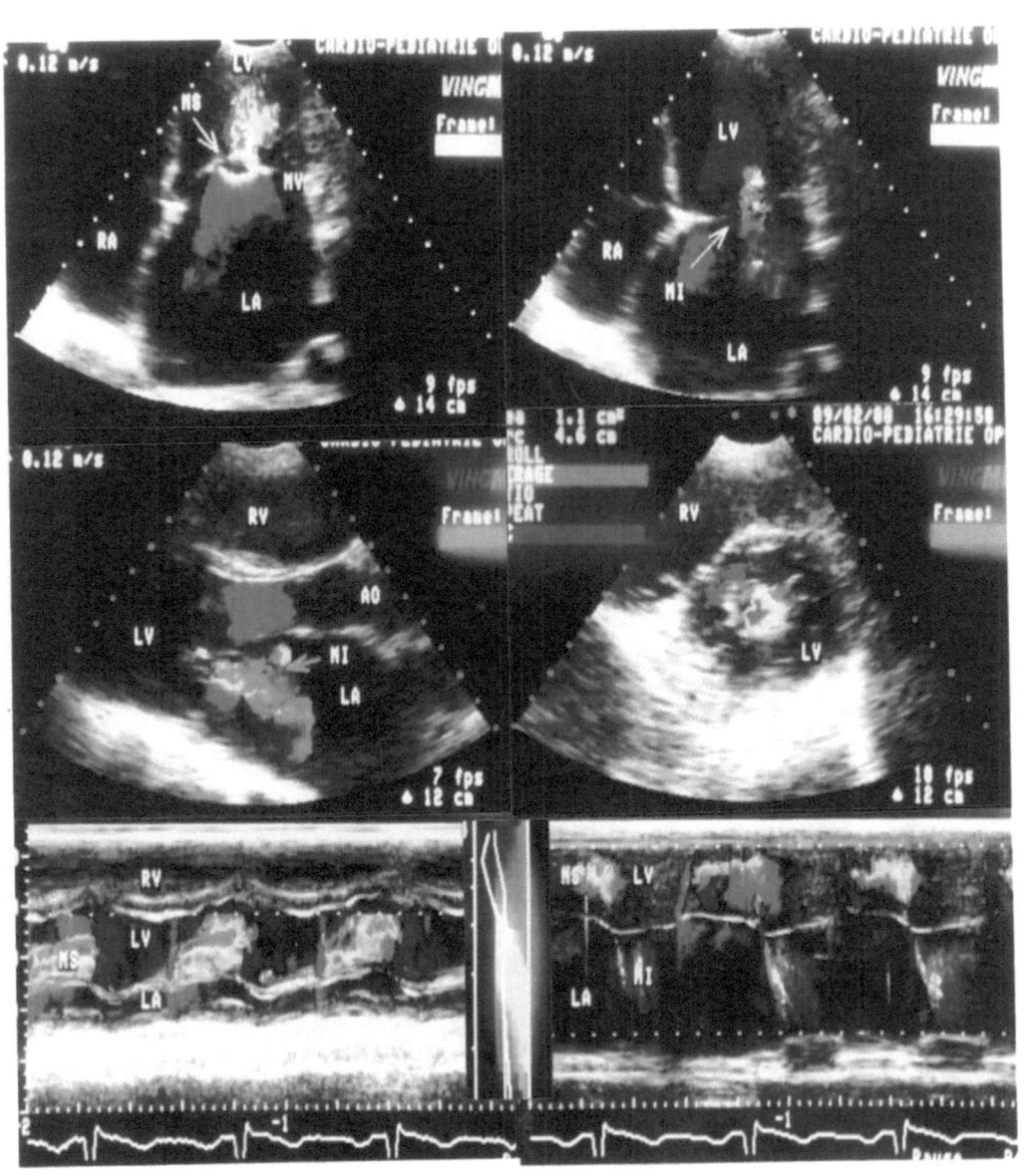

Color Plate 6-4. This figure demonstrates the various means of assessing aortic regurgitation with Doppler, including : the ratio of the jet to outflow tract diameter (top left), the ratio of jet to outflow tract diameter (top right), pulsed Doppler flow mapping (middle), and the pressure halftime measured by continuous wave Doppler (lower).

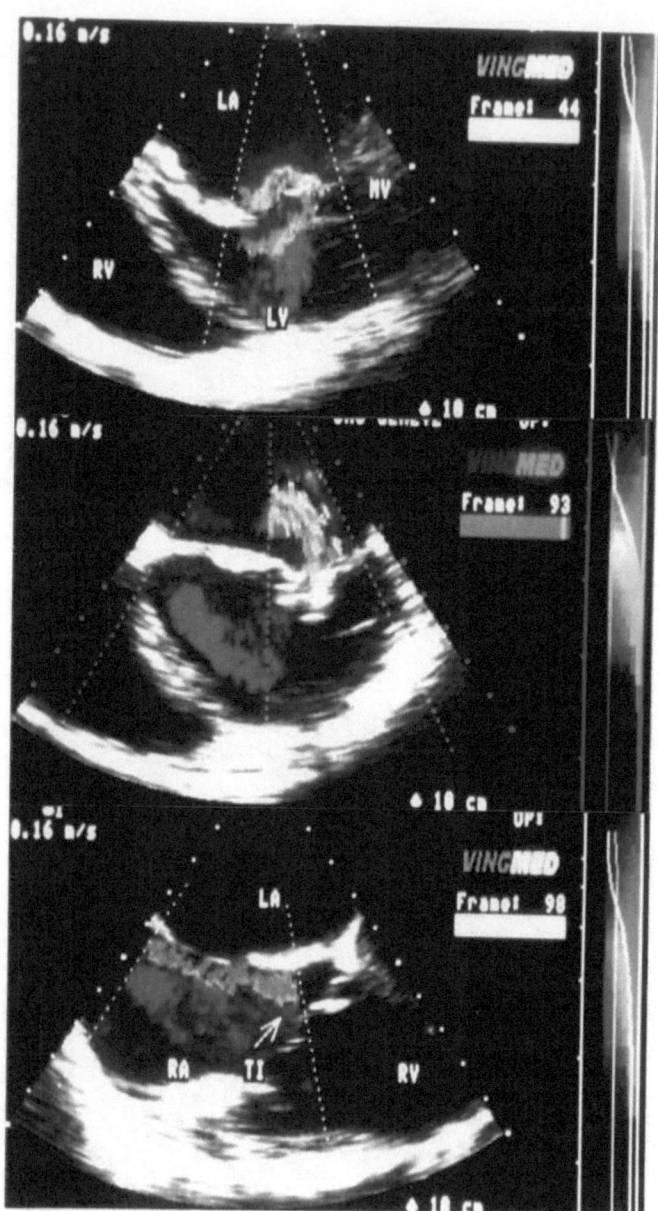

Color Plate 6-5. This series of images is from a thirteen year old girl with mitral stenosis and regurgitation. A high velocity diastolic jet with acceleration of flow originating deep in the left atrium indicates a severe stenosis (top left), the systolic regurgitant jet is noted in the same view (top right). The long axis view in systole demonstrates the regurgitant jet (middle left). The short axis view of the mitral valve permits the stenotic area to be planemetered (middle right). The mitral stenosis and regurgitation can be studied by color TM mode (lower), demonstrates the temporal sequence of the stenotic and regurgitant jets.

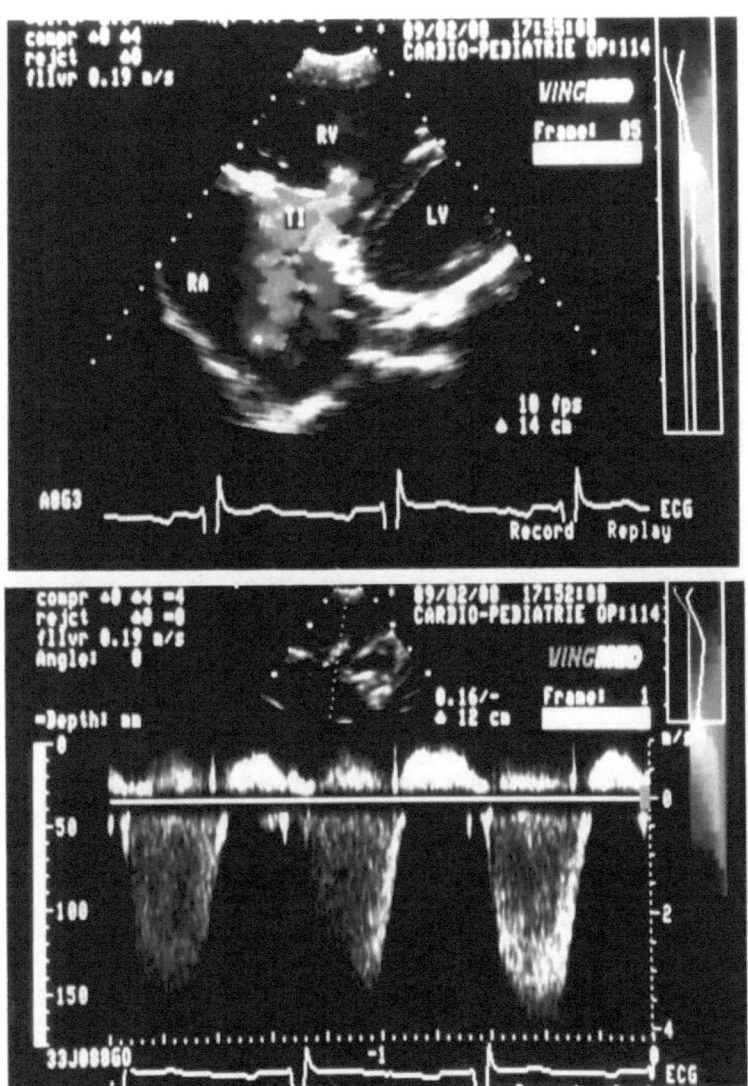

Color Plate 6-6. Preoperative study in the same patient as previous color plate. Transesophageal recording of the mitral stenosis (top), regurgitation (middle), and tricuspid regurgitation (bottom). This method permits the echocardiographer to evaluate the patient before surgery, and post bypass but before chest closure.

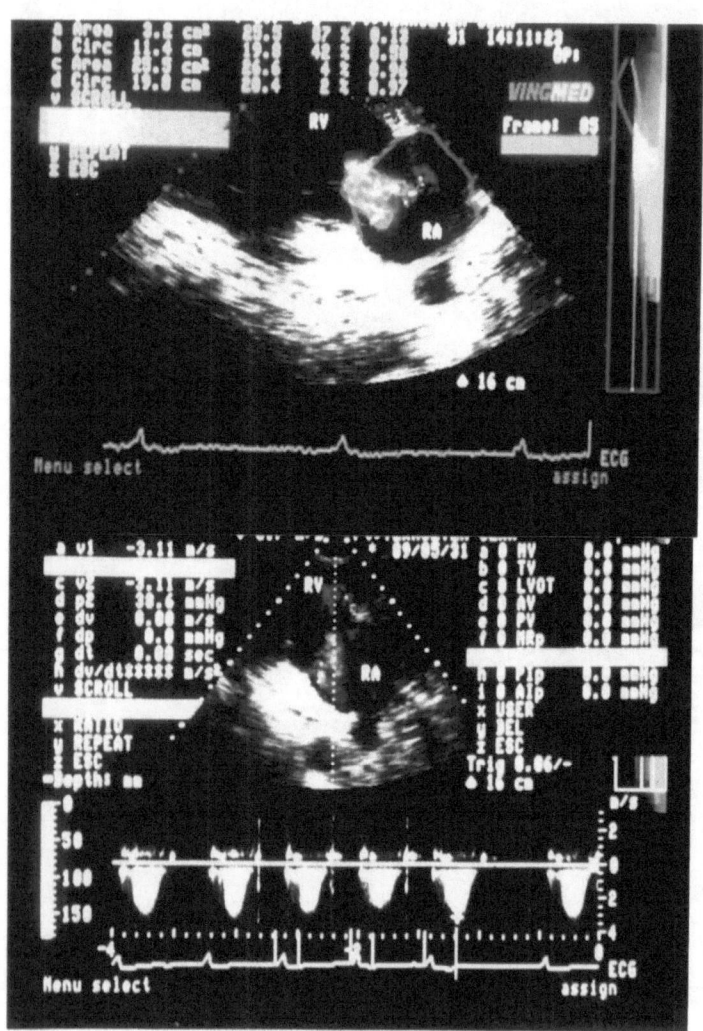

Color plate 6-7. Severe tricuspid regurgitation in a child with severe pulmonic stenosis. The color flow map demonstrates that the regurgitant jet extends to the region of the superior vena cava, and the high velocity jet measured by continuous wave Doppler indicates the presence of pulmonary hypertension (lower).

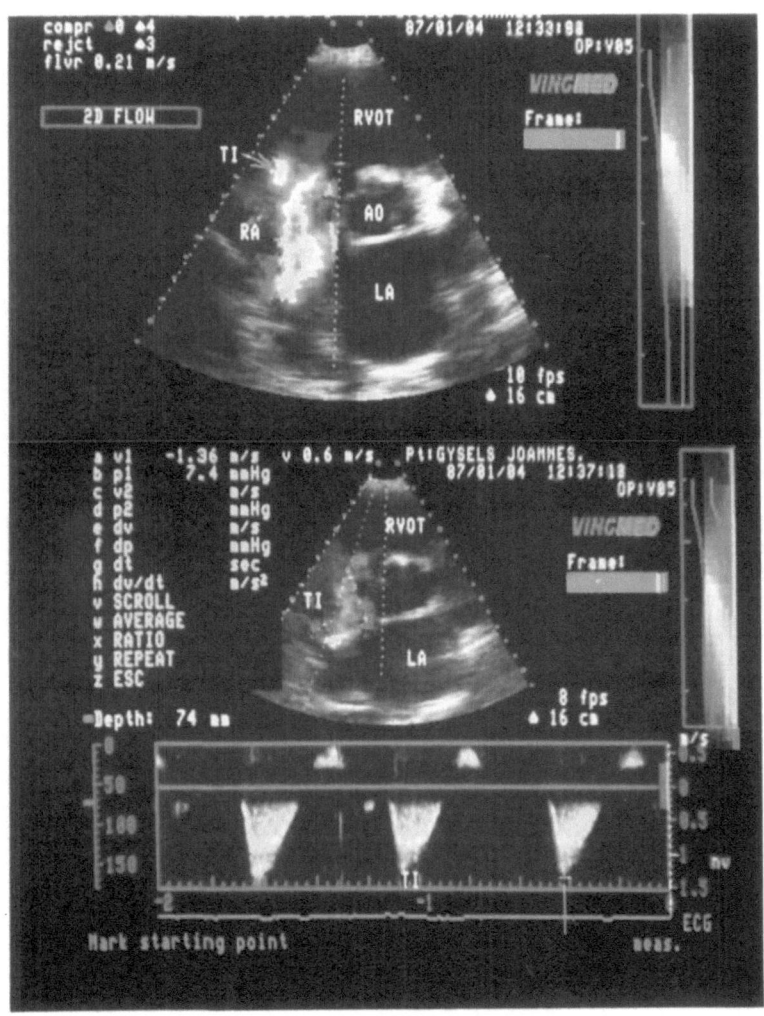

Color plate 6-8. A severe tricuspid regurgitation in an adult with a dilated cardiomyopathy is measured from a parasternal short axis view (top), a large area of regurgitant flow is noted. A low peak velocity of 1.36 m/s is measured using pulsed Doppler (lower), as previously mentioned, the velocity of the regurgitation is related to the pressure drop across the tricuspid valve in systole, not the severity of the regurgitation.

ESTIMATION OF PULMONARY ARTERY PRESSURE

James V. Chapman

The Measurement of Pulmonary Artery Pressure

The ability to measure, and follow changes in the right ventricular and pulmonary artery pressure is of extreme importance in the setting of many congenital lesions such as ventricular and atrial septal defects, patent ductus arteriosus, valvular lesions, and in the setting of various complex abnormalities. The invasive measurement of the pulmonary wedge pressure by insertion of a catheter into the distal region of the main pulmonary artery yields accurate measurements, but has two inherent limitations. First, the invasive nature of the technique compromises its utility for follow-up of patients in the outpatient clinic, and secondly, even monitoring of patients post-operatively and in the intensive care unit carries the risk of damage to the pulmonary arterial wall if the ballon is not deflated after each measurement [1], though this is a minor point. One method which is accurate and circumvents both these limitations is the application of Doppler ultrasound. These methods permit one to measure the pulmonary artery pressure and right ventricular pressure as often as necessary, and without risk or patient discomfort. By using various Doppler techniques, the systolic, diastolic, and mean pulmonary artery pressure can be measured with a clinically acceptable degree of accuracy

There are primarily two approaches which can be applied to measure intracardiac pressures using Doppler ultrasound. First described were methods based on timing measurements of pulmonary artery flow acceleration and ejection time, that is the time from the onset of flow to peak flow velocity, and the systolic flow period [2]. Either the flow acceleration alone, or a ratio between the acceleration and ejection time can be applied. The second group of measurements are based on the ability to measure flow velocities in the setting of tricuspid regurgitation and pulmonary regurgitation. A variation of this technique, which will be reviewed, is based on the measurement of the flow velocity across various intracardiac shunts and estimating the pressure based on these measurements.

The Pulmonary Artery Acceleration Time

This method can be used either qualitatively or quantitatively, as a qualitative technique one can obtain a rough estimation of the pulmonary artery pressure which generally permits patients with elevated pulmonary artery pressures to be separated from those with normal pulmonary artery pressures. The measurement is performed on the right ventricular outflow or main pulmonary artery systolic flow tracing, usually sampled from the parasternal transducer position. The flow measurement obtained from the right ventricular outflow tract appears to yield significantly better correlation to invasive measurements of pulmonary artery pressure than those obtained in the main pulmonary artery [3]. For this reason we use measurements from the main pulmonary artery only for qualitative assessment of the mean pulmonary artery pressure. In the event this window cannot be used, the subcostal window offers a good alternative study position. It is important to localize the flow being interrogated as changes in the sample position can alter the morphology of the flow curve, for this reason pulsed Doppler is generally applied. In Figure 7-1 the effect of sample volume position on the spectral curve is demonstrated. The time required from onset of flow to peak velocity is measured as demonstrated in Figure 7-2, and in the patient with normal pulmonary artery pressure the curve is "rounded" in appearance. When the mean pulmonary artery pressure exceeds ≈ 30 mm Hg the acceleration time is shorter as demonstrated in Figure 7-3. In the setting of severe pulmonary hypertension a notching of the systolic flow curve may actually be noted. In infants and young children a pulmonary acceleration time of less than 80 ms, and in older children and adults less than 100 ms, should be suspected to have an increased pulmonary artery pressure. The measurement of the acceleration time alone is dependent on the heart rate, so a ratio between the ejection time and the acceleration time is used for quantitative measurements. While there is a significant inverse relationship between the main pulmonary artery flow acceleration time alone and the pulmonary artery pressure, the standard error of the measurement precludes its applicability for more quantitative measurements.

For the quantitative measurement of the mean pulmonary artery pressure based on the acceleration time (Acc_t) and ejection time (E_t), the measurements described above are used to calculate a ratio;

$$Acc_t / E_t$$

Equation 7-1

The mean pulmonary artery pressure (PAPm) is then calculated as described by Kitabatake and coworkers[4];

$$PAPm = -2.8 (Acc_t / E_t) + 2.4$$

Equation 7-2

In our experience, the measurement of the right ventricular outflow velocity curve used in conjunction with the Kitabatake method outlined yields the most accurate determination of the mean pulmonary artery pressure. This is in agreement with the findings of Stevenson[2], in which he compared the various Doppler methods of measuring the pulmonary artery pressure in pediatric patients. The clinical utility of the technique is further enhanced by the fact that it is generally quite easy to obtain the required Doppler traces from the right ventricular outflow tract in both children and adults.

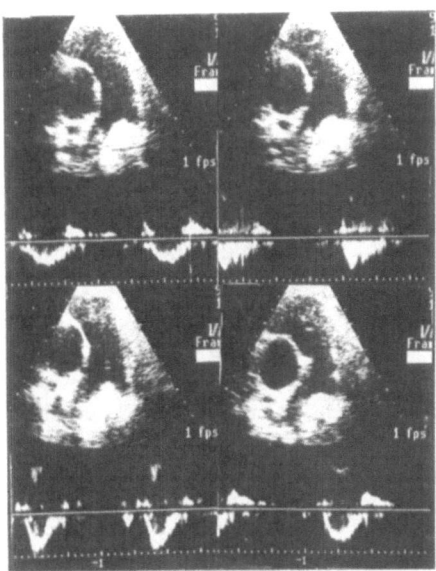

Fig. 7-1. This series of spectral traces from the pulmonary artery of the same patient sampled at different sites in the right ventricular outflow tract and pulmonary artery demonstrates the effect of sampling position on waveform morphology.

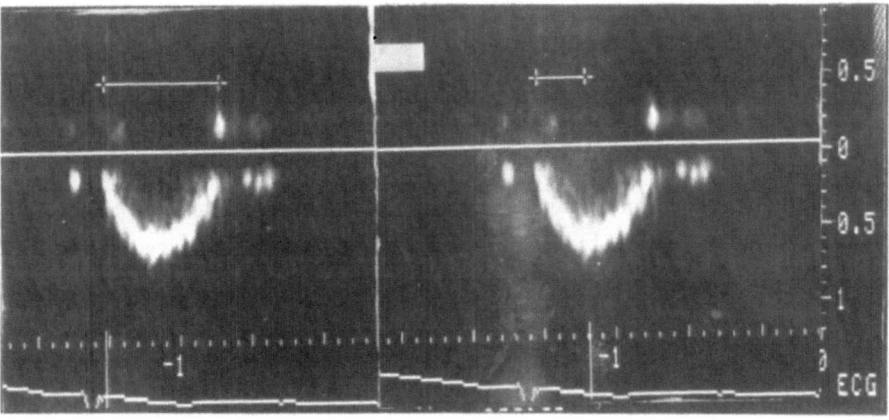

Fig. 7-2. This pulmonary artery flow trace obtained from the parasternal transducer position demonstrates the measurement of the ejection time and acceleration time in a subject with normal pulmonary artery pressure.

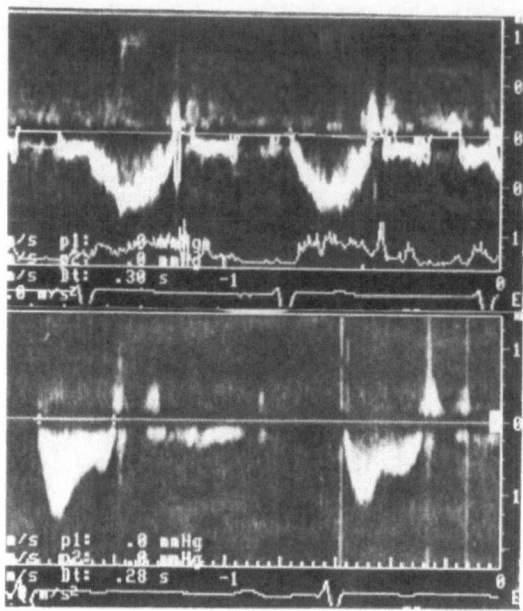

Fig. 7-3. This figure demonstrates the characteristic flow tracings from a patient with a normal pulmonary artery pressure (top), and from a patient with severe pulmonary hypertension (lower). Note the rapid acceleration, and systolic notching of the curve from the patient with pulmonary hypertension. As stated in the text, the position of the sample volume can greatly affect the morphology of the flow curve.

The Bernoulli Equation in Determination of Right Ventricular Pressure

The application of the Bernoulli equation to measure transvalvular pressure gradients has been discussed. This method is quite accurate and correlations to invasively derived measurements are good. In many instances the ability to measure the pressure drop from one cardiac chamber to another in the setting of various regurgitant and shunt lesions permits the investigator to extrapolate intracardiac pressures. Each of these techniques will be discussed in turn, but the theoretical basis for these measurements will first be presented.

The Bernoulli equation yields the pressure drop across a flow circuit. If the gradient is known, and the pressure of the chamber distal to the flow circuit can be measured or estimated, the driving pressure proximal to the flow circuit can be approximated (Fig.7-4). This driving pressure can be used to represent the intracardiac pressure in the chamber from which the flow originated [5].

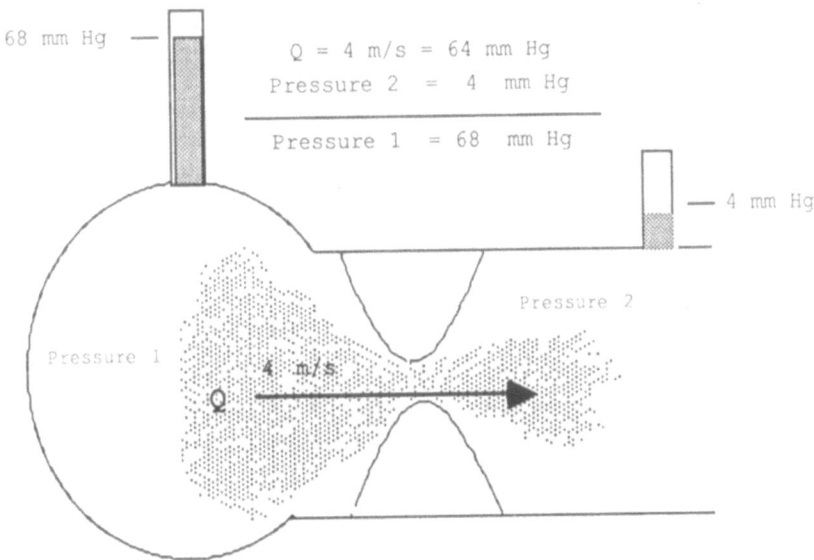

Fig. 7-4. *This figure yields a schematic description of the rationale for quantitative measurement of intracardiac pressures derived from the modified Bernoulli equation. The Doppler measurement of the velocity of flow across the circuit is used to calculate the pressure drop between the chambers. If the measured pressure at the downstream site is 4 mm Hg, this value is added to the pressure drop (64 mm Hg) to yielding the pressure (68 mm Hg) in the chamber proximal to the circuit.*

The accuracy of the estimate is limited by A) the ability to measure the peak velocity across the flow circuit, and B) the ability to measure the pressure at the downstream site. There are various ways to approach this problem which will now be described.

Tricuspid Regurgitation

In the setting of tricuspid regurgitation the velocity of flow across the incompetence can be used to calculate the systolic pressure drop between the right ventricle and the right atrium [5,6,7,8]. During systole the pulmonic valve is open and the pressure difference between the pulmonary artery and the right ventricle is negligible. We can therefore use the pressure drop between the right ventricle and the right atrium to express the pressure drop from the pulmonary artery and right atrium, so long as there is no obstruction to right ventricular outflow. In the setting of pulmonic stenosis this model is no longer valid, as the pressure in the right ventricle is significantly different to that of the pulmonary artery.

The unknown quantity for the calculation of the systolic pulmonary artery pressure from the tricuspid regurgitation velocity measurement is the right atrial pressure. Several means of deducing this missing information have been proposed. The right atrial pressure can be measured from jugular pulsatility, an arbitrary value for right atrial pressure can be inserted, or the term for right atrial pressure can simply be neglected. In an earlier study, we compared the clinically measured right atrial pressure to the catheterization measurement of right atrial pressure and found a poor correlation, and therefore find this technique for deriving the right atrial pressure of little use. Some investigators have used an arbitrary value of 7 to 14 mm Hg for the right atrial pressure which appears to yield acceptable results. However, it is the opinion of the author that the potential error caused by neglecting the right atrial pressure is clinically unimportant, and that one is as likely to introduce an error as correct it with the former methods. We therefore use the gradient measurement alone to represent right ventricular pressure, and assuming there is no obstruction to right ventricular outflow, the systolic pulmonary artery pressure.

As stated in chapters III and V, there is a high incidence of tricuspid regurgitation found in normal valves [7,8], and invariably in the setting of pulmonary hypertension tricuspid regurgitation is present. This permits a reliable, reproducible, and easily applied method for measuring and following the pulmonary artery pressure in patients noninvasively.

The most common method of applying this technique is from the apical four chamber view or the parasternal right ventricular inflow view, both of which have been previously described. In our experience, the right ventricular inflow view generally permits a better alignment between the regurgitant jet and the Doppler beam. Continuous wave Doppler is most frequently applied as the regurgitant velocity usually exceeds the pulse Dopplers' Nyquist limit. It is useful to apply high prf mode in situations where the jet intensity is weak and the Doppler beam must pass through highly dynamic structures (i.e. valves and septum), as the discrete sample cell does not simultaneously sample these strong reflectors which may obscure the regurgitant signal. The velocity of the regurgitant jet does not relate to the severity of the lesion, but to the gradient between the right atrium and ventricle. It is quite possible to find a low velocity flow in a severe regurgitation or a high velocity flow in a mild regurgitation (Figs. 7-5,7-7).

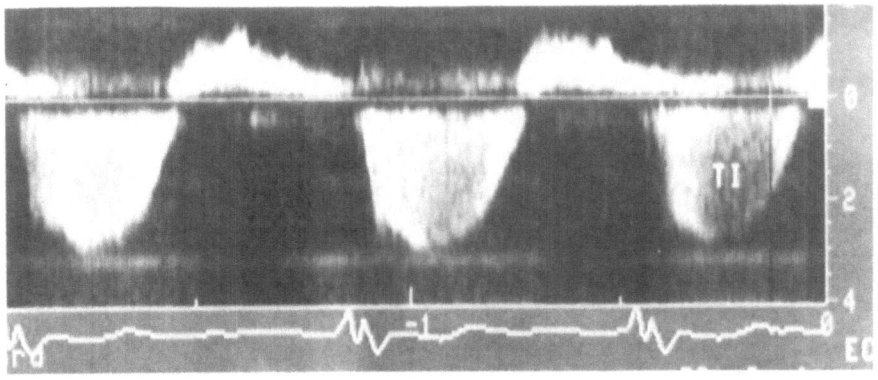

Fig. 7-5. This study was obtained in a subject with a small degree of tricuspid regurgitation and normal right ventricular and pulmonary artery pressure. Note the low velocity regurgitant jet.

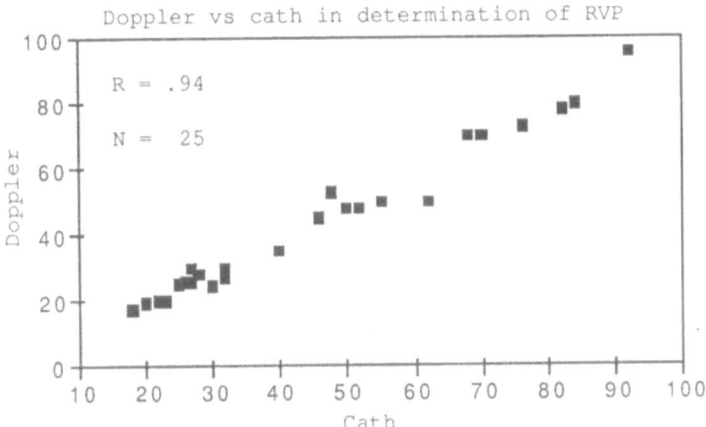

Fig. 7-6. This figure demonstrates the correlation obtained in a comparison of invasive and noninvasive measurement of the systolic right ventricular pressure in children with congenital heart disease.

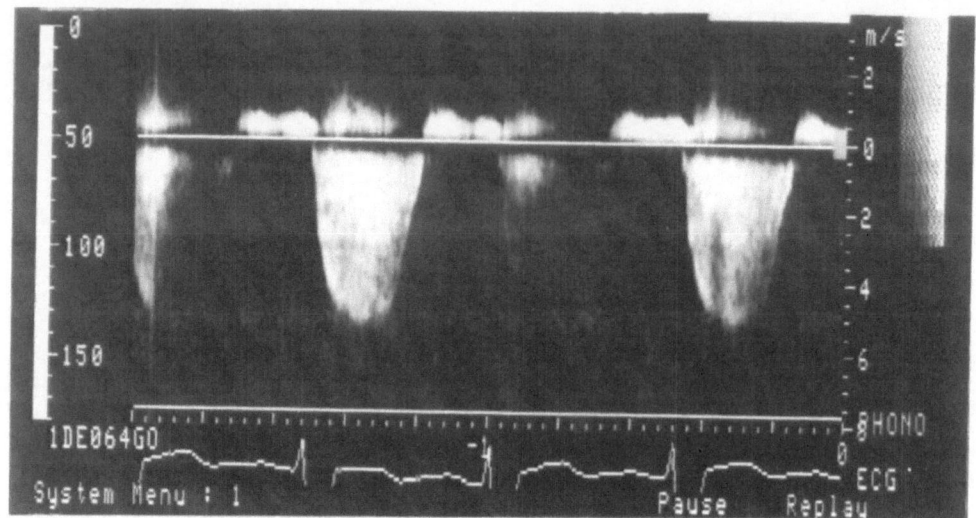

Fig. 7-7. This study was obtained in a subject with a moderate degree of tricuspid regurgitation and elevated right ventricular and pulmonary artery pressure. Note the high velocity systolic regurgitant jet.

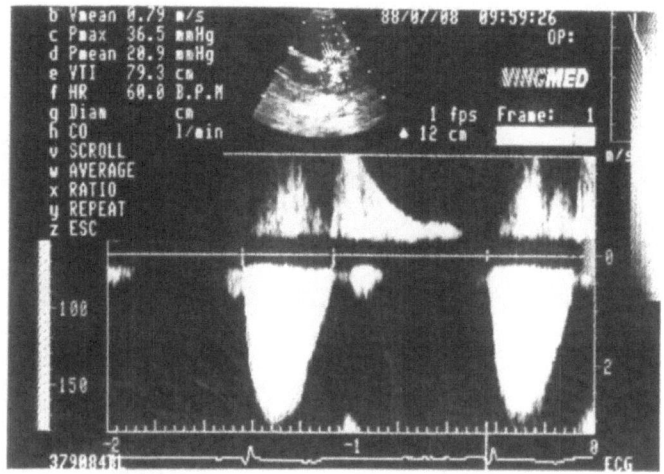

Fig. 7-8. This CW study was obtained in a subject with a moderate degree of pulmonary regurgitation and normal diastolic pulmonary artery pressure. Note the low velocity diastolic regurgitant jet.

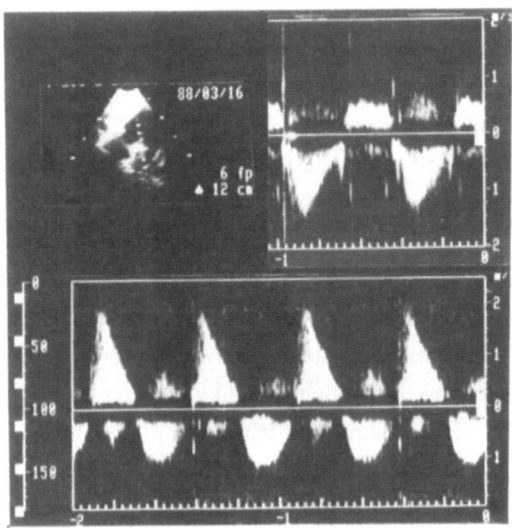

Fig. 7-9. This study was obtained in a subject with a moderate degree of pulmonary regurgitation and a normal diastolic pulmonary artery pressure. Note the low velocity diastolic regurgitant jet.

Pulmonary Regurgitation

The presence of pulmonary regurgitation is frequently found both in the normal and pathologic setting, as is tricuspid regurgitation. The regurgitant flow signal is usually obtainable from the parasternal window in the second to fourth intercostal space, with the patient turned to an extreme left lateral position. The subcostal window can be used as an alternative investigation site when the parasternal window cannot be used. If pulsed Doppler or high prf modes are applied, the sample volume is positioned in the right ventricular outflow tract proximal to the pulmonary valve. Continuous wave Doppler should be used when the velocity is high to circumvent the Nyquist limit. The regurgitant signal can be quite weak, one should increase the high pass filters so that the gain can be increased without saturating the low velocity signals originating from valve and heart motion. It is often helpful to have the patient exhale deeply and hold the breath out to optimize the flow trace.

The measurement of the diastolic regurgitant jet velocity can be used to estimate the diastolic pulmonary artery pressure in much the same manner as previously discussed for tricuspid regurgitation. Though the changes in right ventricular pressure are greater than right atrial pressures, and the pressures change more with time than in tricuspid insufficiency, the technique appears to be an accurate predictor of diastolic pulmonary artery pressure. There is a high frequency of pulmonary regurgitation in normal subjects as previously mentioned, and it is invariably present in the setting of pulmonary hypertension which makes this a useful technique indeed. The end diastolic velocity of the regurgitant jet is used for this measurement, *not the peak diastolic velocity*. The deceleration slope of the regurgitant signal appears to bear a relationship to the severity of hypertension in that a high end diastolic velocity indicates a high pulmonary artery pressure (or a very low right ventricular end diastolic pressure which is not generally the case). However, this needs to be studied more closely before any definitive conclusions can be drawn.

Ventricular Septal Defect

In the setting of ventricular septal defect with a left to right shunt the velocity of flow across the defect in systole can be used to estimate the systolic right ventricular pressure, and the pulmonary artery pressure as long as there is no obstruction to right ventricular outflow [2]. Qualitatively, a high velocity flow across the defect indicates that the right ventricular pressure is low and conversely, a low velocity flow across the defect indicates that the right ventricular pressure is high. The velocity of the trans-defect flow is directly related to the pressure drop from the left ventricle to the right ventricle, and in the normal pressure state will result in quite a large gradient since the left sided pressure is usually several times higher than that on the right side [1]. In the setting of an elevated right ventricular pressure the gradient between the left and right ventricles is reduced, thereby reducing the flow velocity which, as previously stated, is a function of the pressure drop.

A more quantitative measurement can be performed by obtaining the measurement of the flow velocity across the defect and calculating the pressure gradient using the Bernoulli equation. The systemic blood pressure is measured by sphygmomanometer, and the Doppler derived pressure gradient is subtracted from this value. The product represents the right ventricular pressure. There are limitations to this technique i.e. the peak velocity of flow across the defect must be obtained. This can be difficult in ventricular septal defects due to the size of the shunt volume, and due to the eccentric direction of the defect in many patients. Another major limitation in our opinion is the measurement of the cuff pressure. While the cuff measurement is acceptably accurate from the clinical side, the quantitative measurement of pulmonary artery pressure described can be significantly influenced by an error of 10 or 12 mm Hg in the cuff pressure. This error becomes more important in the situations where the right ventricular pressure is moderately elevated and the associated pressure gradient is reduced. If the cuff pressure is 100 mm Hg and the Doppler measurement of the left to right ventricular gradient is 80 mm Hg, the resulting estimation of the right ventricular pressure is 20 mm Hg, and a 10 to 12 mm Hg error is not important. However, if the cuff pressure is 100 mm Hg and the Doppler measurement of the left to right ventricular gradient is 60 mm Hg, the resulting estimation of the right ventricular pressure is 40 mm Hg, a 10 to 12 mm Hg error is significant.

In view of this discussion, we prefer to apply this measurement in a qualitative fashion. It presents the echocardiographer with a rapid, reproducible means of evaluating the presence of increased right ventricular pressure when tricuspid regurgitation is either not present or when the jet cannot be measured.

Patent Ductus Arteriosus

In the setting of a patent ductus arteriosus, the pulmonary artery pressure can be estimated in much the same way as described in the setting of ventricular septal defect, the major difference is that the pulmonary artery pressure is measured directly, and not inferred from the right ventricular pressure. The left to right gradient is calculated from the peak flow velocity across the ductus, and this value is then subtracted from the cuff measurement of systemic systolic pressure to yield the pulmonary artery pressure. The same potential sources of error exist with this method as those described in the setting of ventricular septal defect, but the method does permit separation of those patients with or without pulmonary hypertension.

Conclusion

The application of Doppler ultrasound to qualitatively and quantitatively assess the right ventricular and pulmonary artery pressures in the setting of congenital heart disease has become a very important tool in the management of these patients. The techniques described permit clinically relevant measurements to be made, and offer an ideal way to follow the pulmonary artery pressures in pediatric and adult patients over long periods [8,9]. There are no associated risks with the technique and it can be applied as frequently as required. In the hands of a trained sonographer, it is an easily performed measurement. Each of the methods discussed have advantages and disadvantages, the investigator can obtain highly accurate measurements only as long as these issues are taken into consideration.

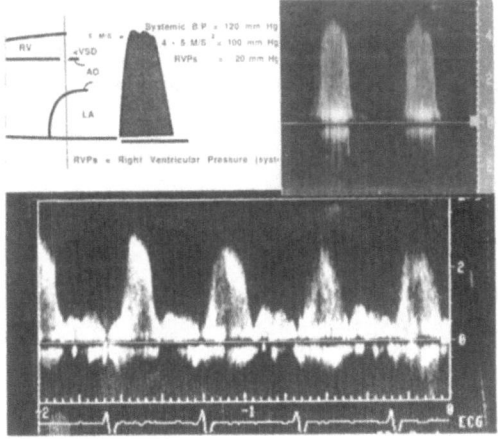

Fig. 7-10. This study was obtained in a subject with a small ventricular septal defect and normal right ventricular pressure and pulmonary artery pressure. Note the high velocity systolic jet across the defect. As mentioned in the text, the velocity of flow across the defect is not a direct indicator of the severity of the lesion. However, the patient with a small isolated ventricular septal defect generally has normal or only slightly elevated right ventricular pressures, so a high velocity jet is usually noted in these subjects.

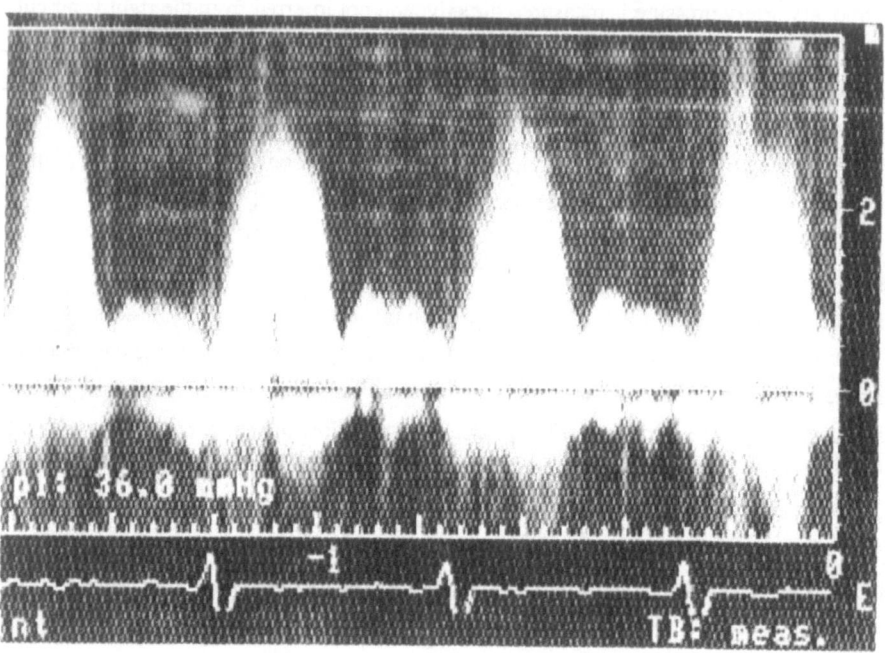

Fig. 7-11. This study was obtained in a subject with a small ventricular septal defect and elevated right ventricular pressure and pulmonary artery pressure due to a coexistent pulmonic stenosis. Note the low velocity systolic jet across the defect.

References

1) Ganz W, et.al. Balloon tipped flow directed catheters pp 79-84 In: Grossman W.(Ed) Cardiac Catheterization and Angiography, Second edition, Philadelphia, Lea and Febiger.

2) Kosturakis D, Goldberg SJ, Allen HD, et al. Doppler echocardiographic prediction of pulmonary arterial hypertension in congenital heart disease. Am. J. Cardiol, 53; 1110-1115, 1984.

3) Stevenson G. Comparison of several noninvasive methods for estimation of pulmonary artery pressure. J Am Soc Echo 1989;2:157-71.

4) Kitabatake A, Inoue M, Asao M, et.al. Noninvasive estimation of pulmonary hypertension by a pulsed Doppler technique. 1983;68:302-9.

5) Chapman JV, Lopez-Sendon JL, Sottillo, Fantidis P, Conrades A. Determinacion con Doppler continuo de la presion sistolica del ventriculo derecho. Rev. Port. Cardiol ,1986; 5:83.

6) Beard JT, Byrd BF. Saline contrast enhancement of trivial tricuspid regurgitation signals for estimating pulmonary artery pressure. Am J Cardiol 1988; 62: 486.

7) Yoshida K, Yoshikowa J, Shakudo M, et al. Color Doppler evaluation of valvular regurgitation in normal subjects. Circulation 1988; 78: 840.

8) Chapman JV, Sgalambro A. Basic Concepts in Doppler Echocardiography pp 155-165, Dordrecht, Martinus Nijhoff Publishers, 1987.

9) Hatle L, Angelsen B, Tromsdal A. Noninvasive assessment of the pulmonary artery systolic pressure with Doppler ultrasound. Br Heart J 1981;45:157.

10) Lynch J, Sagar K, Wann L. Tricuspid regurgitation in normal subjects: Prevalence and possible mechanism (abstr). J Am Coll Cardiol 1986;7,2:145A.

ATRIAL SEPTAL DEFECTS

Alan G. Fraser

Introduction

Cross-sectional echocardiographic imaging was welcomed as the ideal investigative method for diagnosing atrial septal defects, but it has proved to be a less than perfect technique. Most defects and large ones in particular are readily recognised by imaging in appropriate planes, including subcostal views, but demonstration of the thin primum septum at the oval fossa can sometimes be difficult from a precordial approach since the interrogating ultrasound beam may be virtually parallel to the septum. Apparent defects in the middle part of the atrial septum may be false positive findings in normal subjects, due to "drop-out" of reflected echo signals. Thus Doppler techniques should always be used to demonstrate transseptal flow and confirm the diagnosis of an atrial septal defect. In addition, there is still a role for echocardiographic contrast studies in selected patients, such as those with sinus venosus or coronary sinus defects in whom the left to right communication cannot always be demonstrated by cross-sectional imaging and Doppler investigations.

Doppler echocardiography has three main roles in the noninvasive assessment of patients with suspected or proven atrial septal defects. Firstly, by demonstrating associated shunting, color flow mapping can confirm the impression obtained from cross-sectional imaging that there is an anatomical defect. If it fails to demonstrate any transseptal flow, this suggests that a suspected defect was a false positive finding; even in patients with balanced left and right heart pressures, some minor bidirectional shunting can usually be detected. Color flow mapping can also be used to assess the sites of pulmonary venous return, which is particularly important in patients with sinus venosus defects. Secondly, *pulsed Doppler techniques* can be used to study the dynamic velocity profile of flow across a defect. Finally, *Doppler techniques together with imaging* provide an assessment of the hemodynamic consequences of any defect, including an estimate of the degree of shunting. This is especially important if echocardiographic techniques are being used without cardiac catheterization in an individual patient, to establish if surgical closure is required.

This chapter will review briefly the components of the atrial septum and the main types of atrial septal defects. The normal physiological changes which occur after birth, and the significance of a patent foramen ovale in adolescent or adult life, will be discussed. The Doppler echocardiographic assessment of the major types of atrial septal defects including methods of assessing systemic and pulmonary flow ratios will then be reviewed. "Primum" atrial septal defects will not be discussed in detail, since they are included in the chapter on atrioventricular septal defects.

Normal Development of the Atrial Septum

The atrial septum arises early in fetal life as part of the process of septation and valve leaflet formation by which adjacent segments of the primitive heart tube become separated from each other. The primum septum develops from dorsal mesocardial tissue in the posterior atrial wall[1] which extends downwards and outwards, towards what will be the anterior and inferior borders of the atrial septum. At its inferior edge, the primum septum fuses with the endocardial cushions at the atrioventricular junction. During its development, the septum primum is shaped as a crescent, with an aperture in its lower part which is called the ostium primum. With further development the ostium primum closes, and in order to allow continued right to left shunting in utero a second aperture appears higher up in the primum septum, by breakdown of tissue. This is the ostium secundum.

The secundum septum develops as a ridge which is involuted from the outer aspect of the right atrium, between the venous valves and the septum primum. It spreads to overlap the right atrial aspect of the primum septum but it grows more rapidly around the borders of the septum than towards the centre, and so a defect persists in the middle of the secundum septum which is called the foramen ovale. The edge of the septum secundum which bounds the upper aspect of the foramen ovale is the limbus, and after birth the area of the foramen ovale in which primum septum is not covered by secundum septum is called the oval fossa. It occupies almost one third of the total area of the atrial septum.[2]

In utero, oxygenated blood returns from the inferior vena cava across the foramen ovale and through the ostium secundum to the left atrium. After birth the "valve" of the patent foramen ovale closes once the left atrial pressure exceeds the right atrial pressure, because this apposes the primum septum to the limbus of the secundum septum. The atrial septum is thus functionally closed in the majority of term infants within a few days of birth. However, a potential communication remains, and right to left shunting may occur if the right atrial pressure should again become elevated above the left atrial pressure, for example during crying or in infants with respiratory problems.

Primum atrial septal defects occur if there is excessive resorption of the primum septum, or incomplete closure of the ostium primum. They can occur as part of the spectrum of atrioventricular septal defects which arise because of failure of fusion of the endocardial cushions. Secundum atrial septal defects lie partially or completely at the site of the oval fossa, and are bounded by a rim of atrial septum. They occur when the secundum septum fails to develop sufficiently to cover gaps in the primum septum such as the ostium secundum, or when the ostium secundum is misplaced.[3] It is possible that some further downward growth of the septum secundum may occur after birth this has been suggested as one mechanism which would account for the observation that there is a significant incidence of spontaneous closure of secundum atrial septal defects during the first year of life, but apparently not thereafter.[4]

The true atrial septum is composed of its primum and secundum components as already described, but the barries between the atria, is pastly formed in addition by contributions from adjacent structures. The upper and posterior rim of the right atrium develops from the right horn of the sinus venosus, and the components of the great veins as these become incorporated into the right atrium. Abnormal or incomplete absorption leads to atrial septal defects adjacent to the junctions of the caval veins; strictly speaking, such defects lie adjacent to rather than in the atrial septum. A deficiency in the upper part of the septum, at the orifice of the superior caval vein, is more common, and such a sinus venosus atrial septal defect is usually associated with abnormal drainage of the right upper pulmonary vein. Sinus venosus defects next to the orifice of the inferior caval vein are also possible, but very uncommon.

The coronary venous circulation develops from the cardinal veins which leave the left sinus horn and develop to drain the myocardium alone.[1] The coronary sinus lying in the posterior atrioventricular groove is separated by its roof from the left atrium, and the coronary venous return is established into the right atrium. If this process is incomplete, there may be a small defect in the atrial septum in the region of the coronary sinus orifice. The left to right shunt associated with such a coronary sinus defect may be directly across the atrial septum just above the orifice of the coronary sinus, or more frequently routed from the left atrium via an unroofed coronary sinus to the right atrium. Coronary sinus defects are usually associated with a persisting left superior caval vein.

Patent Foramen Ovale

In most normal children the primum and secundum septa become firmly adherent to each other during infancy or early childhood (usually after the age of one year)[5], so that it is impossible thereafter even at cardiac catheterization to find a communication between the atria. However, in many healthy people the foramen ovale stays patent, so that right to left shunting can develop when the right atrial pressure becomes elevated. Autopsy studies suggest that a patent foramen ovale may be present in up to one third of normal subjects up to the age of 30 years, and in up to one quarter of older people.[6] A contrast echocardiographic study in 127 children with structurally normal hearts identified a patent foramen ovale in 37% of them[7], but studies in adults have found a much lower prevalence. For example, contrast echocardiography during a Valsalva maneuver, which has been proposed as the most useful diagnostic test of the competence of the atrial septum because right to left shunting develops as a normal event during forced expiration, revealed a patent foramen ovale in only 8.5% of 176 adults studied in two series.[8,9]

Echocardiographic imaging alone cannot usually discriminate between a normal atrial septum and a septum which appears normal but incorporates a patent foramen ovale, nor in small children can Doppler studies distinguish between a patent foramen ovale and a secundum atrial septal defect.[10] The average size of the potential communication through a patent foramen ovale is only 5 mm.[6] Even transesophageal echocardiographic imaging with its higher resolution and better image quality cannot always help, since it is now recognised that there may be an echo free space between the primum and secundum septa near the oval fossa in normal individuals, without this necessarily being associated with an actual or a potential shunt. However, transesophageal echocardiography does provide very accurate delineation of the primum and secundum septa and the region of the oval fossa, so that it may prove to be the most sensitive investigation for detecting minor shunts. At present, if a patent foramen ovale is suspected or needs to be excluded, a small volume of ultrasound contrast medium or of hand-agitated saline should be injected into a peripheral vein in the upper limbs, during continuous transthoracic echocardiographic imaging. When the patient is asked to perform a Valsalva maneuver, if there is a patent foramen ovale some contrast will appear in the left atrium.[11] The same test can be performed during a transesophageal study, and a small transseptal jet can also be seen when using color flow mapping in the region of the oval fossa during a Valsalva maneuver. However, contrast echocardiography is a better technique than color flow mapping for demonstrating right to left shunting.[12]

These investigations are important in patients with suspected paradoxical embolism[9], and they should be performed before it is reported in any patient that echocardiographic studies have failed to detect any possible source or cause of systemic embolism. In addition, they have assumed greater importance in normal subjects since it was discovered that a patent foramen ovale may be a risk factor for the development of complications of diving such as decompression sickness.[13] During decompression, it is common for nitrogen bubbles to develop in the systemic venous circulation, even after diving only to relatively minor depths. Usually, these bubbles are filtered or reabsorbed in the pulmonary microcirculation, but in the presence of a patent foramen ovale they may cross into the systemic circulation and cause gas emboli. In future, therefore, such relatively simple diagnostic tests may become important for the medical screening of individuals who want to dive for either recreational or occupational reasons.

It has now been demonstrated that paradoxical embolism through a patent foramen ovale can occur in a wide variety of circumstances. During general anesthesia, it may be found in patients receiving positive end-expiratory pressure; thus there may be a role for assessing the patency of the foramen ovale as part of the intraoperative transesophageal echocardiographic monitoring of patients at risk of paradoxical embolism, for example of air during neurosurgery[14] or of fat during orthopedic operations. Patients are also at risk in medical conditions associated with high right heart filling pressures, such as right ventricular infarction[15], heart failure, or chronic respiratory disease.

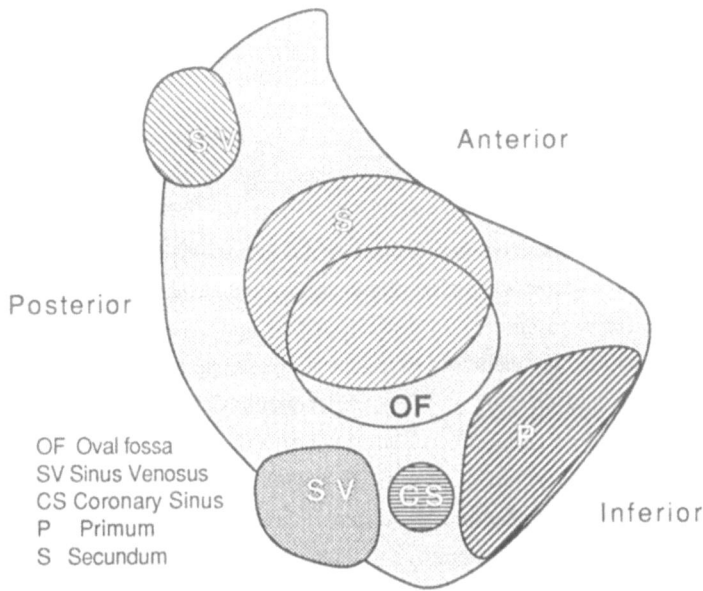

Fig. 8-1. Diagram of the atrial septum, as viewed from the right side, showing the sites of the different types of septal defects. OF = oval fossa, S = site of secundum defects, P = site of primum defects, SV = site of superior or inferior sinus venosus defects, CS = site of coronary sinus defects.

Types of Atrial Septal Defects

The majority of defects, probably more than two thirds, are secundum defects involving the oval fossa.[16] The next most common group are primum defects, which are relatively common in pediatric practice where they may be seen as part of more complex disease. The precise proportions of patients in each group vary considerably according to the selection and age of patients reported. In adults primum defects are found infrequently, for example in 10% of one series.[16] Sinus venosus defects account for a small proportion only (about 3% in one study)[17], and coronary sinus defects are rarest. The different types of atrial septal defects can coexist; patients with three separate communications between the atria have been described.

The sites of the common defects are illustrated in Figure 1. The borders of the septum which are depicted in this diagram were defined by an anatomical study in which the septum was transilluminated.[2] The anterior border is adjacent to the aortic arch and follows its curvature. The inferior border of the true *interatrial* septum is defined by the mitral annulus. Below this level on the right side, the apparent interatrial septum seen on inspection consists of a portion of the free wall of the right atrium, and the atrioventricular membranous septum.

The presence of an atrial septal defect associated with significant right ventricular volume and/or pressure overload can be suspected when a patient with the appropriate clinical signs has evidence on echocardiographic imaging of a dilated right ventricle. There may in addition be abnormal motion of the ventricular septum, which is most apparent on M-mode traces of the ventricles obtained from a parasternal approach. Once a defect is suspected, special care is required during the imaging studies to minimize the chance of diagnostic uncertainty caused by drop-out of echoes from the atrial septum. The best ultrasound imaging plane in which to study the atrial septum is the subxiphoid one[18], because it is approximately perpendicular to the atrial septum. If satisfactory images cannot be obtained, then the atrial septum can also be identified in parasternal short axis images.

Even with optimal imaging including subcostal views, not all atrial septal defects can be seen. All primum defects and the vast majority of secundum defects are usually identified, but subcostal scanning misses about 50% of sinus venosus defects.[19] These are furthest from the chest wall and may be small. Color flow mapping has improved the sensitivity of echocardiography to detect all atrial septal defects including fenestrated secundum defects which can be missed on imaging alone[20], and it appears to have very high specificity, but sinus venosus defects remain a problem.[21] The false negative rate can be reduced by using contrast echocardiographic studies, which should be performed whenever suspicion remains that a patient has an atrial septal defect but it has not been possible to prove this either with imaging or color flow mapping. Although contrast studies may not always localize the site of a left to right shunt, the demonstration of a negative contrast effect improves the diagnostic sensitivity of echocardiographic studies considerably, to virtually 100% in all types of defects.[19]

Transesophageal echocardiography represents a major advance in the ultrasound diagnosis of atrial septal defects.[22] Since the oesophagus lies adjacent to the posterior left atrial wall, the technique is ideal for detecting small sinus venosus defects, and for detecting the sites and analysing the patterns of pulmonary venous blood flow. It is also able to demonstrate the fine anatomical details of the components of the atrial septum in considerably greater detail than is possible from the precordium or the subxiphoid approach. Nevertheless, the technique is not usually necessary in children, and it should only be performed when doubt remains after a standard precordial ultrasound study.

Secundum Defects

These are imaged best in subcostal planes, which should also be used for color flow mapping. Usually, a broad and laminar jet is seen passing from the left to the right atrium, and it may extend directly through the tricuspid valve into the right ventricle in diastole. If there is high flow across the defect, or if the velocity map is adjusted to demonstrate lower velocities, there may be aliasing on the color flow map at the site of the septal defect (Figure 8-2). However, secundum defects are usually unrestrictive, so this is unusual. In the presence of a large shunt, some turbulence may be detected in the right ventricle or the pulmonary artery.

Pulsed Doppler studies should be performed to confirm the diagnosis of an atrial septal defect. If color flow mapping is available, it can be used to position the sample volume within the jet on both sides of the atrial septum; otherwise, the right surface of the septum should be scanned carefully with pulsed Doppler, and if a jet is detected the abnormal flow signal should be followed through the defect into the left atrium. If the velocity is found to increase as blood flows across the septum, the defect is almost certainly restrictive and the shunt is likely to be less than 2:1. If the subcostal approach is difficult in any particular patient, pulsed Doppler studies can be performed from a right parasternal approach.[23] Sampling at the defect shows the typical flow pattern of interatrial shunting (Figure 8-3).

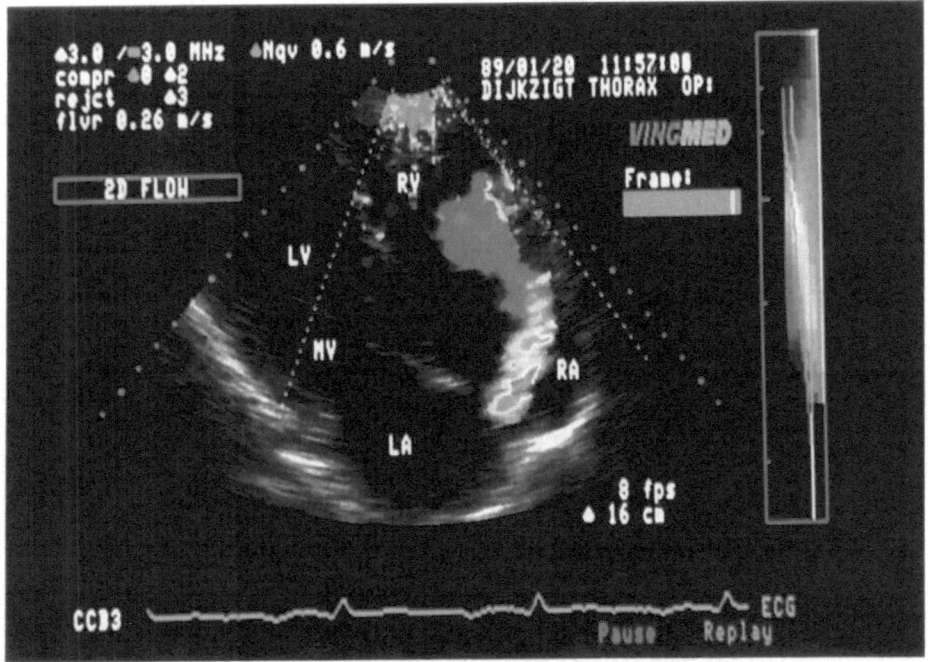

Fig. 8-2. Color flow map obtained in a four chamber-view in a patient with a large secundum atrial septal defect. The transseptal jet is demonstrated in diastole and extends into the right ventricle. There is aliasing because of high velocity flow through a relatively restricted defect.

In a patient with a small atrial septal defect which is restrictive, the velocity of flow across the septum is influenced mainly by the pressure difference between the left and right atria. However, most atrial septal defects are large and there is only a minimal pressure gradient between the atria. Atrial septal defects which exceed 2 cm^2 in area are essentially unrestrictive[24], so that transseptal velocities are determined mainly by flow and the degree of shunting. In a patient with a large atrial septal defect there is the equivalent of a common venous return from all the pulmonary veins and the caval veins, and in diastole all four cardiac chambers are in communication with each other through the open atrioventricular valves and the atrial septal defect. The major share of blood flow from both atria returns to whichever ventricle is the most compliant.[24] Since the right ventricle is more thin walled than the left and since, at least until extremely late in the natural history of the disease, it has a lower diastolic pressure, most blood returns to the right ventricle. At birth, there is little shunting across an atrial septal defect because the right ventricle is hypertrophied after functioning in utero at systemic pressures. As the right ventricular wall thickness declines, the distensibility of the right ventricle increases[25], and gradually left to right shunting develops. This is usually not significant until several months after birth.

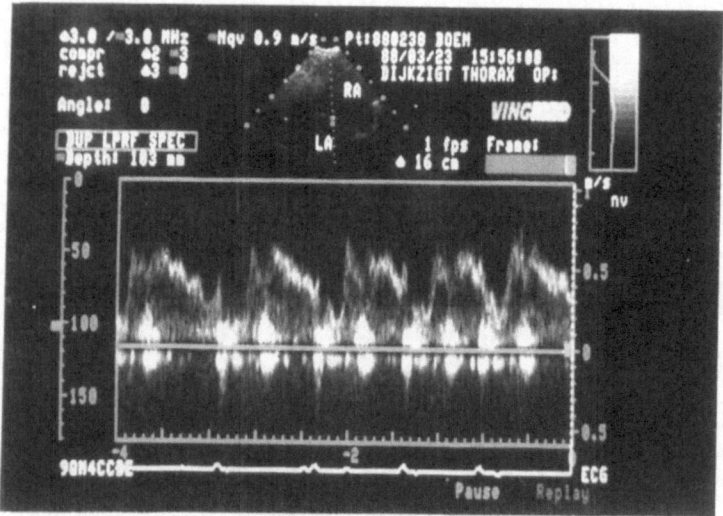

Fig. 8-3. Pulsed Doppler trace of flow across a secundum atrial septal defect.

The patterns of flow across the atrial septum are influenced not only by the relative compliances of the ventricles but also by minor differences in pressure, or in the timing of changes of pressure, between the atria.[26] The right atrium is more compliant than the left[27], so during ventricular systole when the atrioventricular valves are closed, left to right shunting is facilitated by its greater distensibility.[28] The left atrial pressure is higher than the right atrial pressure throughout the cardiac cycle, except for a short period at the beginning of atrial relaxation.[29] However, these pressure differences are small - for example, an average of 0.7 mmHg at the end of diastole[24] - and so the peak velocities lie within the range of pulsed Doppler sampling which does not cause aliasing. Thus, pulsed Doppler recordings of flow across an uncomplicated secundum atrial septal defect (Figure 8-3) show predominant low velocity left to right shunting throughout most of the cardiac cycle. This increases in velocity during systole, and reaches a peak at the end of systole or early in diastole, coinciding with the peak of the atrial *v* wave. The maximum velocity is usually of the order of 1 m/sec.[30] During atrial contraction there is a second peak of flow across the septum from left to right, corresponding to the *a* wave of the atrial pressure trace. In addition, transient (and trivial) right to left shunting often occurs in uncomplicated atrial septal defects. It may occur at the beginning of ventricular systole, because left atrial pressure falls more prominently than does right atrial pressure during early atrial relaxation (corresponding to the *x* descent of the atrial pressure wave), perhaps because there is greater contraction and movement of the base of the left ventricle. Usually, right to left shunting also occurs early in ventricular diastole (at the trough of the *y* descent) when the right atrial pressure is again momentarily higher than the left.[29] Significant right to left shunting (greater than 0.7 l/min), however, is found in only 15% of patients with uncomplicated atrial septal defects, and predominantly in the older ones.[31]

Exact measurement of the peak velocity of flow across an atrial septal defect is not important for most clinical purposes, since there is no clear relationship between it and the degree of shunting. However, analysis of the patterns of flow does convey clinically useful information. The second forward flow signal following atrial contraction is reduced in infants and small children until the right ventricular hypertrophy present at birth has regressed.[30] It is also less obvious in patients with pulmonary hypertension and right ventricular hypertrophy. In patients with pulmonary or tricuspid stenosis coexisting with an atrial septal defect, there may even be reversed flow from right to left during atrial systole, because of the elevated right atrial pressure.[30] This can be present at the same time that a patient has a left to right shunt during ventricular systole. When an atrial septal defect occurs in a patient with more complex disease, the flow pattern may be quite different. For example, there is predominant right to left shunting in patients with tricuspid atresia, and a similar pattern may be the only echocardiographic clue to the diagnosis of obligatory right to left shunting found in a patient with total anomalous pulmonary venous drainage.[32] When there is absence of the left atrioventricular connection, obligatery shunting is from left to right (Figure 8-4).

Sometimes diagnostic difficulties arise during color flow mapping when the inflow from the superior caval vein and the flow across a septal defect lie adjacent to each other in the right atrium, and during pulsed Doppler studies if the sample volume is placed in the flow from the superior caval vein, rather than in a jet arising from a defect high in the secundum septum. In such circumstances, it is helpful to analyse the Doppler waveforms during respiration. In uncomplicated atrial septal defects, the pressure difference between the atria decreases on inspiration and increases on expiration.[29] Thus forward (or left to right) flow and peak velocities across an atrial septal defect decrease on inspiration.[30] At the same time, forward flow from the superior caval vein increases. The left to right shunt across an atrial septal defect also decreases on exercise, because left ventricular filling is increased as an indirect consequence of the fall in systemic vascular resistance.

Pulmonary venous drainage in secundum defects is usually anatomically normal, but even so the blood returning from the right pulmonary veins may drain preferentially into the right atrium because their orifices lie very close to the posterior rim of a large secundum defect. Nevertheless, some patients with secundum defects (perhaps 5%) have coexisting partial anomalous pulmonary venous drainage.[33] Color flow mapping should therefore be used to confirm that venous drainage is normal. The right upper pulmonary venous orifice is relatively easy to identify in infants or children, when using an apical four-chamber view.[34]

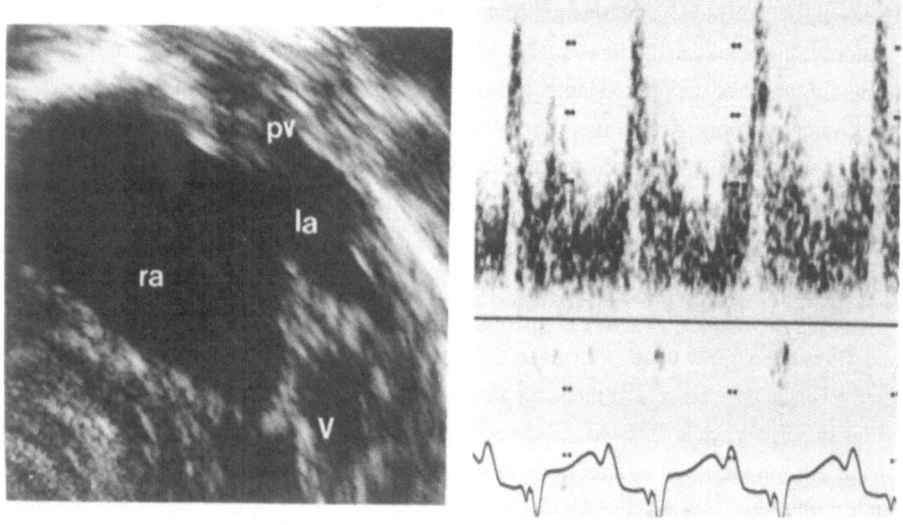

Fig 8-4 · Obligatory right to left shunting found in a patient with total anomalous pulmonary venous drainage. PV=Pulmonary Vein, LA=Left Atrium, RA=Right Atrium, V=Ventricle.

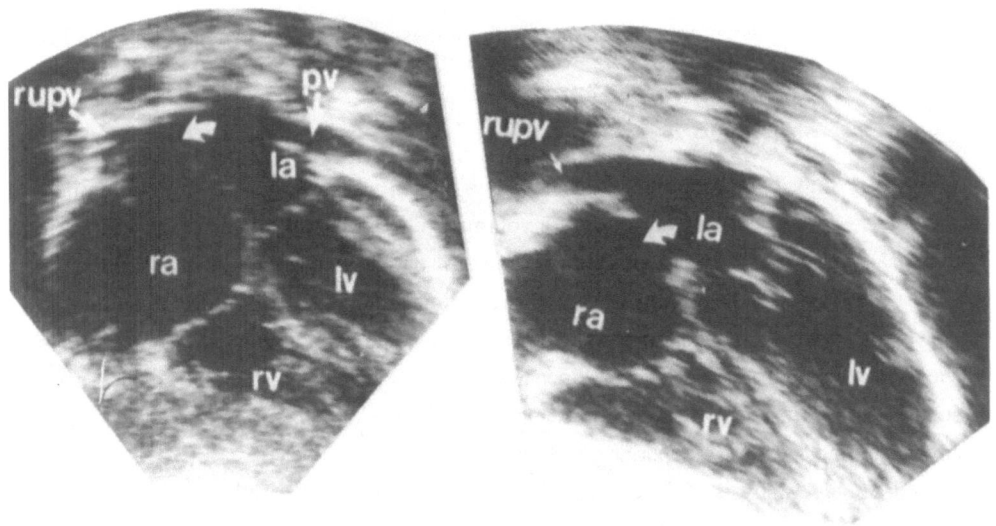

Fig. 8-5 (a) (left) Sinus Venosus defect (arrows). This lies posteres to the atrial septum. (b) (right) Secundum (os oval fossa) defect (arrows) due to deficiency of the septum primum in the middle of the atrial septum.

Sinus Venosus Defects

In the more common type of sinus venosus defect, imaging may reveal the defect in the upper or posterior atrial septum (Figure 8-5), adjacent to the posterior interatrial groove on four chamber views, and immediately inferior to the orifice of the superior caval vein.[35] Strictly speaking, this type of defect lies outwith the true atrial septum and is an abnormality of the systemic venous connections. Color flow maps show shunting at this level, although the left to right shunt can occasionally be confused with inflow from the superior caval vein or the right upper pulmonary vein. In the uncommon type of sinus venosus defect, the hole in the atrial septum is located inferior to the oval fossa, merging with the floor of the inferior caval vein. If there is any doubt about the presence of a sinus venosus defect, especially in older patients, the investigation of choice now is a transesophageal echocardiographic study. Since small transesophageal probes have been developed for pediatric use, such investigations can also be performed in children.

The sites of pulmonary veins are usually abnormal in patients with sinus venosus defects, and this can best be confirmed with color flow mapping. In particular, the right upper pulmonary vein drains directly into the right atrium in most patients (86% in one series)[17], as does the middle lobe pulmonary vein in about two thirds of patients, and the lower lobe vein in about one third.[17]

Pulsed Doppler flow patterns across the septum are essentially the same as those found in patients with secundum defects.

Coronary Sinus Defects

A coronary sinus defect should be suspected in a patient who has right heart flow murmurs and evidence of right ventricular pressure or volume overload, but no suggestion of a defect in the central portion of the atrial septum, if standard parasternal long axis scans show the coronary sinus to be considerably dilated. In such circumstances, the abnormal anatomy may not be demonstrated by transthoracic imaging studies, but an injection of contrast into a vein in the left arm will confirm the diagnosis. Since there is an associated persisting left superior caval vein, this test will demonstrate that contrast enters the right atrium via the coronary sinus rather than via a normal right sided superior caval vein.

Pulsed Doppler analysis of the coronary sinus flow pattern is difficult but may be possible from a parasternal tricuspid inlet view. If there is shunting through the coronary sinus, the peak velocities of flow are increased compared with normal. It is important if this is found, to distinguish a coronary sinus atrial septal defect from total anomalous pulmonary venous drainage with the pulmonary venous flow returning to the coronary sinus. In patients with an atrial septal defect, it should be possible to image the defect directly, or to locate an unroofed coronary sinus.[36]

Assessment of Pulmonary and Systemic Blood Flow

The traditional criterion for judging the severity of an atrial septal defect, or indeed any other intracardiac shunt, has been the ratio of pulmonary to systemic blood flow. Before the development of echocardiography this was measured at cardiac catheterization, but now patients may be referred for surgery without invasive investigation. It has been reported that the prognosis of patients who have atrial septal defects with a very small shunt (less than 2 : 1) is excellent, with no deterioration being seen at a mean follow up of 11.6 years.[37] It is clear therefore that some patients with atrial septal defects do not require treatment perhaps those with a shunt of 1.5 to 1, or less, and normal right ventricular dimensions and function. However, without a good non-invasive method of estimating a shunt and confidently identifying such patients, it is possible that some will be submitted to operation unnecessarily.

There have been numerous studies of echocardiographic techniques for the non-invasive estimation of systemic and pulmonary blood flows. In essence, these require calculations of volumetric flow from Doppler velocity profiles and cross-sectional areas, at points in the pulmonary and systemic circulations. They usually make the assumption that flow velocity profiles across the vessel or valve orifice at which the Doppler information is being derived, are flat. Although this is not strictly true, the errors introduced by such assumptions are probably quite small, and no greater than those of comparable invasive methods.[38]

The degree of shunting associated with an atrial septal defect is not caused by the size of the defect per se. Instead, as already mentioned, it is related to the distensibility of the right ventricle in diastole[24], and of the right atrium in systole.[28] Since compliance is similar in both ventricles after birth, little shunting occurs until the right ventricular pressure and wall thickness start to fall. Babies who develop considerable shunting before this has happened constitute a distinct group, who have a less favorable prognosis and who may require early operation.

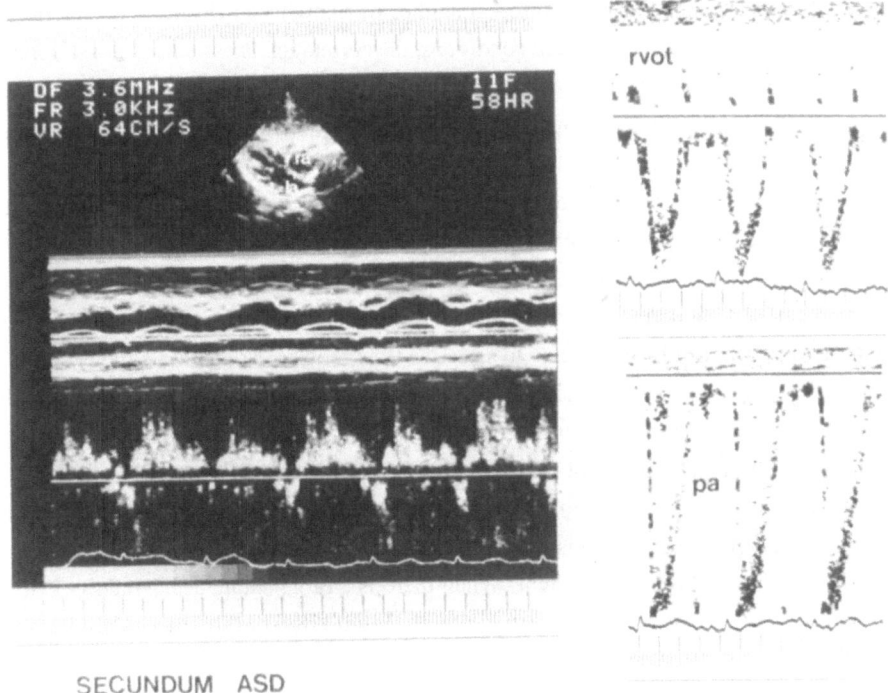

SECUNDUM ASD

Fig. 8-6. Left handed panel; Pulsed Doppler sampling of flow across a secundum defect. In the same patient, due to a large left- to right shunt, there is a considerable increase in the velocity of flow in the right heart as blood accelerates from the right ventricular outflow tract (RVOT) into the pulmonary artery (PA). There is no pulmonary stenosis.

Pulmonary blood flow is usually estimated by pulsed Doppler analysis of flow at the orifice of the pulmonary valve, obtained in a parasternal short axis view. Systemic flow is estimated at the aortic valve, often from a suprasternal approach. If there is disease of either of these valves, such as significant valvar regurgitation, then alternative sites for the Doppler measurements have to be used.[38] If flow across the mitral valve is studied to calculate left ventricular output, it is usually assumed that the dimensions and area of the annulus are constant, and that the annulus is circular, when in fact the annulus shortens its circumference by about 30% in systole, and it is ellipsoid in shape. The timing and precise location of measurements is therefore critical. Similar difficulties are encountered at the aortic valve, in deciding which measurement is most useful for calculating aortic cross-sectional area; usually the diameter is recorded from a parasternal long axis image at the level of the base of the cusps. Nevertheless, flow ratios calculated by these methods correlate well with those calculated using the Fick principle from data obtained by dye dilution studies or oximetry at cardiac catheterization. Under carefully controlled experimental conditions, the correlation is extremely close[39], and in clinical studies it is also excellent.[39,40]

Doppler analysis of pulmonary and systemic blood flow is quite time-consuming, and so alternative, more simple approaches have been suggested. For example, Cloez et al calculated the square of the ratio of pulmonary to aortic luminal diameters and multiplied this by the ratio of pulmonary to aortic peak flow velocities, instead of using the respective areas and time velocity integrals, and reported that the resulting estimate of the flow ratio was as accurate as the more detailed technique.[41] Marx et al found that the mean transatrial septal velocity correlates quite well with the pulmonary to systemic flow ratio.[42] As an even simpler Doppler screening test for the presence of a significant left to right shunt, it is possible to measure the peak velocities of inflow across the atrioventricular valves, as long as these are neither stenotic nor regurgitant. If one assumes that the filling periods of the ventricles are not significantly different, then because the tricuspid valve orifice is larger than the mitral orifice, the peak velocity of tricuspid flow should always be lower than the peak velocity of mitral flow. If it is higher, this implies a considerable shunt. When there is a large shunt, acceleration of flows will be observed across the pulmonary valve (Figure 8-6). Finally, in adults with uncomplicated secundum atrial septal defects, the width of the jet across the atrial septum determined by color flow mapping correlates reasonably well with the size of the shunt, so that it has been suggested that surgery should be recommended when the transatrial jet width exceeds 15 mm.[43] Jet area also correlates with the degree of shunting, but not closely enough for its measurement to be of any practical value for clinical decisions. The size of an atrial septum defect is also not useful for estimating the degree of shunting.[20]

Cross-sectional Imaging and M-mode Echocardiography

Before cross-sectional echocardiography was introduced, much energy was devoted to the recognition of abnormal patterns of motion of the ventricular septum in patients with atrial septal defects. Since Doppler estimates of a small left to right shunt are only reliable as indicators of an unimportant atrial septal defect if right ventricular function is normal, it is still important to assess right ventricular function as part of the routine echocardiographic examination in all patients with atrial septal defects.

There is abnormal rapid anterior motion of the ventricular septum at the beginning of systole, as found also in patients with right ventricular diastolic volume overload from other causes, and there is brisk posterior motion of the septum in diastole.[44] These changes are most prominent in the upper, thinner part of the ventricular septum. It is now appreciated that diastolic flattening of the ventricular septum is the result of right ventricular volume overload; this causes the posterior motion of the ventricular septum in early diastole. If the range of this motion is more than 0.5 cm, it is likely that the left to right shunt exceeds 2.5 to 1.[45] In patients with uncomplicated atrial septal defects, the left ventricle generates higher pressures during systole than does the right, and so the normal relative configuration of the ventricles is restored. The anterior septal motion in systole is thought to represent the restitution of the normal circular shape of the left ventricle[44], compared with the abnormal crescentic shape seen in these patients during diastole.[46] In older patients with chronic right ventricular volume and pressure overload, the ventricular septum bulges towards the left throughout diastole and systole, and the variations in septal motion are not seen. The degree of curvature of the ventricular septum correlates with the right ventricular systolic pressure[47], and eccentricity of the left ventricle persisting into systole indicates right ventricular pressure overload.[48]

Septal motion in patients with atrial septal defects sometimes appears to be paradoxical. Recently, it has been suggested that this impression is artefactual since even in patients with considerable shunts, the pattern of contraction of the left ventricle appears to be normal if it is analysed from a parasternal short axis cross-section by using an algorithm incorporating a floating centroid. Paradoxical septal motion is apparent only when analytic techniques are used which employ a fixed centroid.[49]

Alternative methods of assessing the significance of an intracardiac shunt have been reported, based only on cross-sectional imaging studies. In patients with large shunts, the left atrial and left ventricular volumes are reduced compared with normal, and right ventricular volume is increased. The relationship between right ventricular dimensions and pulmonary blood flow is weak[50] or non-existent[51], but the ratio of pulmonary trunk to aortic root dimensions correlates quite well with the degree of shunting. In one study, all patients with a shunt of > 1.5 : 1 had an abnormal ratio.[50]

Doppler Analysis of Complications of Atrial Septal Defects

The cross-sectional area of the pulmonary circulation needs to decrease by more than two thirds before pulmonary arterial pressure increases or pulmonary arterial flow is reduced. Nevertheless, pulmonary vascular resistance does increase in response to a chronic volume overload, and then pressures of course rise in the pulmonary artery and right ventricle. In patients with atrial septal defects, this is uncommon before the age of twenty, and usual after the age of forty. The ventricle is already dilated because of the chronic volume load, and so the addition of pressor stress results in a high prevalence of tricuspid regurgitation. The regurgitant jet can be sampled with continuous wave Doppler techniques, and the right ventricular systolic pressure and by extrapolation the pulmonary arterial systolic pressure can be estimated by applying the modified Bernoulli equation.[52] If the central venous pressure cannot be estimated by examining the neck veins, for example in small children, then it is reasonable to assume for such calculations that the right atrial pressure is about 5 mmHg, although in patients with an atrial septal defect and pulmonary hypertension it may be as much as 20 mmHg.[24] Pulmonary artery pressure can also be estimated non-invasively by measuring the right ventricular isovolumic relaxation time, which becomes prolonged.[53] The presence of a prominent jet from tricuspid regurgitation may make it difficult to record transseptal pulsed Doppler flow signals, and it may also cause increased right to left shunting during systole.[30]

Analysis of the pattern of flow across an atrial septal defect may be helpful in indicating the onset of right ventricular dysfunction.[28] Since a failing ventricle is less compliant than normal, the left to right shunt will decline as right ventricular failure develops. This should not be construed as an improvement in a patient's condition, since the reduction of the left to right shunt presages the later development of a reversed shunt, nor should a small shunt be accepted as satisfactory in a patient who has other features on complete echocardiographic assessment which suggest that right ventricular function is abnormal. A sustained right to left shunt during atrial systole is the clue to reduced right ventricular compliance, even if the pulmonary arterial pressure is not significantly elevated. If the right ventricular diastolic pressure is elevated, indirect evidence may be available from the Doppler derived waveform of pulmonary regurgitation, since the regurgitant jet will show attenuation of its velocity in diastole. In the presence of right heart failure, flow reversal is present in the inferior caval vein and the hepatic veins.

In patients with atrial septal defects, the hemodynamic consequences of failure developing in the left and right ventricles are different. In left heart failure, the diastolic pressure in the left ventricle rises, but left ventricular stroke volume is more or less maintained. In right heart failure, however, the right ventricular diastolic pressure usually does not increase, but the stroke volume and output fall.[24]

Eisenmenger Syndrome

A small proportion (about 9%) of those patients who have an undetected and untreated atrial septal defect will develop the Eisenmenger syndrome, with predominant right to left shunting.[54] The etiology of this complication is not understood but it seems to be an idiosyncratic reaction, since its incidence is roughly the same in all age groups[54], and many older patients do not develop it. In patients with the Eisenmenger syndrome, there may be very little flow across the atrial septum at rest because the pulmonary and systemic pressures are equalised. During exercise, however, there may be a further increase in pulmonary arterial pressures and right ventricular dysfunction which will exacerbate right to left shunting across the defect. Doppler sampling across the defect is unlikely to be possible during dynamic exercise, but a similar phenomenon may be observed during isometric exercise such as handgrip or during a Valsalva maneuver. In general, the smaller the right ventricular output, the greater the right to left shunt.

Atrial Septal Aneurysm

This is an uncommon abnormality which seems to be being recognised more frequently now, perhaps because of the increased use of transesophageal imaging. It probably represents an extreme degree of redundancy of the valve of the foramen ovale and it may be a normal variant, at one end of the spectrum of mobility of the atrial septum. This conclusion is supported by an autopsy study which reported a prevalence of atrial septal aneurysm of 1% in adults, none of whom had had symptoms which might be attributed to it.[55] However, thrombus has been found in such patients[55], and more marked degrees of ballooning or deviation of the atrial septum have been reported to be associated with systemic embolism.[56]

The main significance of atrial septal aneurysms in the context of this chapter, however, is that they are also associated with atrial septal defects. Brand et al found an atrial septal aneurysm in 1% of 3,500 children undergoing echocardiographic examination, and in 69% of them it was associated with a secundum atrial septal defect.[57] It is unclear whether an aneurysm represents the cause or the result of a defect, but if a localized protrusion of the atrial septum is observed then an atrial septal defect should be suspected. In such circumstances, however, the incidence of spontaneous closure is probably high.[57]

Monitoring of Therapeutic Interventions

A new context for the echocardiographic study of atrial septal defects has arisen in recent years with the development of interventional cardiology. Now color flow mapping is an extremely simple, rapid and helpful means of monitoring the increase in flow across the atrial septum achieved after a Rashkind balloon atrial septostomy in a baby with transposition of the great arteries, and it can equally well be used after the insertion of an umbrella device to check that an atrial septal defect has been closed. In adults, too, the technique is being used to study the closure of atrial septal defects produced by transseptal puncture during mitral balloon valvotomy in patients with rheumatic mitral stenosis.

References

1. Wenink ACG. Embryology of the heart. In: Anderson RH, Macartney FJ, Shinebourne EA, Tynan M. Paediatric Cardiology. Edinburgh, Churchill Livingstone, 1989: 83-107.

2. Sweeney LJ, Rosenquist GC. The normal anatomy of the atrial septum in the human heart. Am Heart J 1979; 98: 194-199.

3. Hudson R. The normal and abnormal inter-atrial septum. Br Heart J 1955; 17: 489-495.

4. Mody MR. Serial hemodynamic observations in secundum atrial septal defect with special reference to spontaneous closure. Am J Cardiol 1973; 32: 978-981.

5. Patten BM. The closure of the foramen ovale. Am J Anat 1931; 48: 19-44.

6. Hagen PT, Scholz DG, Edwards WD. Incidence and size of patent foramen ovale during the first 10 decades of life: an autopsy study of 965 normal hearts. Mayo Clin Proc 1984; 59: 17-20.

7. Van Hare GF, Silverman NH. Contrast two-dimensional echocardiography in congenital heart disease: techniques, indications and clinical utility. J Am Coll Cardiol 1989; 13: 673-686.

8. Lynch JJ, Schuchard GH, Gross CM, Wann LS. Prevalence of right-to-left atrial shunting in a healthy population: detection by Valsalva maneuver contrast echocardiography. Am J Cardiol 1984; 53: 1478-1480.

9. Lechat PH, Mas JL, Lascault G, Loron P, Theard M, Klimczac M, Drobinski G, Thomas D, Grosgogeat Y. Prevalence of patent foramen ovale in patients with stroke. New Eng J Med 1988; 318: 1148-1152.

10. Oberhoffer R, Lang D. Diagnostic criteria of interatrial defects: a single gate pulsed Doppler echocardiographic study. Int J Cardiol 1989; 25: 167-171.

11. Kronik G, Mösslacher H. Positive contrast echocardiography in patients with patent foramen ovale and normal right heart hemodynamics. Am J Cardiol 1982; 49: 1806-1809.

12. Suzuki Y, Kambara H, Kadota K, Tamaki S, Yamazato A, Nohara R, Osakada G, Kawai C. Detection of intracardiac shunt flow in atrial septal defect using a real-time two-dimensional color-coded Doppler flow imaging system and comparison with contrast two-dimensional echocardiography. Am J Cardiol 1985; 56: 347-350.

13. Moon RE, Camporesi EM, Kisslo JA. Patent foramen ovale and decompression sickness in divers. Lancet 1989; 1: 513-514.

14. Cucchiara RF, Seward JB, Nishimura RA, Nugent M, Faust RJ. Identification of patent foramen ovale during sitting position craniotomy by transesophageal echocardiography with positive airway pressure. Anesthesiology 1985; 63: 107-109.

15. Manno BV, Bemis CE, Carver J, Mintz GS. Right ventricular infarction complicated by right to left shunt. J Am Coll Cardiol 1983; 1: 554-557.

16. Bedford DE. The anatomical types of atrial septal defect. Their incidence and clinical diagnosis. Am J Cardiol 1960; 6: 568-574.

17. Davia JE, Cheitlin MD, Bedynek JL. Sinus venosus atrial septal defect: analysis of fifty cases. Am Heart J 1973; 85: 177-185.

18. Bierman FZ, Williams RG. Subxiphoid two-dimensional imaging of the interatrial septum in infants and neonates with congenital heart disease. Circulation 1979; 60: 80-90.

19. Shub C, Dimopoulos IN, Seward JB, Callahan JA, Tancredi RG, Schattenberg TT, Reeder GS, Hagler DJ, Tajik AJ. Sensitivity of two-dimensional echocardiography in the direct visualization of atrial septal defect utilizing the subcostal approach: experience with 154 patients. J Am Coll Cardiol 1983; 2: 127-135.

20. Forfar JC, Godman MJ. Functional and anatomical correlates in atrial septal defect. An echocardiographic analysis. Br Heart J 1985; 54: 193-200.

21. Khanderia BK, Shub C, Tajik AJ, Taylor CL, Hagler DJ, Seward JB. Utility of color flow imaging for visualizing shunt flow in atrial septal defect. Int J Cardiol 1989; 23; 91-98.

22. Hanrath P, Schlüter M, Langenstein BA, Polster J, Engel S, Kremer P, Krebber H-J. Detection of ostium secundum atrial septal defects by transoesophageal cross-sectional echocardiography. Br Heart J 1983; 49: 350-358.

23. Minagoe S, Tei C, Kisanuki A, Arikawa K, Nakazono Y, Yoshimura H, Kashima T, Tanaka H. Noninvasive pulsed Doppler echocardiographic detection of the direction of shunt flow in patients with atrial septal defect: usefulness of the right parasternal approach. Circulation 1985; 71: 745-753.

24. Dexter L. Atrial septal defect. Br Heart J 1956; 18: 209-225.

25. Mathew R, Thilenius OG, Arcilla RA. Comparative response of right and left ventricles to volume overload. Am J Cardiol 1976; 38: 209-217.

26. Alexander JA, Rembert JC, Sealy WC, Greenfield JC. Shunt dynamics in experimental atrial septal defect. J Appl Physiol 1975; 39: 281-286.

27. Little RC, Opdyke DF, Hawley JG. Dynamics of experimental atrial septal defects. Am J Physiol 1949; 158: 241-250.

28. Joffe HS. Effect of age on pressure-flow dynamics in secundum atrial septal defect. Br Heart J 1984; 51; 468-472.

29. Levin AR, Spach MS, Boineau JP, Canent RV, Capp MP, Jewett PH. Atrial pressure-flow dynamics in atrial septal defects (secundum type). Circulation 1968; 37: 476-488.

30. Hatle L. Flow velocity patterns across atrial septal defects recorded with Doppler echocardiography. Acta Paediatr Scand 1986; Supp 329: 68-77.

31. Galve E, Angel J, Evangelista A, Anivarro I, Permanyer-Miralda G, Soler-Soler J. Bidirectional shunt in uncomplicated atrial septal defect. Br Heart J 1984; 51; 480-484.

32. Stevenson JG. Doppler evaluation of atrial septal defect, ventricular septal defect, and complex malformations. Acta Paediatr Scand 1986; Supp 329: 21-43.

33. Gotsman MS, Astley R, Parsons CG. Partial anomalous pulmonary venous drainage in association with atrial septal defect. Br Heart J 1965; 27: 566-571.

34. Smallhorn JF, Freedom RM, Olley PM. Pulsed Doppler echocardiographic assessment of extraparenchymal pulmonary vein flow. J Am Coll Cardiol 1987; 9: 573-579.

35. Nasser FN, Tajik AJ, Seward JB, Hagles DJ. Diagnosis of sinus venosus atrial septal defect by two-dimensional echocardiography. Mayo Clin Proc 1981; 56: 568-572.

36. Hamada Y, Ebihara H, Tanimoto Y, Kobayashi Y, Matsuda Y. Unroofed coronary sinus demonstrated by two-dimensional echocardiography. Am Heart J 1984; 108: 1558-1560.

37. Andersen M, Lyngborg K, Møller I, Wennevold A. The natural history of small atrial septal defects: long-term follow-up with serial heart catheterizations. Am Heart J 1976; 92: 302-307.

38. Sanders SP, Yeager S, Williams RG. Measurement of systemic and pulmonary blood flow and Q_P/Q_S ratio using Doppler and two-dimensional echocardiography. Am J Cardiol 1983; 51: 952-956.

39. Valdes-Cruz LM, Horowitz S, Mesel E, Sahn DJ, Fisher DC, Larson D. A pulsed Doppler echocardiographic method for calculating pulmonary and systemic blood flow in atrial level shunts: validation studies in animals and initial human experience. Circulation 1984; 69: 80-86.

40. Kitabatake A, Inoue M, Asao M, Ito H, Masuyama T, Tanouchi J, Morita T, Hori M, Yoshima H, Ohnishi K, Abe H. Noninvasive evaluation of the ratio of pulmonary to systemic flow in atrial septal defect by duplex Doppler echocardiography. Circulation 1984; 69: 73-79.

41. Cloez J-L, Schmidt KG, Birk E, Silverman NH. Determination of pulmonary to systemic blood flow ratio in children by a simplified Doppler echocardiographic method. J Am Coll Cardiol 1988; 11: 825-830.

42. Marx GR, Allen HD, Goldberg SJ, Flinn CJ. Transatrial septal velocity measurement by Doppler echocardiography in atrial septal defect: correlation with Qp:Qs ratio. Am J Cardiol 1985; 55: 1162-1167.

43. Pollick C, Sullivan H, Cujec B, Wilansky S. Doppler color-flow imaging assessment of shunt size in atrial septal defect. Circulation 1988; 78: 522-528.

44. Weyman AE, Wann S, Feigenbaum H, Dillon JC. Mechanisms of abnormal septal motion in patients with right ventricular volume overload. A cross-sectional echocardiographic study. Circulation 1976; 54; 179-186.

45. Chazal RA, Armstrong WF, Dillon JC, Feigenbaum H. Diastolic ventricular septal motion in atrial septal defect: analysis of M-mode echocardiograms in 31 patients. Am J Cardiol 1983; 52: 1088-1090.

46. Hung J, Uren RF, Richmond DR, Kelly DT. The mechanism of abnormal septal motion in atrial septal defect. Circulation 1981; 63: 142-148.

47. King ME, Braun H, Goldblatt A, Liberthson R, Weyman AE. Interventricular septal configuration as a predictor of right ventricular systolic hypertension in children: a cross-sectional echocardiographic study. Circulation 1983; 68: 68-75.

48. Ryan T, Petrovic O, Dillon JC, Feigenbaum H, Conley MJ, Armstrong WF. An echocardiographic index for separation of right ventricular volume and pressure overload. J Am Coll Cardiol 1985; 5: 918-924.

49. Vincent RN, Saurette RH, Pelech AN, Collins GF. Interventricular septal motion and left ventricular function in patients with atrial septal defect. Pediatr Cardiol 1988; 9:143-148.

50. Denef B, Dumoulin M, van der Hauwaert LG. Usefulness of echocardiographic assessment of right ventricular and pulmonary trunk size for estimating magnitude of left-to-right shunt in children with atrial septal defect. Am J Cardiol 1985; 55: 1571-1575.

51. Radtke WE, Tajik AJ, Gau GT, Schattenberg TT, Giuliani ER, Tancredi RG. Atrial septal defect: echocardiographic observations. Studies in 120 patients. Ann Int Med 1976; 84: 246-252.

52. Yock PG, Popp RL. Noninvasive estimation of right ventricular systolic pressure by Doppler ultrasound in patients with tricuspid regurgitation. Circulation 1984; 70: 657-662.

53. Hatle L, Angelsen BAJ, Tromsdal A. Non-invasive estimation of pulmonary artery systolic pressure with Doppler ultrasound. Br Heart J 1981; 45: 157-165.

54. Cherian G, Uthaman CB, Durairaj M, Sukumar IP, Krishnaswami S, Jairaj PS, John S, Krishnaswami H, Bhaktaviziam A. Pulmonary hypertension in isolated secundum atrial septal defects: high frequency in young patients. Am Heart J 1983; 105: 952-957.

55. Silver MD, Dorsey JS. Aneurysms of the septum primum in adults.Arch Pathol Lab Med 1978; 102: 62-65.

56. Gallet B, Malergue MC, Adams C, Saudemont JP, Collot AM, Druon MC, Hiltgen M. Atrial septal aneurysms - a potential cause of systemic embolism. An echocardiographic study. Br Heart J 1985; 53: 292-297.

57. Brand A, Keren A, Branski D, Abrahamov A, Stern S. Natural course of atrial septal aneurysm in children and the potential for spontaneous closure of associated septal defect. Am J Cardiol 1989; 64: 996-1001.

CHAPTER IX

DOPPLER ECHOCARDIOGRAPHY IN VENTRICULAR SEPTAL DEFECTS

George R. Sutherland

Naryswamy Sreeram

Introduction

In a suprisingly short period of time, cardiac ultrasound has become accepted as an accurate and reproducible technique for the noninvasive evaluation of many aspects of both morphology and hemodynamics of ventricular septal defects. High resolution cross-sectional imaging can visualize virtually all moderate to large sized defects. Small defects (i.e. <3 mm. maximal diameter) normally lie beyond the powers of resolution of even the most modern cross-sectional imaging systems. However, such isolated small defects are virtually always associated with restrictive hemodynamics (i.e. a high trans-septal gradient with low right ventricular pressure), and although they are frequently missed by cross-sectional imaging, their high velocity trans-septal turbulent jet is easily picked up by continuous wave Doppler interrogation. From a combined complete continuous pulsed wave Doppler study both the right heart systolic pressures and the relative volume flows in the aorta and pulmonary artery can be calculated. The addition of colour flow mapping plays an important part in identifying the site (or sites) of trans-septal flow and defining the location of small restrictive defects. However, problem areas in the ultrasound evaluation of ventricular septal defects do exist: i) the presence of multiple ventricular septal defects can be missed (especialy if non-restrictive hemodynamics are present); ii) precise intra-cardiac shunt calculations in young infants are fraught with problems; iii) poor alignment with the high velocity trans-septal jet can lead to serious overestimation of right ventricular peak systolic pressure. Wrong diagnoses can occur despite the use of all three ultrasound modalities if these important pitfalls are not appreciated. In this chapter we will attempt to review the current understanding and use of cardiac ultrasound in the evaluation of the complex morphology and frequently changing hemodynamics in this important group of lesions.

Morphology and Classification of Ventricular Septal Defects

Any complete ultrasound study of a ventricular septal defect must first take into account the type of defect being studied, as different defect types have both differing natural histories and associated malformations. The intact ventricular septum has both membranous (small) and muscular (large) components. The fibrous membranous septum occupies part of the area enclosed by the fibrous annuli of the tricuspid, mitral and aortic valves and is divided into an atrioventricular and an interventricular component by the attachment of the septal leaflet of the tricuspid valve which runs oblique across it. When viewed from its right ventricular aspect the muscular component of the ventricular septum can be subdivided into inlet, trabecular and outlet portions. The smooth inlet muscular septum is sited in the inlet of the ventricles and lies under the septal leaflet of the tricuspid valve. It merges inferiorly with the trabecular septum, which extends to the apex of the heart. The trabecular septum in turn merges with the smooth outlet septum. The interventricular portion of the membranous septum is therefore bound posteriorly by the inlet septum, inferiorly by the trabecular septum and anteriorly by the outlet septum.

Ventricular septal defects can be classified into three main groups based on the structures forming their margins (Fig. 9-1): 1) perimembranous defects are defects which are always roofed in part by the central fibrous body and which involve, wholly or in part, the area normally occupied by the membranous septum; 2) muscular defects which are bound on all aspects by muscle tissue, and 3) doubly committed subarterial defects which lie directly beneath both great vessels and are roofed by the conjoint aortic and pulmonary valves [1]. Perimembranous defects almost invariably are not confined to the area normally occupied by the membranous septum, but extend to involve the adjacent muscular portions of the interventricular septum. Depending on the predominant sub-unit of the septum involved, perimembranous ventricular septal defects can be subclassified into perimembranous inlet, trabecular and oulet defects. Large "confluent" perimembranous defects extend to involve all three muscular sub-units of the interventricular septum. Muscular defects are subdivided into inlet, trabecular and outlet muscular defects, depending on their location within the muscular septum. Doubly committed subarterial defects can be divided into two types: 1) those which involve the membranous septum and 2) those which have entirely muscular rims. The above classification of ventricular septal defects is equally applicable wheter the defect exists as an isolated cardiac lesion or is part of a more complex malformation.

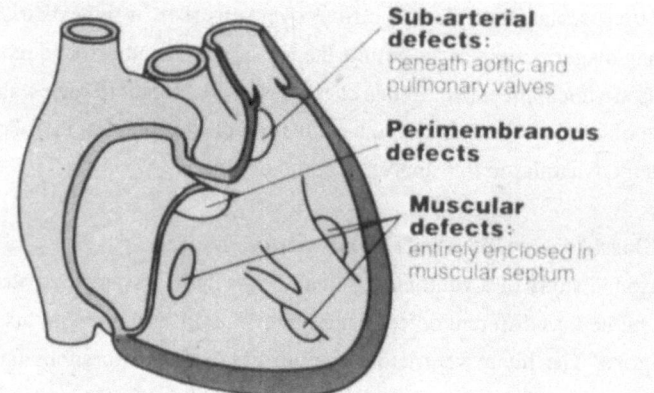

Fig. 9- 1. *Classification of Ventricular Septal Defects: A diagrammatic representation of the three main types of ventricular septal defects. a) Perimembranous defects are always roofed in part by the central fibrous body. They can be subclassified into perimembranous inlet, trabecular, outlet or confluent perimembranous defects depending on their extension into the adjacent muscular septum.b) Muscular defects have a complete rim of muscle tissue, and are divided into muscular inlet, trabecular and outlet defect depending on their location. c) Doubly committed subarterial defects are directly beneath both outflow tracts and are roofed by the conjoint aortic and pulmonary valves. They may extend posteriorly and inferiorly to involve the membranous septum.*

The Use of Cross-Sectional Imaging to Define Ventricular Septal Defect Morphology

With the resolution of currently used imaging systems, cross-sectional echocardiography permits visualization of the location, size and the structures forming the margins of the majority of moderate and large ventricular septal defects, thus allowing accurate classification of defect morphology. A complete scan of the ventricular septum requires the analysis of multiple intracardiac planes by the ultrasound beam. A standard scanning protocol should be adopted which includes apical and subcostal four-chamber plus aortic root views, parasternal long axis view, parasternal short axis view at the level of the ventricles and the great arteries, and a subcostal outflow tract view (the latter being the only view which consistently images the muscular outflow septum) (Figs.9-2,3). The aim of such a scanning technique should be to create as near a three-dimensional reconstruction of the heart as is possible. From the location of the defect in each of the imaging planes, the identification of the structures which form its margins and its extension into adjacent scanning planes, a composite picture of defect morphology can be obtained [2]. Small ventricular septal defects (<3mm diameter) are usually missed by cross-sectional imaging alone [3]. The majority of these small defects occur in the trabecular septum, and are restrictive. Similarly, multiple muscular defects ("Swiss cheese" ventricular septal defects) of the trabecular septum are also poorly identified by cross-sectional echocardiography, as they fail to create a complete ultrasound window across the septum.

Serial follow-up of unoperated defects by cross-sectional imaging has been used as a means of studying prospectively the natural history of isolated ventricular septal defects [4]. It is known from previous clinical and angiographic studies that a significant proportion of such defects either close spontaneously, or diminish in size with time [5,6]. Specific mechanisms and rates of closure have been shown to differ depending on defect type. A precise morphologic assessment by cross-sectional imaging therefore helps to distinguish between hemodynamically significant ventricular septal defects that are likely to close spontaneously and those that will almost certainly require surgical closure. The precise mechanisms of closure can also be assessed [4]. Imaging has demonstrated perimembranous inlet defects to close or reduce in size by the involvement of accessory tissue outgrowths from the septal leaflet of the tricuspid valve in the defect; perimembranous outlet defects may be partially closed by the prolapse of an aortic valve cusp into the defect. Trabecular defects have been shown to close spontaneously by direct muscle ingrowth. This muscle ingrowth usually commences on the right ventricular aspect of the defect and may be accelerated by the development of right ventricular outflow tract obstruction or banding of the pulmonary artery. Subarterial defects never close spontaneously but are associated with a significant incidence of aortic valve cusp prolapse, producing aortic regurgitation [7].

While cross-sectional imaging can define both the size and location of a septal defect, it does not predict the associated hemodynamics. Particularly in infants and young children and where surgical intervention is being contemplated, the cardiologist needs to know the degree of left to right shunting, the right ventricular and pulmonary artery systolic pressures, the pulmonary vascular resistance, the nature and severity of any associated outflow tract obstruction and the degree of any related semilunar valve incompetence. Doppler echocardiography can provide invaluable additional information to complement cross-sectional imaging in each of these respects. The role of each of the Doppler modalities in the assessment of ventricular septal defects will now be considered in turn.

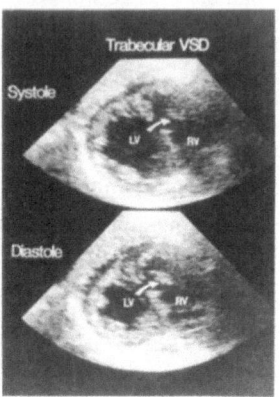

Fig. 9-2. Cross-sectional echocardiogram: Parasternal short axis view at the level of the ventricles showing a trabecular ventricular septal defect. The dropout in the interventricular septum persists through all phases of the cardiac cycle. Abbreviations: LV=left ventricle; RV=right ventricle.

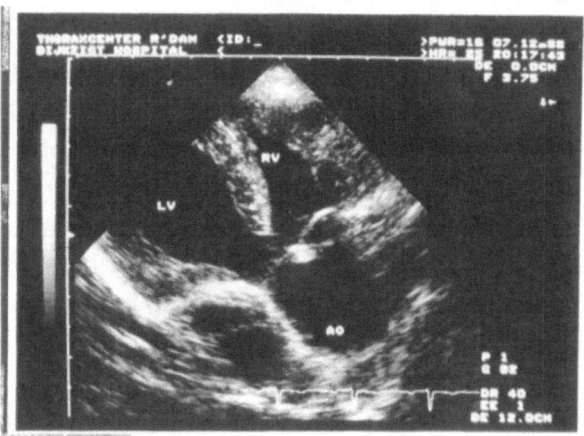

Fig. 9-3. Cross-sectional echocardiogram: Parasternal long axis view from a patient with tetralogy of Fallot, demonstrating the outlet ventricular septal defect with the aortic valve overriding the defect. Abbreviations: LV=left ventricle; RV=right ventricle; AO=aorta.

Pulsed Doppler Echocardiography

Pulsed wave Doppler has been shown to be an extremely sensitive, and specific technique for the identification of either the high velocity trans-septal jet or the associated right ventricular intracavitary turbulence associated with an isolated restrictive ventricular septal defect [8]. It should be used in conjunction with cross-sectional imaging to allow accurate positioning of the interrogating sample volume. A restrictive ventricular septal defect is detected using pulsed Doppler by identifying a characteristic widespread "aliased" pan-systolic flow disturbance within the septum or body of the right ventricle. A sequential pulsed Doppler "mapping technique" can be used to attempt to localize both origin of the turbulent jet from the right ventricular aspect of the septum and the region of trans-septal flow within the cross-sectional image.

While a "blind" pulsed Doppler examination may consistently detect a diagnostic flow disturbance within either the inlet or apical portions of the right ventricle, in our experience it rarely defines the septal exit point of many defects. Furthermore, problems exist if there is associated mid-ventricular or (more commonly) right ventricular outflow tract obstruction, as both these entitles produce indentical "aliased" systolic flow disturbances within the right ventricle. With this combination it may be impossible to determine if there is a coexisting outlet ventricular septal defect on the basis of the pulsed Doppler examination due to limitations of the technique in distinguishing between two abnormal turbulent flows within the one cardiac chamber. Similarly, pulsed Doppler is also of limited value in detecting multiple ventricular septal defects even in the presence of restrictive hemodynamics; spatial separation of the individual systolic turbulent jets within the body of the right ventricle is not normally possible as the regions of disturbed flow normally coalesce with each other. Problems also arise with pulsed Doppler in the situation where a large defect (associated with non-restrictive hemodynamics) has been missed on cross-sectional imaging. In such defects where left and right ventricular peak systolic pressures are equal, there is no turbulent flow within the right ventricle. However, when such defects are visualized, placement of the pulsed Doppler sample within the defect will define multiphasic to and fro low velocity laminar flow across the septal defect.

Several patterns of trans-septal flow may be detected across such non-restrictive defects; the specific pattern for a given ventricular septal defect depends on ventricular function, any associated conducting tissue abnormality, and the relative systemic and pulmonary vascular resistance. With low pulmonary vascular resistance (PVR) and in the absence of right ventricular outflow tract (RVOT) obstruction, left to right shunting across such defects starts in early systole. The left to right flow persists unchanged in direction throughout systole and normally extends with a low velocity through most of diastole, only stopping for a short period at end diastole. However, with increasing pulmonary vascular resistance (but with pulmonary vascular resistance less than or equal to systemic resistance), multiphasic low velocity trans-septal flow will be seen to occur within the defect in systole. The initial direction of flow is from left to right, particularly if there is coexisting right bundle branch block. Later in systole, flow reversal is evident from the change in the direction of flow across the defect, and oscillation of the trans-septal flow pattern may occur several times during systole. When the pulmonary vascular resistance becomes greater than the systemic resistance (Eisenmenger reaction), the major component of flow across the defect will be from right to left. These complex patterns of trans-septal flow are best discerned using either pulsed Doppler or the velocity time mode of the colour flow map.

It should be remembered that in restrictive defects the apparent area of turbulence within the right ventricular cavity is indicative not of the size of a ventricular septal defect, but rather of the pressure difference between the two ventricles in systole. With large non-restrictive defects (i.e. equal systolic pressures in the ventricles), it is impossible to identify the presence of a ventricular septal defect using PW Doppler examination alone as right ventricular turbulence is absent. Such defects however are usually readily imaged by cross-sectional imaging. When the ventricular septal defect is associated with a large left to right shunt, higher than normal peak systolic flow velocities and turbulent flow may also be recorded in the right ventricular outflow tract and pulmonary artery, and across the mitral valve, reflecting the increased flow across these structures.

Pulsed wave Doppler is normally a sensitive means of detecting both "physiologic" and pathologic tricuspid valve regurgitation (TR) over the whole spectrum of the population. "Physiologic" tricuspid regurgitation is a common finding in normal individuals in the pediatric age group. Coexisting tricuspid regurgitation is similarly present in the majority of patients with ventricular septal defects. A search of the floor of the right atrium around the point of tricuspid leaflet coaptation will normally identify a pansystolic aliased flow disturbance indicative of a high velocity jet entering the right atrium through the tricuspid valve in patients with non-restrictive defects and raised RV pressure. This will in the majority of cases be due to the tricuspid regurgitation. However, with some inlet VSDs, the detection of the jet of TR may be complicated by the presence of a left to right atrium shunt whereby the VSD jet is directed through a cleft in the septal leaflet of the tricuspid valve into the right atrium rather than into the right ventricle. Pulsed Doppler cannot distinguish between TR and a left ventricle to right atrium shunt. Pulsed Doppler is also limited in its ability to record peak velocities of regurgitation, particularly with non-restrictive defects and raised right ventricular pressures, where the peak velocity of TR will be high. High pulse repetition frequency (prf) Doppler is the technique to use in this situation, as it avoids the problem of frequency aliasing, and higher velocities of flow can consequently be accurately recorded. Another advantage of the use of high prf Doppler to identify and record the TR waveform in restrictive VSDs is that it is not affected by the anterior widespread flow disturbance in the right ventricle caused by the VSD jet. This contrasts markedly with continuous wave Doppler, with which the TR waveform is virtually impossible to record as the widespread anterior turbulence of the VSD jet will be superimposed on and thus mask the TR waveform. In our experience, an interpretable TR velocity envelope is only recordable in some 12% of restrictive ventricular septal defects, even with high prf Doppler.

Volume Flow Considerations

In theory it is possible using PW Doppler to calculate the ratio of pulmonary to systemic blood flow (QP:QS), and thus evaluate the degree of left to right shunting [9,10]. To determine the relative volumes of pulmonary and systemic flow, the maximum systolic diameters of the pulmonary artery and the left ventricular outflow tract are measured from the appropriate cross-sectional images. The respective cross-sectional areas are then calculated. From the systolic velocity profiles in these vessels (obtained by appropriate placement of the PW Doppler sample volume) the velocity time integrals (VTI) of both pulmonary artery and left ventricular outflow tract flow are derived. The stroke volume is then the product of the respective cross-sectional area and the VTI of flow at each sampling site. However, such measurements are beset with inherent methodological problems as discussed below. These are particularly relevant in the presence of large left to right shunts. Firstly, in young children where high pulmonary blood flow and pulmonary hypertension coexist, the pulmonary artery diameter frequently varies widely through the cardiac cycle [11]. Thus, the maximal systolic diameter which is normally used in the calculation of the cross-sectional area is an approximation. Second, with high velocity turbulent flow, spectral dispersion of the velocity wave-form normally occurs, introducing major errors in the measurement of the VTI of flow. Similar errors also result in the presence of right ventricular outflow obstruction, due to turbulent flow in the pulmonary artery. The existence of pulmonary or aortic valve incompetence also creates major problems with such calculations.

Calculating the volume of flow across the mitral valve in diastole (from the measured maximum diameter of the valve orifice in diastole, and deriving the VTI for diastolic flow across it) has been suggested as an alternative method of measuring pulmonary blood flow, provided there is neither associated mitral regurgitation nor a shunt at atrial or duct level [12]. Corrections have to be made however for phasic variations in diastolic mitral valve diameter. Despite many practical difficulties, it has been shown that this method (using mitral valve VTI) can consistently distinguish large shunts from small ones (QP:QS<2:1)[13].

In summary, standard PW Doppler is a sensitive technique for detecting small restrictive ventricular septal defects. It can aid in identifying defects in unusual locations (for example apical trabecular defects). It also can provide valuable estimations of the systemic to pulmonary flow ratios. However, due to the inherent problem of frequency aliasing it is of virtually no value in measuring the peak jet velocities associated with restrictive ventricular septal defects, or of high velocity tricuspid regurgitant jets occurring with non-restrictive defects and pulmonary hypertension. It is of limited value in determining the site of a ventricular septal defect. High prf Doppler is of greater value in the study of ventricular septal defects. It can both determine higher peak jet velocities and record the complete TR velocity waveform. Despite the use of both pulsed Doppler modalities, less than optimal information may be obtained. A complete pulsed Doppler scan of the right ventricle requires skill and is time consuming. It fails to distinguish between single and multiple ventricular septal defects. It cannot distinguish an outlet ventricular septal defect from right ventricular outflow tract obstruction, without concomitant imaging. Though it can confirm multiphasic low velocity flow or right to left shunting in non-restrictive defects, peak jet velocity of tricuspid regurgitation (and therefore the right ventricular systolic pressure) can only be measured by high prf Doppler. Major problems also exist with volume calculations in small children.

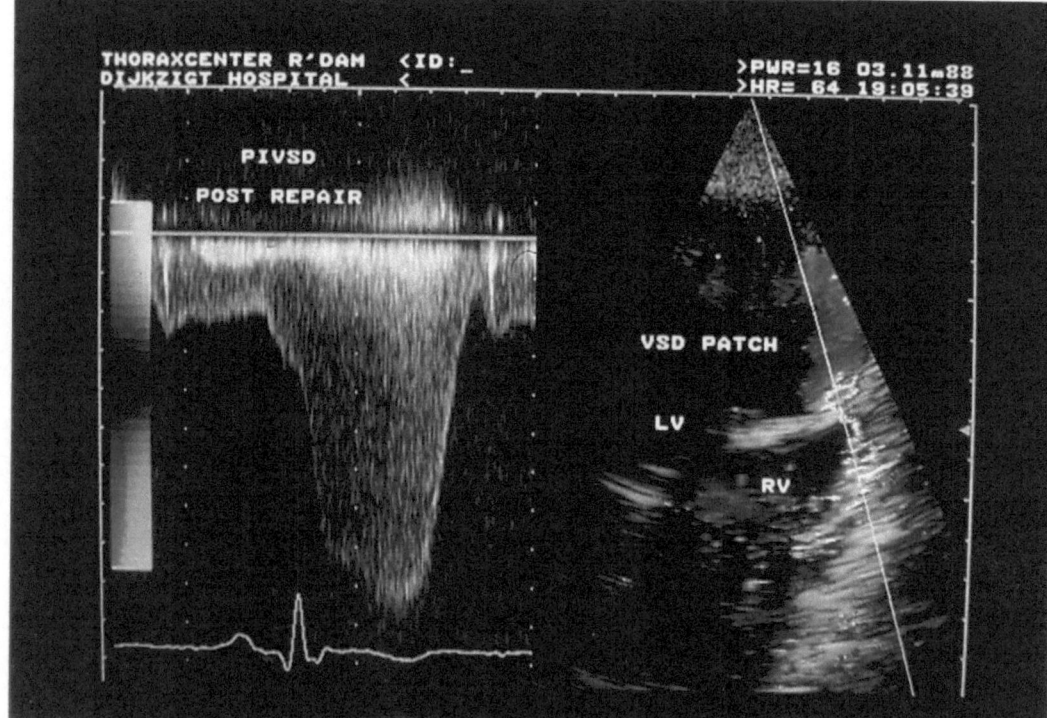

Fig. 9- 4. Continuous wave Doppler (CW) and color flow mapping from a patient who had patch closure of a perimembranous ventricular septal defect. There is a restrictive residual interventricular communication in the region of the trabecular septum. The VSD jet is therefore directed away from the transducer. The CW recording also shows low velocity interventricular shunting in diastole. LV=left ventricle; RV=right ventricle.

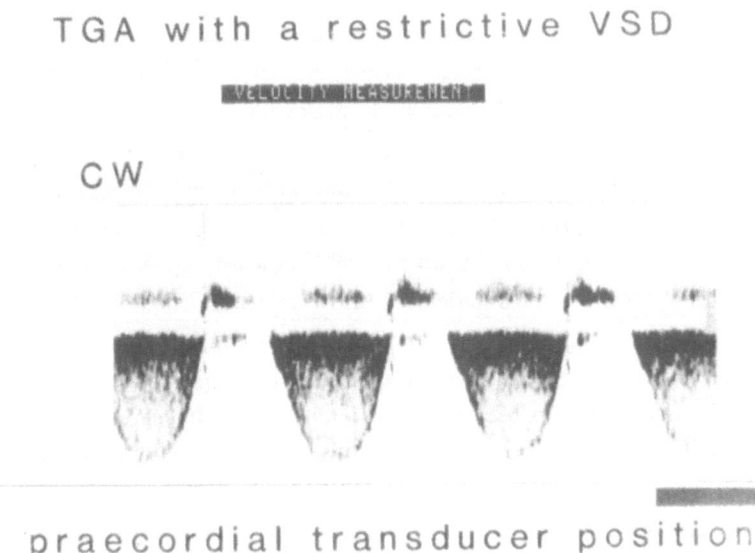

Fig. 9- 5. Continuous wave Doppler velocity profile from a VSD in a patient with transposition of the great arteries. The VSD jet is directed away from the transducer, as the left ventricle is the low-pressure ventricle. The high velocity of the jet also suggests that the VSD is restrictive.

Continuous Wave Doppler

In the investigation of a ventricular septal defect, continuous wave Doppler assessment can be performed either as a stand alone technique or in the duplex mode with concomitant imaging. As with pulsed Doppler, the value of CW Doppler will vary depending on whether the defect is restrictive or non-restrictive.

Parasternal and subcostal transducer positions should be used to detect the characteristic high velocity trans-septal jet associated with restrictive ventricular septal defects. Using a combination of the audio signal and the spectral display, and by varying the transducer position and angle, a near-optimal ventricular septal defect wave-form can be obtained. The peak systolic velocity of flow across the defect can then be calculated. The typical flow profile derived from a restrictive defect is one of high velocity in systole (i.e.>3m/sec), with an early to mid systolic peak and low velocity flow (i.e.<1.5m/sec) continuing into early and mid-diastole in virtually every case. This diastolic flow only stops very late in diastole. Thus flow is virtually continuous across the defect in both systole and diastole. The normal direction of the ventricular septal defect jet is anterior (towards a transducer placed on the praecordium). Exceptions to this rule are the jets associated with apical trabecular defects, and those of restrictive ventricular septal defects coexisting with transposition of the great arteries (Fig. 9-4,5). In both these cases the ventricular septal defect jet is directed away from the transducer - medially in the case of an apical trabecular defect interrogated from an apico-lateral transducer position and posteriorly in transposition of the great arteries where the left ventricle is the low pressure ventricle. When the full spectral waveform of the high velocity systolic component has been obtained, the instantaneous pressure drop across the ventricular septal defect can be calculated from the peak velocity of flow using the modified Bernoulli equation (Fig. 9-6). From a knowledge of the systolic arterial blood pressure, and with the exclusion of aortic valve or left ventricular outflow tract obstruction by imaging and Doppler studies, the right ventricular systolic pressure can be calculated. The right ventricular systolic pressure is the difference between the systolic arterial pressure (which is presumed to be the peak left ventricular systolic pressure as left ventricular outflow tract obstruction has been excluded) and the calculated pressure drop across the ventricular septal defect. Estimates of the right ventricular systolic pressure using the derived peak instantaneous trans-septal gradient obtained from CW Doppler examination have been found to correlate well with cardiac catheterization measurements of peak interventricular gradients in a very large number of correlative series[14] (Fig. 9-7).

As stated previously, "physiologic" or pathologic tricuspid regurgitation commonly coexists with ventricular septal defects. In theory CW Doppler can be used to measure the peak velocity of regurgitant flow (Fig. 9-8). The calculated peak systolic pressure drop across the tricuspid valve plus the mean venous pressure will derive the right ventricular systolic pressure. This has been validated in many series by simultaneous right ventricular pressure measurement at cardiac catheterization [15]. In practice, restrictive ventricular septal defects are associated with a widespread pansystolic flow disturbance within the body of the right ventricle. The turbulence associated with the VSD jet will therefore be superimposed on any tricuspid regurgitation waveforms that may be recorded. It is therefore impossible to record the complete TR waveform (see pulsed Doppler section).

Non-restrictive ventricular septal defects are associated with a raised pulmonary artery pressure, and hence a raised right ventricular systolic pressure. This results in low velocity trans-septal flow profiles in systole. Under these conditions it is possible to record the entire velocity profile of tricuspid regurgitation. However, in our experience only some 70% of patients with non-restrictive ventricular septal defects have recordable tricuspid regurgitation using the CW technique. (This finding correlates well with the color flow mapping information in the presence of TR in the same patient group). When low velocity trans-septal flow is detected, it may not be possible to decide whether the low velocity is due to poor alignment with flow, or to pulmonary hypertension. An independent noninvasive technique for confirming the right ventricular systolic pressure is therefore required. The detection of tricuspid regurgitation (when present), and measurement of peak velocity of the regurgitant jets makes it possible to assess right ventricular systolic pressure accurately. Where good correlation between the two methods of deriving RV peak systolic pressure is not acquired, then this should be confirmed by cardiac catheterization where clinically indicated.

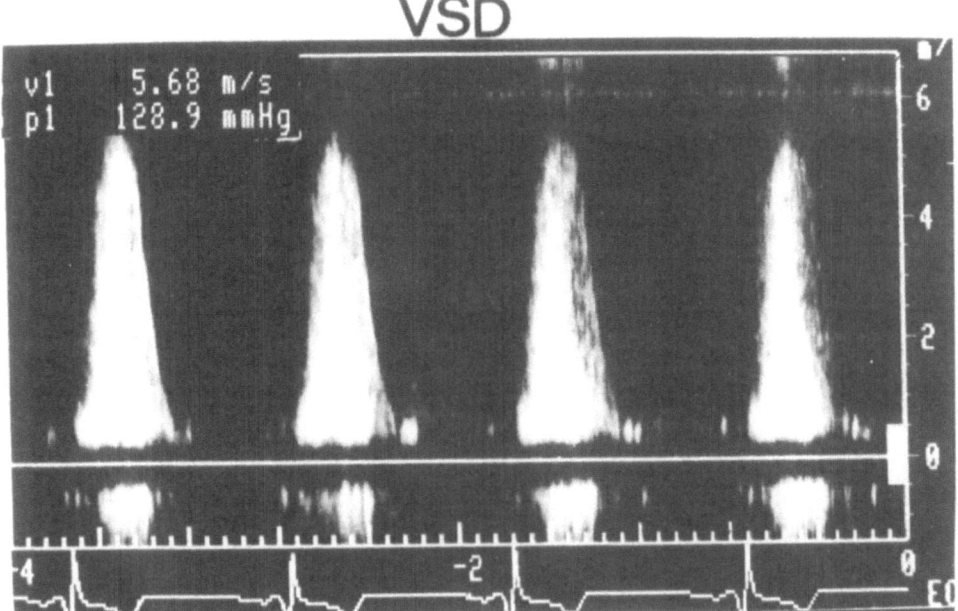

Fig. 9-6. *Continuous wave Doppler velocity profile from a restrictive VSD. The high peak velocity of flow in systole confirms the restrictive nature of the defect. The calculated pressure drop across the defect is over 120 mm.Hg. From a knowledge of the systolic arterial pressure, the right ventricular systolic pressure can easily be calculated.*

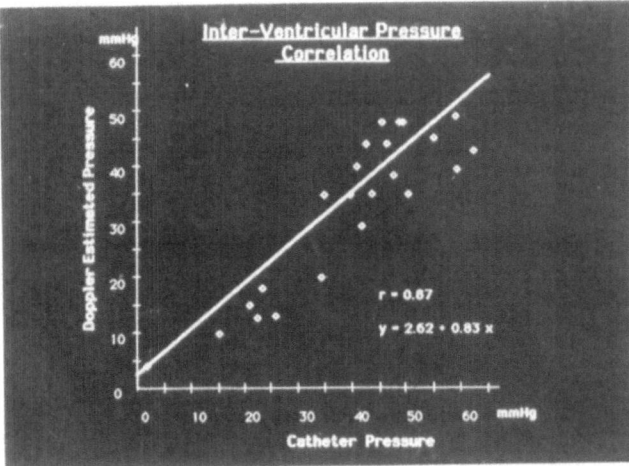

Fig. 9-7. *A graph showing the relation between the right ventricular systolic pressure measured at cardiac catheterization and that estimated from the peak velocities of the VSD jet using continuous wave Doppler, in a group of patients with VSD who underwent cardiac catheterization at our institution. There was excellent correlation between the two methods.*

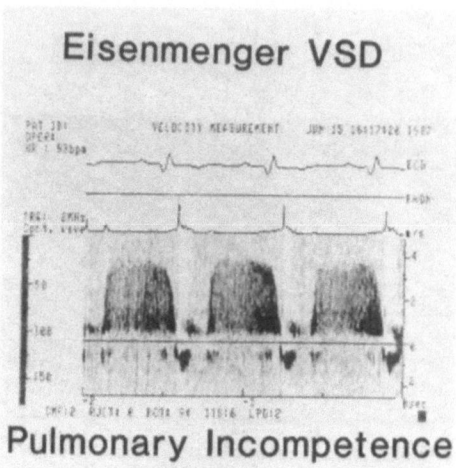

Fig. 9-8. Continuous wave Doppler recording of tricuspid regurgitation on a patient with ventricular septal defect. The regurgitant jet is directed away from the transducer (into the right atrium). The peak velocity of the jet is over 4m/sec. This confirms that the right ventricular systolic pressure (and, therefore the pulmonary artery systolic pressure) is very high.

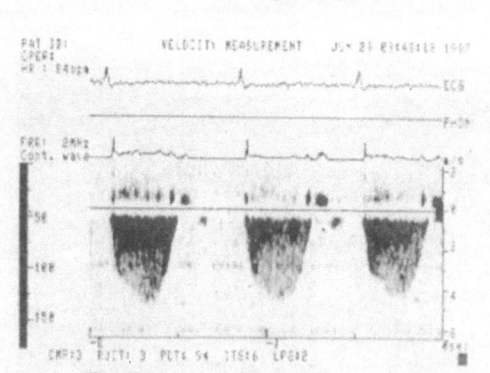

Fig. 9-9. Continuous wave Doppler recording of pulmonary regurgitation in a patient with a ventricular septal defect: The regurgitant jet is directed towards the transducer, and is of very high velocity (approximately 4m/sec). This confirms a very high pulmonary artery diastolic pressure. The high velocity of regurgitation is sustained throughout diastole, and this is characteristic of pulmonary vascular disease.

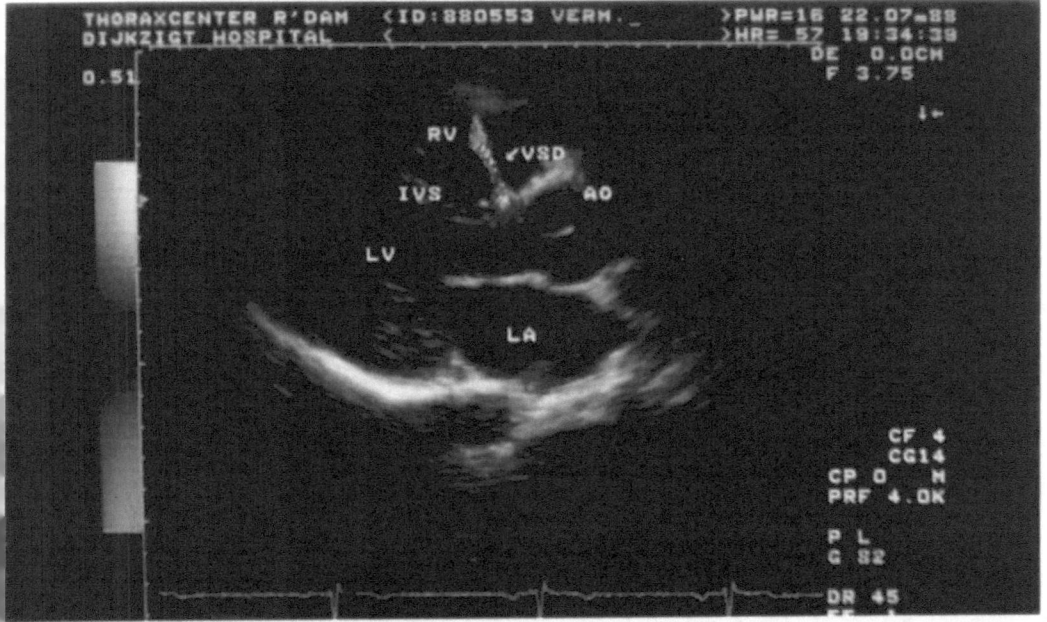

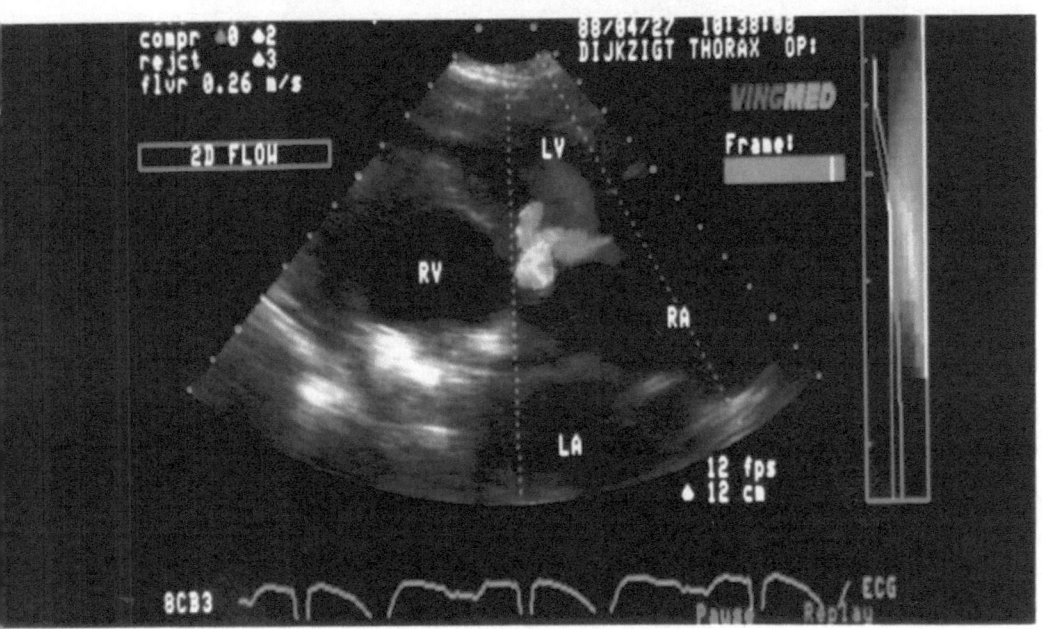

Fig. 9-10. Doppler Color Flow Mapping (CFM) of a restrictive perimembranous outlet VSD in the parasternal long axis view. There is high velocity turbulent flow. LA=left atrium; LV=left ventricle; IVS=interventricular septum; RV=right ventricular; AO=aorta.

Fig. 9-11. Doppler CFM: Parasternal four-chamber view showing the VSD jet going in three different directions. This may happen when there are muscle bundles traversing the defect. This picture is from a patient with congenitally corrected transposition of the great arteries (atrio-ventricular discordance). LA=left atrium; RA=right atrium; LV=left atrium; RV=right ventricle.

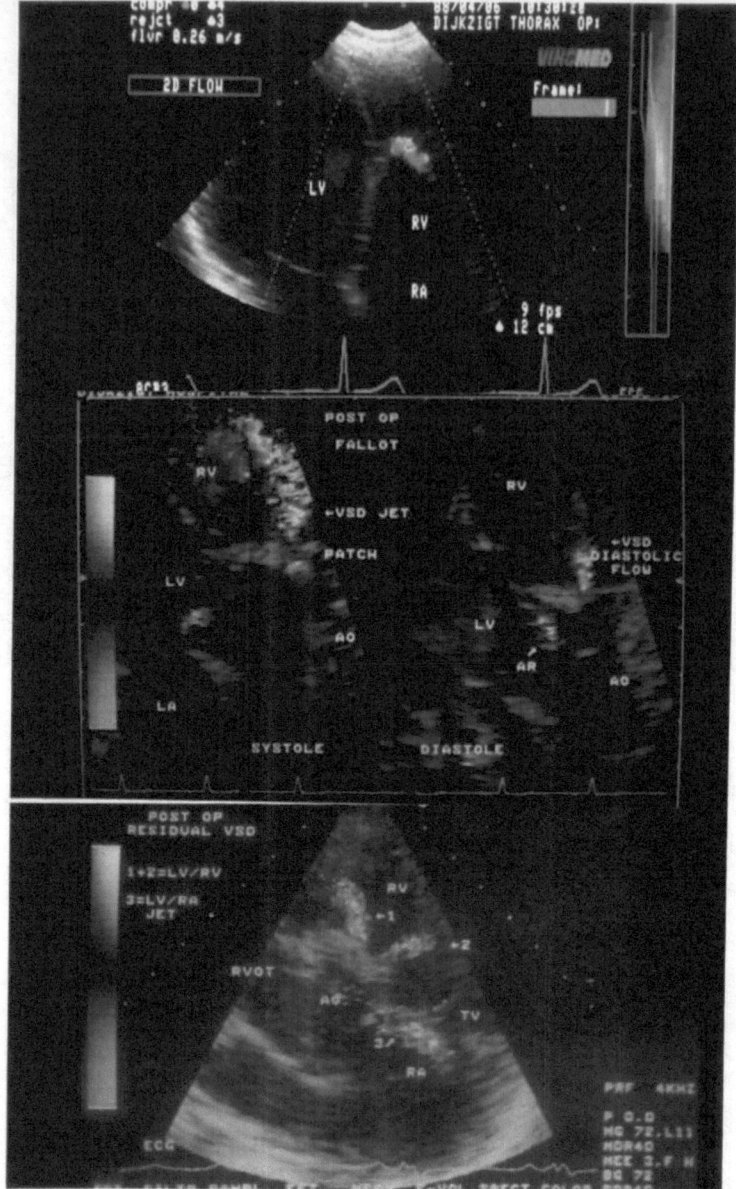

Fig. 9-12. Doppler CFM: Parasternal four-chamber view of a trabecular ventricular septal defect, which clearly demonstrates that the VSD jet is direct medially.

Fig. 9-13. Doppler CFM showing a residual peri-patch VSD following correction of tetralogy of Fallot. CFM confirms left to right shunting in both systole and diastole. Diastolic shunting is characterized by low velocity laminar flow. The diastolic frame also shows mild aortic valve regurgitation. LA=left atrium; LV=left ventricle; RV=right ventricle; AO=aorta; AR=aortic regurgitation.

Fig. 9-14. Post-operative residual VSD, following attempted closure of a perimembranous defect. Doppler CFM shows three discrete peri-patch jets, two of them directed into the right ventricle, and the third from the left ventricle to the right atrium. RA=right atrium; RV=right ventricle; TV=tricuspid valve; RVOT=right ventricular outflow tract; AO=aorta.

The ability to calculate peak right ventricular pressure with reasonable accuracy has important implications for patient management. The majority of defects fall into one of two groups [16]: - A) those with high peak velocities of flow in systole, e.g.>4m/sec. These are restrictive defects, and the instantaneous gradient derived by CW Doppler has been shown to correlate well with the pulmonary and systemic resistance ratios (Rp:Rs) measured at catheterization [17] B) defects with a low peak velocity of systolic flow e.g. <2.5m/sec associated with a high velocity tricuspid regurgitation jet. In the absence of pulmonary valve stenosis or right ventricular outflow tract obstruction, this is indicative of pulmonary hypertension. Further invasive investigation and surgical closure may therefore be required.

Some ventricular septal defects fall into an intermediate category in terms of the peak systolic velocities of flow across the defect. The peak velocity of tricuspid regurgitation (where detected and accurately recorded) will frequently provide an estimate of pulmonary artery systolic pressure in such cases. CW Doppler information may also be misleading with perimembranuous inlet defects. This is due to the occasional association of a left ventricle to right atrium shunt with such defects. Such a shunt is always of high velocity, and can be mistaken for tricuspid regurgitation. Doppler Color Flow Mapping is of value in indentifying these complex flow disturbances and can even simultaneously demonstrate both TR and LV to RA shunt within the right atrium. Subsequent alignment of a steerable CW beam to each flow disturbance in turn will allow the respective velocity waveforms to be recorded.

Additional causes of high velocity turbulent systolic flow into the right ventricle need to be distinguished from a ventricular septal defect. One such lesion is an aorta to right ventricle fistula through the sinus of Valsalva. In this situation, continuous flow occurs through the defect with a high velocity jet into the RV persisting throughout the cardiac cycle, owing to the continuing high pressure difference between aorta and right ventricle. This contrasts markedly with interventricular shunting where diastolic flow is of low velocity.

The presence of right ventricular outflow tract pressure gradient (whether due to a true morphologic obstruction or to a flow gradient due to intracardiac shunting) needs to be taken into account when attempting to derive the pulmonary artery peak systolic pressure from the peak velocity of the ventricular septal defect jet. CW Doppler when used in conjunction with cross-sectional imaging can accurately record peak velocities of systolic flow in the right ventricular outflow tract. The direction of the recorded velocity of flow in the outflow tract (away from the transducer) will distinguish it from the jet associated with the ventricular septal defect. Large shunts are also associated with an increased velocity of flow in the pulmonary artery. In such cases, by using PW Doppler, turbulent high velocity flow be shown to originate in the right ventricle itself, with no localized increase of flow velocity in the outflow tract.

In the presence of pulmonary hypertension, pulmonary regurgitation is virtually always present. This can be identified using PW Doppler from the parasternal short-axis view, with the sample volume in the RVOT below the pulmonary valve, as diastolic flow towards the transducer. From the peak velocity of regurgitation derived by CW Doppler, the pulmonary artery early diastolic pressure can be estimated. The velocity profile of the pulmonary regurgitation jet also can give some indication of the mean pulmonary artery pressure [18]. The presence of a sustained high velocity regurgitant jet throughout diastole indicates a raised mean PA pressure and raised pulmonary vascular resistance (Fig. 9-9).

Continuous wave Doppler therefore allows the estimation of pulmonary artery systolic pressure in the majority of restrictive ventricular septal defects, from the derived interventricular pressure gradient. With non-restrictive defects, the peak velocity of tricuspid regurgitation (where recorded) will provide correlative information. Serial estimates of both peak pulmonary artery systolic pressure and the pulmonary regurgitation waveform can therefore provide valuable information for the long-term follow-up of restrictive ventricular septal defects.

Doppler Color Flow Mapping

The use of color flow mapping (CFM) has considerably enhanced the ability to noninvasively diagnose ventricular septal defects. A standard technique whose aim is to produce a three dimensional reconstruction of the heart (as described in the section on the cross-sectional echocardiographic evaluation of ventricular septal defects) should be utilized to scan all components of the ventricular septum and obtain the CFM information. Restrictive ventricular septal defects are characterized by aliased high velocity trans-septal turbulent jets exiting from the septum into the right ventricle in systole (Fig. 9-10). The entry point on the left ventricular aspect of the septum (with its area of accelerating flow into the defect - the "Venturi effect" normally well seen on the color flow map), the septal exit point into the right ventricle and the subsequent direction of the jet are easily defined (Fig. 9-11). The jets associated with apical trabecular defects or with transposition of the great arteries (where the right ventricle is the systemic ventricle) will be directed away from the transducer, in the apical or parasternal four-chamber views (Fig. 9-12). Flow is not restricted to systole in such defects; diastolic flow also exists through the majority of restrictive defects. This diastolic component is of low velocity and the flow laminar (Fig. 9-13). Even when it is not possible to directly visualize trans-septal flow e.g.with small apical trabecular ventricular septal defects that may take a tortuous course through the septum, the presence of a defect can be inferred from the occurrence of turbulence at its exit point on the right ventricular aspect of the septum, as seen in the color flow map. CFM is a very sensitive technique for the diagnosis of isolated restrictive ventricular septal defects - being in our experience more sensitive than either PW or CW Doppler.

Non-restrictive ventricular septal defects, with equal peak systolic pressures in the two ventricles, are characterized by low velocity laminar flow across the defect. With large left to right shunts, some degree of systolic flow acceleration (normally with laminar flow persisting) may occur, as indicated by the appropriate change in the color map [19]. With the majority of non-restrictive defects however, bi-directional shunting will be evident, with the predominant direction of shunting depending on the relative systemic and pulmonary vascular resistance.

CFM may be a useful method for assessing the natural history of a ventricular septal defect [19]. An estimate of the defect size may be made on the largest color flow diameter measured at the exit point of the defect. Such measurements have been found to correlate well with angiographic measurements of defect diameter [19]. Serial assessment of defect size is therefore possible. With perimembranous defects, decreases in defect size by tricuspid pseudoaneurysm formation may be documented. Spontaneous closure of trabecular defects may also be determined by serial CFM studies. Estimates of absolute defect size, or defect diameter/aortic root diameter ratios have also been found to correlate well with cardiac catheterization derived Qp/Qs ratios [19].

It is in the detection of multiple ventricular septal defects however, that CFM has proved to be particularly useful [20,21]. Pulsed Doppler is limited in its ability to detect multiple restrictive ventricular septal defects, as the systolic turbulence within the right ventricle arising from one ventricular septal defect cannot usually be distinguished from that caused by an adjacent defect. In a recently reported series of patients with multiple ventricular septal defects, occurring both as isolated lesions and in the setting of complex cardiac defects, CFM accurately identified the multiple defects in 24/31 (77%) of patients, compared with 20/31 (65%) by left ventricular angiography [21]. The ability of CFM to detect multiple defects depends on whether they are restrictive or non-restrictive. CFM is a very sensitive technique for detecting multiple restrictive ventricular septal defects, as it is usually easy to recognize the mosaic pattern of turbulent trans-septal flow associated with individual defects, provided there is adequate spatial separation between the defects (>0.5cm. between adjacent defect) (Fig. 9-14). Thus in the series of Sutherland et al CFM correctly identified multiple restrictive ventricular septal defects in 16/18 (89%) patients compared with 15/18 patients by angiography [20].

Color flow imaging is less useful in identifying multiple ventricular septal defects in the presence of non-restrictive hemodynamics. With a large, low resistance interventricular communication and rapid equalization of ventricular pressures in systole, the volume of flow through additional smaller defects is probably very limited so that they cannot be separately identified. In addition, it is more difficult to recognize the laminar flow patterns through small defects in the presence of non-restrictive hemodynamics (as opposed to the turbulent mosaic pattern seen with restrictive defects [20,22]. Color M-mode scanning (M/Q mode) may be of value in these cases, as it allows a higher sampling rate than color flow imaging alone. Color M-mode scanning of the ventricular septum may be performed at multiple levels, to detect the systolic flow acceleration at the right ventricular exit point of the defect, even in the absence of turbulent flow. In practice, even with the addition of color M-mode scanning CFM accurately diagnosed multiple non-restrictive defects in only 8/13 (62%) patients in the series of Sutherland et al [20]. With such defects, similar limitations also apply to left ventricular angiography as a diagnostic technique. A combination of the two investigative techniques considerably increased the diagnostic accuracy for multiple non-restrictive ventricular septal defects.

The ability to detect even restrictive ventricular septal defects is limited in the presence of concomitant morphologic right ventricular outflow tract obstruction, as the increased right ventricular peak systolic pressure will result in low velocity laminar flow across the ventricular septal defect. Additionally, certain areas of the septum are difficult to image - e.g. the muscular outflow septum, and it is likely that multiple defects occurring in this area will be missed [20].

CFM is also a sensitive method for detecting tricuspid regurgitation. Visualization of the direction of the TR jet within the right atrium enables accurate alignment and measurement of its peak velocity with CW Doppler. The peak RV systolic pressure can thus be accurately estimated. Left ventricle to right atrium shunts that may coexist with perimembranous inlet defects can also be clearly distinguished from tricuspid regurgitation.

CFM has also been used to obtain semi-quantitative estimates of shunt size with restrictive ventricular septal defects. The maximum area of the right ventricle occupied by turbulent systolic jet has been shown to correlate reasonably well with QP:QS ratios calculated at cardiac catherization [23]. Such calculations however do not take into account the existence of diastolic left to right shunting that is a feature of some defects.

Intraoperative Color Flow Mapping

Intraoperative Doppler CFM has been utilized to detect the presence of residual interventricular shunting after patch closure of a ventricular septal defect. Hemodynamically significant residual defects have been shown to exist in a significant proportion of patients undergoing surgery for ventricular septal defect closure [24]. These may be additional ventricular septal defects that were missed preoperatively (see section for color flow mapping in multiple ventricular septal defects), true residual defects at the original site, or due to patch dehiscence. Cross-sectional epicardial imaging alone is usually unsatisfactory in this setting, as the patch material may be echo-dense, and produces masking of the image behind it in the plane of scanning. Color flow mapping of the entire ventricular septum provides valuable information about residual shunts. Left to right shunting of minor degree occurring in early systole along the suture lines of the patch is a common finding using CFM, and in the majority of cases, tends to disappear within a few days after surgery [25]. Such peri-patch jets are usually of low velocity, and do not extend far into the right ventricular cavity. Minor degrees of systolic turbulence within the right ventricle on the CFM may be due to the patch itself, and this is also of no consequence. Semi-quantitative estimates of the degree of any residual shunting may be made, based on the extension of the turbulent ventricular septal defect jet into the cavity of the right ventricle.

Major limitations to this technique exist, particularly with equal peak systolic pressures in the ventricles. In this situation the low velocity laminar flow across the defect may be difficult to recognize. The presence of residual right ventricular outflow tract obstruction imposes similar restrictions in detecting residual ventricular septal defects based on the pattern of flow across the defect. Contrast echocardiography (using agitated blood) may be useful in some cases; the appearance of contrast within the right ventricular cavity following injection into the left atrial line is indicative of a residual shunt. The technique may also provide an estimate of the degree of shunting based on the contrast density within the right ventricle. It provides however only limited information about the exact location of the defect . A combination of CFM and contrast echocardiography may improve the diagnostic accuracy of hemodynamically significant residual defects. Despite its limitations, intraoperative post bypass CFM is thus a useful technique for immediate assessment of the surgical repair, and the recognition of significant residual defects.

Post Operative Follow-up

Pulsed Doppler studies in the immediate post-operative period following ventricular septal defect closure have shown that flow disturbances around the patch associated with residual shunting is a common finding [26]. As discussed above, the experience with CFM has been similar, and peri-patch turbulent flow can usually be seen in the early post-operative period. In the majority of patients, these flow disturbances disappear, and shunting can no longer be detected within a few days or weeks of operation. Semi-quantitative estimates of the shunt size by pulsed Doppler (based on the width and extension of the flow disturbances into the right ventricle), with CFM (based on the area of the right ventricle occupied by the shunt jet), or actual calculation of QP:QS as described with PW Doppler all provide information on which management decisions can be made.

In summary, the reasons for invasive investigation of a ventricular septal defect are based on a need to know the size and location of a defect, the magnitude of the left to right shunt, the pulmonary artery pressure and pulmonary vascular resistance. Cross-sectional imaging when combined with Doppler echocardiography provides much of this information, and with experience, such a noninvasive assessment can now form the basis for clinical decisions in the majority of patients with isolated ventricular septal defects.

References

1) Soto B, Becker AE, Moulaert AJ, Andersen RH. Classification of ventricular septal defects. Br heart J. 1980; 43: 332-43.

2) Sutherland GR, Godman MJ, Smallhorn JF, Guiterras P, Anderson RH, Hunter S. Ventricular septal defects. Two dimensional echocardiographic and morphological correlations. Br Heart J. 1982; 47:316-28.

3) Cheatham JP, Latson LA, Gutgesell HP. Ventricular septal defect in infancy: detection with two-dimensional echocardiography. Am J Cardiol. 1981; 47:85-9.

4) Sutherland GR, Bain HH, Anderson RH, Hunter S. Natural history of ventricular septal defects - long term prospective two dimensional study (abstr). Br Heart J. 1983; 49:293-4.

5) Hoffman JIE. Natural history of congenital heart disease: Problems in its assessment with special reference to ventricular septal defects. Circulation 1968; 37:97-125.

6) Moe DG, Guntheroth WG. Spontaneous closure of uncomplicated ventricular septal defect. Am J Cardiol. 1987; 60:674-8.

7) Merrick SH, Verrier ED, Hanley FA, Turley KT, Ebert PA. Doubly - committed subarterial ventricular septal defect: an eleven-year experience. J Am Coll Cardiol 1989; 13: 74A (abstr).

8) Stevenson JG, Kawabori I, Dooley T, Guntheroth WG. Diagnosis of ventricular septal defect by pulsed Doppler echocardiography: specificity and limitations. Circulation 1978; 58: 322-6.

9) Vargas Barron J, Sahn DJ, Valdes-Cruz LM, Lima CO, Goldberg SJ, Grenadier E, Allen HD. Clinical utility of two-dimensional Doppler echocardiographic techniques for estimating pulmonary to systemic blood flow ratios in children with left to right shunting atrial septal defect, ventricular septal defect or patent ductus arteriosus. J Am Coll Cardiol. 1984; 3:169-78.

10) Stevenson JG, Kawabori I. Noninvasive determination of pulmonic to systemic flow ratio by pulsed Doppler echo. Circulation 1982; 66(suppl.II):232.

11) Greenfield JC, Griggs DM. The relation between pressure and diameter in main pulmonary artery of man. J Appl Physiol. 1963; 557-9.

12) Fisher DC, Sahn DJ, Friedman MJ, et al. The mitral orifice method for noninvasive two-dimensional echo Doppler determinations of cardiac output. Circulation 1983: 67:872-7.

13) Vargas Barron J, Sahn DJ, Valdes-Cruz LM, Lima CO, Grenadier E, Allen HD, Goldberg SJ. Quantification of the ratio of pulmonary: systemic blood flow (QP:QS) in patients with ventricular septal defect by two-dimensional range gated Doppler echocardiography. Circulation 1982: 66(suppl.II): 318.

14) Silbert DR, Brunson SC, Schiff R, Diamant S. Determination of right ventricular pressure in the presence of a ventricular septal defect using continuous wave Doppler ultrasound. J Am Coll Cardiol. 1986; 8:379-84.

15) Currie PJ, Seward JB, Chan KL, Fyfe DA, Hagler DJ, Mair DD, Reeder GS, Nishimura RA, Tajik AJ. Continuous wave Doppler determinations of right ventricular pressure: a simultaneous Doppler-catheterisation study in 127 patients. J Am Coll Cardiol. 1985; 6:750-6.

16) Houston AB, Lim MK, Doig WB, Reid JM, Coleman EN. Doppler assessment of the interventricular pressure drop in patients with ventricular septal defects . Br Heart J. 1988; 60:50-6.

17) Murphy DJ, Ludomirsky A, Huhta JC. Continuous wave Doppler in children with ventricular septal defect: noninvasive estimation of pressure gradient. Am J cardiol. 1986; 57:428-32.

18) Miyatake K, Okamoto M, Kinoshita N, Matsuhisa M, Nagata S, Beppu S, Park YD, Sakakibara H, Nimura Y. Pulmonary regurgitation studied with the ultrasonic pulsed Doppler technique. Circulation 1982; 65:969-76.

19) Hornberger LK, Sahn DJ, Krabill KA, Sherman FS, Swensson R, Pesonen E, Hagen-Ansert S, Chung KY. Elucidation of the natural history of ventricular septal defects by serial Doppler color flow mapping studies. J Am Coll Cardiol 1989; 13: 1111-8.

20) Sutherland GR, Smyllie JH, Ogilvie BC, Keeton BR. Colour flow imaging in the diagnosis of multiple ventricular septal defects. Br Heart J 1989. (in press).

21) Ludomirsky A, Huhta JC, Vick GW, Murphy DJ, Danford DA, Morrow WR. Color Doppler detection of multiple ventricular septal defects. Circulation 1986; 74:1317-22.

22) Chin A, Alboliras E, Barber G, Murphy J, Helton G, Pigott J, Norwood W. Does color Doppler echocardiography detect additional small muscular defects in infants with a large ventricular septal defect? J Am Coll Cardiol. 1989; 13:206A (abstr).

23) Harlamert E, Harrison M, Smith M, Booth D, Moffett C, Kwan OL, DeMaria A. Quantitative evaluation of ventricular septal defects by color Doppler flow imaging. J Am Coll Cardiol. 1989; 13:24A (abstr).

24) Yeager SB, Freed MD, Keane JF, Norwood WI, Castaneda AR. Primary closure of ventricular septal defects in the first year of life: results in 128 infants. J Am Coll Cardiol 1984; 3:1269-76.

25) Sutherland GR, Smyllie J, Roelandt J, van Daele M, Quaegebeur J. Colour flow imaging as intra-operative angiography in ventricular septal defects - advantages and pitfalls? J Am Coll Cardiol. 1989; 13:75A (abstr).

26) Stevenson JG, Kawabori I, Stamm SJ, Bailey WW, Hall DG, Mansfield PB, Rittenhouse EA. Pulsed Doppler echocardiographic evaluation of ventricular septal defect patches. Circulation 1984; 70(suppl I), I-38.

CHAPTER X

COMBINED CROSS-SECTIONAL IMAGING AND DOPPLER ECHOCARDIOGRAPHY IN ATRIOVENTRICULAR SEPTAL DEFECTS

George R. Sutherland

Naryswamy Sreeram

Morphological Considerations - What We Need to Know

Atrioventricular septal defects are characterized by loss of normal septal continuity between the atria and ventricles. The inherent absence of the atrioventricular septum (both the fibrous and muscular components) produces an atrioventricular junction sited at a common level, with associated deficiencies of the atrial and ventricular septa. In addition, all such lesions are characterized by a left ventricular outflow tract and aorta which are displaced from their normal wedged position between the right and left atrioventricular orifices in the normal heart [1].

The "unspringing" of the atrioventricular junction produces what is in effect a single ovoid atrioventricular orifice guarded by a five leaflet valve. This five leaflet valve arrangement is common to all forms of atrioventricular defects. Three of the leaflets are confined to one ventricle only- two to the right and one to the left ventricle. The remaining two leaflets cross the ventricular septum and have attachments to both ventricles. These are termed the anterior and posterior bridging leaflets. The area between the bridging leaflets has been referred to in the past as a "cleft" of the mitral valve, but the atrioventricular valve morphology in these defects cannot be compared with that of normal mitral and tricuspid valves.

When the two bridging leaflets are connected to each other, thereby forming two separate valve orifices, the defect is termed a partial one (Fig. 10-1). This definition does not take into account the presence or absence of an interventricular communication beneath either bridging leaflet. In a "complete" defect, the bridging leaflets are not joined to one another, resulting in a common atrioventricular valve orifice (Fig. 10-2) [2]. Further subclassification of complete defects is based on the extent to which the anterior bridging leaflet crosses the ventricular septum, and the variations in its commissural attachments to the septum or right ventricular wall [3].

Hemodynamic Considerations

Atrioventricular septal defects are commonly associated with complex shunting patterns at both atrial and ventricular level. Prolonged intracardiac shunting of severe degree, associated with pulmonary hypertension, can cause irreversible pulmonary vascular disease. There is some evidence that this sequence of events occurs sooner with complete atrioventricular septal defects that have a large ventricular component, than with isolated VSDs of similar size.

Right and left atrioventricular valve regurgitation occurs in the majority of atrioventricular defects, as well as an obligatory left ventricle to right atrium shunt through the area of the deficient atrioventricular septum.

Therefore, before any surgical intervention can be considered, the following hemodynamic factors need to be established: a) the degree and site(s) of left to right shunting; b) the severity of atrioventricular valve regurgitation, particularly of the left atrioventricular valve; c) the degree of obligatory left ventricle to right atrium shunting and d) an accurate estimate of the pulmonary artery pressure and vascular resistance. Commonly associated anomalies of systemic or pulmonary venous drainage, or coexistent outflow tract obstructions or semilunar valve stenoses should be identified. Finally, it is important to be able to assess the amount of atrioventricular valve cusp tissue available for surgical reconstruction of competent, non stenotic right and left atrioventricular valves. Until recently, only some of this morphologic and hemodynamic information was available from cardiac catheterization, but it is now readily available from the combined use of different ultrasound modalities.

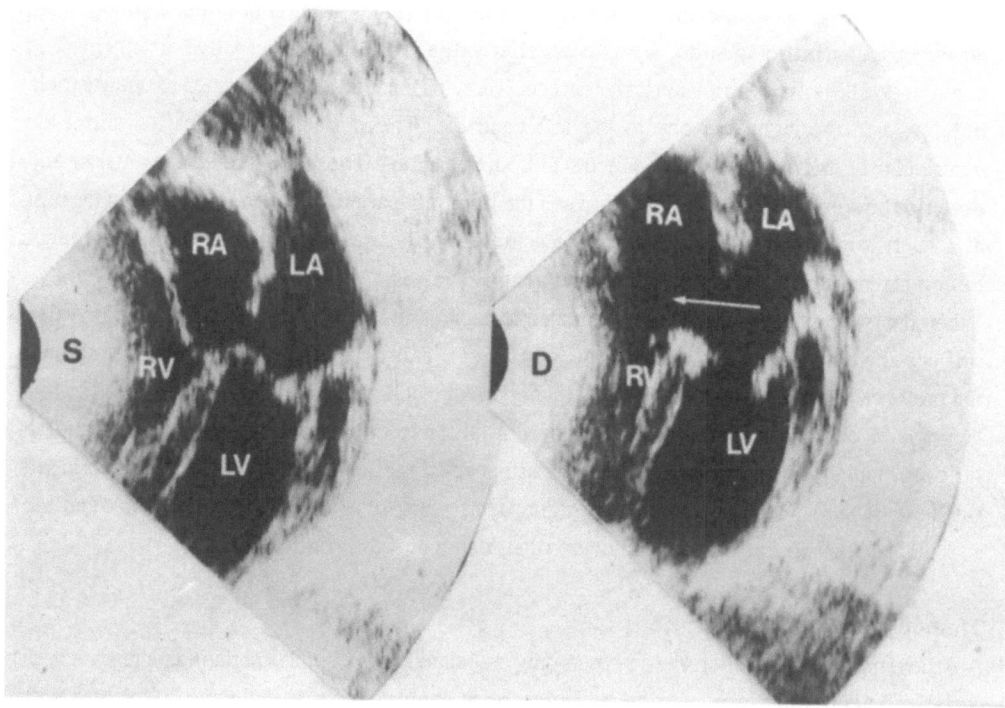

Fig. 10-1 . Cross-sectional echocardiographic appearance of a partial atrioventricular septal defect ("ostium primum ASD") in the apical four-chamber view. The common level of the atrioventricular junction is clearly seen. There is an atrial septal defect in the region of the primum septum. The anterior bridging leaflet appears firmly tethered to the crest of the ventricular septum, with no interventricular communication beneath it. The arrow marks the defect in the primum atrial septum. RA=right atrium; LA=left atrium; RV=right ventricle; LV=left ventricle.

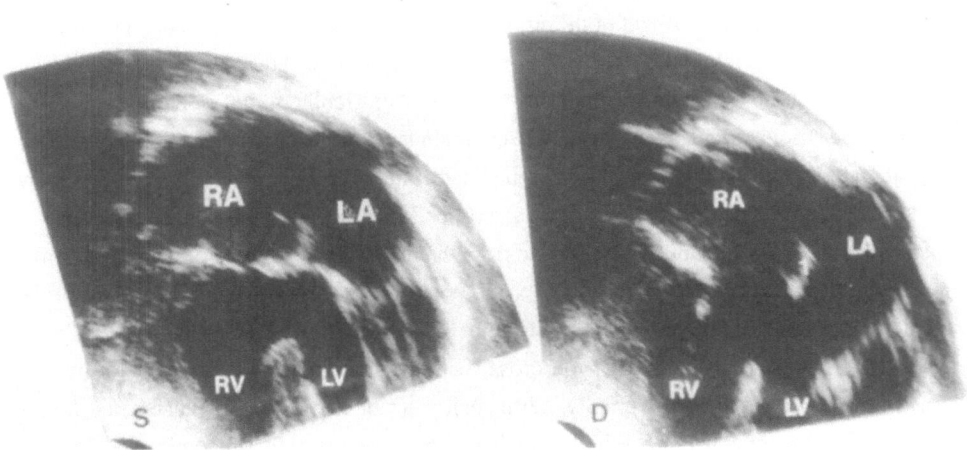

Fig. 10-2. Cross-sectional echocardiographic appearance of a complete atrioventricular septal defect in the apical four-chamber view. There is a large ventricular septal defect beneath the anterior bridging leaflet. The septal defect is more evident in diastole, as the leaflet moves away from the plane of the scan. The anterior bridging leaflet appears to float freely above the crest of the ventricular septum. A part of the primum atrial septum is still present (1), and there is a large atrial septal defect higher up. RA= right atrium; LA=left atrium; RV=right ventricle; LV=left ventricle.

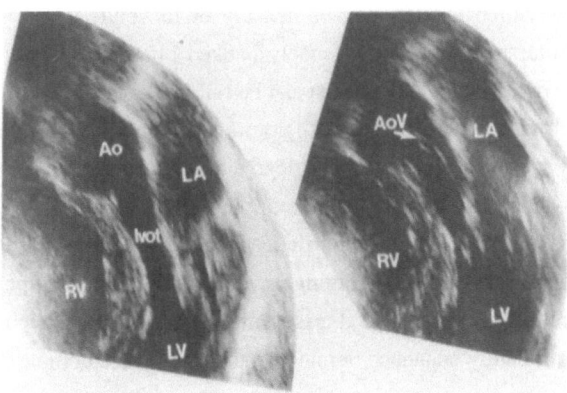

Fig. 10-3. Parasternal long axis scan in a partial atrioventricular septal defect, showing the characteristic "goose neck" deformity of the LVOT. The anterior displacement of the LVOT in this defect can produce potential narrowing of the outflow tract. This may sometimes only be unmasked after surgical repair. LA=left atrium; LV=left ventricle; RV=right ventricle; LVOT=left ventricular outflow tract; Ao=aortic valve.

Cross-Sectional Imaging

Detailed morphologic assessment of the atrioventricular junction can be made noninvasively by cross-sectional echocardiography. The apical four-chamber view will demonstrate virtually all of the typical morphologic features common to all atrioventricular septal defects, such as the absence of the atrioventricular septum and the common level of the atrioventricular junction [4]. In the great majority of cases there is an atrial septal defect in the region of the primum septum, and the inlet portion of the ventricular septum is scooped out to a variable degree. The anterior displacement of the aortic root will be evident from the inability to obtain a normal four-chamber plus aortic root cut from the apical or subcostal positions [5]. This anterior displacement also produces the characteristic "goose neck" deformity of the ventricular outflow tract (LVOT) seen in the long axis left ventricular view on cross-sectional imaging and equivalent to the view defined by left ventricular angiography. With such anterior aortic root displacement, there is always some degree of apparent LVOT narrowing with a potential for anatomic and functional LVOT obstruction (Fig. 10-3) [6].

The leaflet and papillary muscle arrangements can be seen clearly in short axis parasternal and subcostal views. Subcostal views are particularly useful in differentiating partial from complete defects [7]. The parasternal short axis view enables one to distinguish the space between the bridging leaflets from true clefts of the mitral valve [8].

Interventricular communications occurring beneath the anterior bridging leaflet are best seen in the apical four-chamber view, and those beneath the posterior bridging leaflet in subcostal views [4]. The bridging leaflets may be directly attached to the crest of the ventricular septum, or may be tethered to it by chordae, which in turn may be densely or loosely packed. Interventricular communications in the interspaces between densely packed chordae will not be adequately imaged. All the additional defects that may coexist can be reliably categorized by cross-sectional imaging which has been found to be superior to angiography in defining atrioventricular valve morphology and papillary muscle architecture. The degree of left atrioventricular valve dysplasia determined by imaging correlates well with operative findings [9].

Imaging does not predict the amount of atrioventricular valve cusp tissue present, and this is a major failing. In addition, cross-sectional imaging provides only morphological information. Other techniques are required for detailed assessment of the hemodynamics. Doppler echocardiography has significantly enhanced our understanding of these complex defects.

Doppler Echocardiography

Pulsed wave (PW) and continuous wave (CW) Doppler, and more recently Color Flow Mapping (CFM) have been integrated to provide a complete hemodynamic assessment of these defects. Cardiac catheterization provides additional information only in the assessment of pulmonary vascular resistance. In young children, irreversible pulmonary hypertension can usually be ruled out on clinical grounds, and so operative referral may frequently be made on clinical plus ultrasound findings only.

Pulsed Wave Doppler

The pulsed wave Doppler examination is best used in conjunction with cross-sectional imaging. When there is an interatrial communication of small or moderate size in the area of the primum septum, pulsed wave Doppler will confirm the presence of an atrial shunt, and show the direction of flow. The velocity profile of the left to right shunt will have all the characteristics of any atrial septal defect. With the sample volume positioned on the right atrial side of the defect, low velocity flow will be detected towards the transducer, commencing in early systole and with late systolic acceleration of flow. A second velocity peak in the same direction may also be seen during the 'a' wave of atrial contraction. In most cases, a smaller right to left shunt with flow away from the site of the sample volume will also be detected in early systole. The diastolic flow velocities across the right atrioventricular valve and pulmonary valve will be higher than normal, in keeping with increased volume of flow across these valves.

There is usually evidence of right atrioventricular valve regurgitation. This will be detected as a turbulent pansystolic jet directed into the right atrium. Its origin can best be detected with the sample volume within the right atrium, immediately above the right atrioventricular orifice. The area of systolic flow disturbance associated with this "tricuspid" incompetence may be followed back into the right atrium and hepatic veins using a PW Doppler mapping technique. In general, the distance from the right atrioventricular valve at which this flow disturbance is still detectable and the intensity of the regurgitant flow signals within the atrium give some indication of the degree of regurgitation [10]. However, a major problem exists in atrioventricular septal defects with the interpretation of any right atrial systolic turbulence as right atrioventricular valve incompetence, as a significant proportion of such patients have associated obligatory left ventricle to right atrium pansysolic turbulent shunts. The flow disturbance associated with such shunting cannot usually be distinguished from that of right atrioventricular valve regurgitation by pulsed Doppler alone.

Left atrioventricular valve regurgitation, if present, will be detected by placement of the pulsed Doppler sample volume in the left atrium above the left atrioventricular valve. This may occur via the central orifice or via the "cleft" between the bridging leaflets. Pulsed Doppler cannot normally distinguish one from the other. A semi-quantitative estimate of the volume of regurgitation can be attempted based both on the extension of the regurgitant jet in the left atrium and into pulmonary veins using a mapping technique, and from the intensity of the Doppler signal [11]. In addition, with significant regurgitation, the velocity of forward flow in diastole across the left atrioventricular valve will also be higher than normal. The value of this increased velocity of forward flow across the left atrioventricular valve as a guide to the regurgitant volume is limited in the presence of a large volume left to right shunt.

Pulsed Doppler has been shown to be extremely sensitive and specific for diagnosing isolated restrictive ventricular septal defects [12]. The diagnosis is based on the detection of a systolic flow disturbance within the right ventricular cavity. The disturbed flow can be shown to orginate from the right ventricular aspect of the interventricular septum, and can frequently be mapped backwards through the septum to its left ventricular aspect. The ability to detect such shunts depends on the presence of turbulent flow across the defect, which in turn is a function of the pressure difference between the two ventricles and is therefore related to the size of the defect. In the complete form of atrioventricular septal defect, the perimembranous inlet ventricular septal defect is virtually always non-restrictive. As a result, the ventricular peak systolic pressures are equal, and no turbulent flow exists across the defect. Even with restrictive VSDs, a defect located in the inlet portion of the septum can cause difficulties in diagnosis if one relies on PW Doppler detection of ventricular turbulence alone. This is due to the frequent coexistence of a high velocity left ventricle to right atrium shunt. Previous pulsed Doppler studies of ventricular septal defects have demonstrated that it is impossible to distinguish the two flow disturbances [12,13]. Furthermore, in the presence of non-restrictive ventricular septal defect hemodynamics, additional distal VSDs may also be missed on account of the equal ventricular pressures and absence of turbulent flow.

Pulsed wave Doppler has been used to calculate the systemic and pulmonary flow volumes (QP:QS) and shunt ratios in a variety of cardiac defects [14,15,16]. Such volumetric calculations are dependent on accurate measurement of the diameters of the left ventricular outflow tract and pulmonary artery, and the subsequent calculation of their cross-sectional area. Then, by taking the velocity time integrals of flow across these vessels (derived by pulsed Doppler), the stroke volumes can be calculated as the product of the cross-sectional area and the velocity time integral. However, large left to right shunts normally produce turbulent flow in the pulmonary artery, with inherent spectral dispersion of the Doppler signal thus preventing accurate measurement of the velocity time integral. In addition, in young children with raised pulmonary artery pressure, the diameter of the pulmonary artery can vary considerably during the cardiac cycle, with systolic expansion and diastolic contraction [17]. This introduces significant errors of measurement of pulmonary artery cross-sectional area, and thus inaccuracies in volume calculations.

To circumvent these problems, the velocity-time integral of flow across the mitral valve in diastole, and the maximum diastolic diameter of the valve have been used for calculating pulmonary blood flow, in the presence of large left to right shunts [18]. Such volumetric calculations are possible only if there is no mitral regurgitation. The velocity time integral of flow for the left atrioventricular valve in diastole cannot therefore be used to calculate pulmonary blood flow either, in the presence of the left atrioventricular valve regurgitation. The abnormal atrioventricular valve morphology common to all atrioventricular septal defects also prevents accurate measurement of valve diameter in diastole from cross-sectional images.

Thus, while PW Doppler is potentially capable of detecting the presence both of intracardiac shunts and atrioventricular valve regurgitation, the hemodynamic information it can provide is limited. It is also a time-consuming process in atrioventricular septal defects, in view of the multiplicity of hemodynamic abnormalities that need to be analysed.

Continuous Wave Doppler

Continuous wave (CW) Doppler examination provides additional information to pulsed wave in this spectrum of defects. Frequency aliasing, which limits the accurate measurement of peak velocities of flow by the pulsed mode is not a problem with CW Doppler and there is no limit to the maximum peak velocities that can be recorded. In theory therefore, the spectral velocity profiles and peak velocities of regurgitant jets can be accurately recorded (Fig. 10-4). From these recordings, the peak instantaneous pressure drop across either atrioventricular valve in systole can be calculated using the modified Bernoulli equation. In the absence of right ventricular outflow obstruction, the calculated systolic pressure drop across the right atrioventricular valve plus the estimated mean venous pressure will give the pulmonary artery peak systolic pressure. Although this does not provide an estimate of the pulmonary vascular resistance, knowledge of the pulmonary artery systolic pressure and the ability to measure it serially by a reliable non-invasive technique provides useful information which can be used to decide on the timing of surgical repair (Fig. 10-5).

In the presence of a restrictive ventricular septal defect, similar information on right ventricular peak systolic pressure may be obtained by measuring the peak systolic flow velocity across the defect from either the parasternal or subcostal positions. With knowledge of both the systolic arterial blood pressure and the calculated interventricular pressure drop, the right ventricular systolic pressure can be derived (Fig. 10-6). With non-restrictive defects and equal peak systolic pressures in the ventricles, the peak velocity of trans-septal flow will be low. It may not be possible from transeptal flow velocity alone to decide whether the raised RV systolic pressure is due solely to the ventricular septal defect or whether there is coexisting pulmonary vascular disease.

The degree of any associated outflow tract obstruction (either left or right), or semilunar valve stenosis can also be assessed by similar appropriate measurements of the peak velocities of flow across the narrowing, and subsequent calculation of the pressure drop. Increased velocity of flow in the right ventricular outflow tract also occurs in the presence of a large volume associated with left to right shunting. In these situations, the velocity of flow is increased both in the right ventricular outflow tract and the pulmonary artery, and a localized area of increased velocity will not be seen using PW Doppler.

CW Doppler has the problem of range ambiguity. All flows occurring within the direction of the ultrasound beam are profiled. Thus, the detection of a high velocity atrioventricular regurgitant signal in systole does not permit one to differentiate right atrioventricular valve regurgitation from a left ventricle to right atrium shunt, or from a left ventricle to left atrium shunt through the cleft between the bridging leaflets. The velocity profiles associated with all the above regurgitant flows may be superimposed, and spatial separation may not be possible despite concomitant cross-sectional imaging. Misinterpretation of the LV to RA jet for "tricuspid" regurgitation can lead to gross overestimation of the RV systolic pressure. This is a major problem in the use of CW Doppler in atrioventricular septal defects.

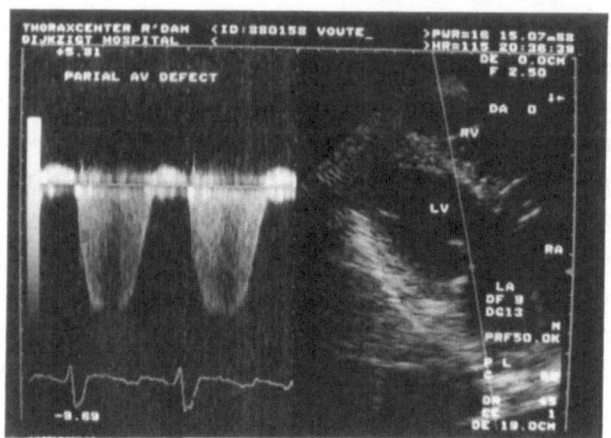

Fig. 10-4. Continuous wave Doppler examination of a partial atrioventricular septal defect: With the transducer in the apical position and directed upwards and medially, the high velocity jet of left atrioventricular valve regurgitation is recorded.

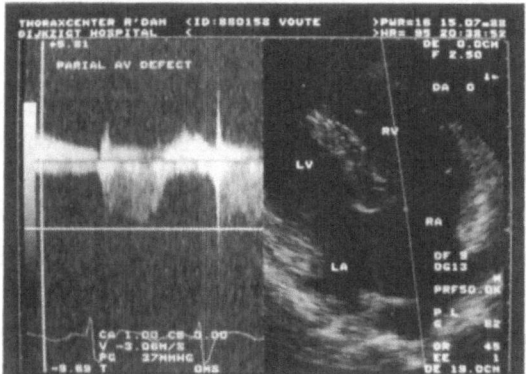

Fig. 10-5. Continuous wave Doppler examination of a partial atrioventricular septal defect, with the transducer in the parasternal position (midway between the apex and the left sternal edge), and angulated slightly upwards, posteriorly and medially. The velocity profile of right atrioventricular valve regurgitation is recorded. From the peak velocity of this regurgitant jet, the pressure drop across the right atrioventricular valve has been calculated and suggests moderate elevation of RV systolic pressure.

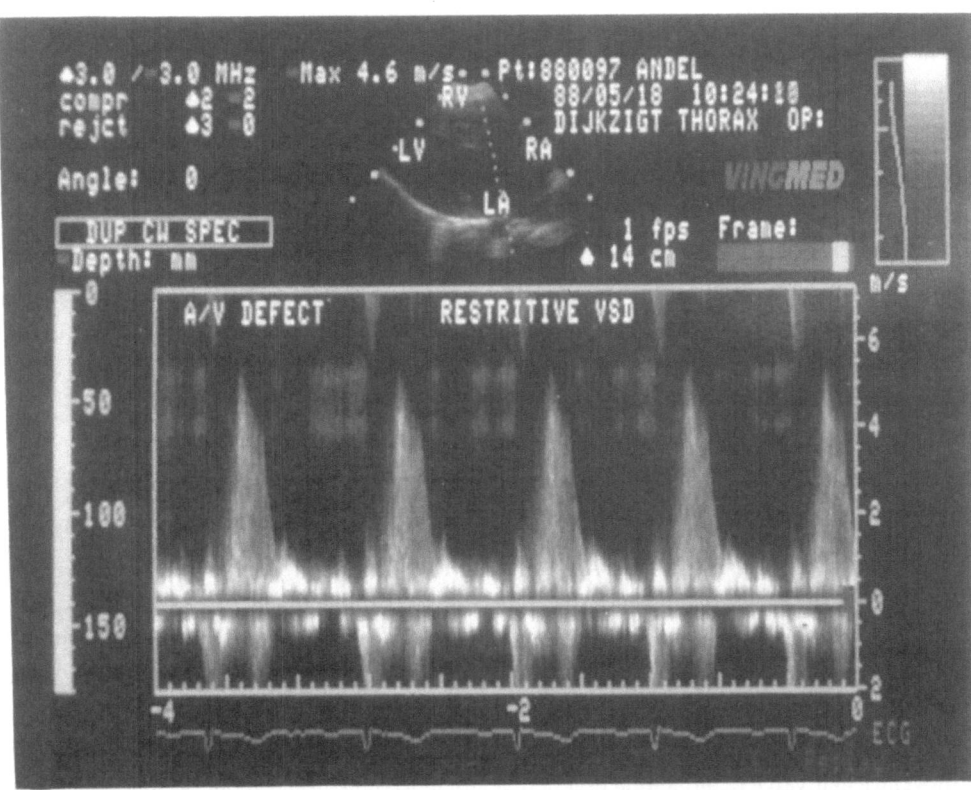

Fig. 10-6. Complete atrioventricular septal defect: CW Doppler flow profile in a restrictive ventricular septal defect from the parasternal position. The direction of shunting is from left to right, as evidenced by the anterior direction of flow. The high peak velocity of flow confirms a significant pressure difference between the two ventricles, and hence normal RV systole pressure.

Pulmonary regurgitation can be detected in a large number of patients with atrioventricular septal defects, using pulsed and continuous wave Doppler. With placement of the PW Doppler sample volume in the right ventricular outflow tract just below the pulmonary valve, the diastolic regurgitant jet will be directed towards the transducer. With high velocities of regurgitant flow, CW Doppler may be used to record the peak velocity. The waveform associated with pulmonary regurgitation will give some indication of both pulmonary diastolic pressure and mean pulmonary artery pressure [19]. A high peak velocity of regurgitation indicates that the pulmonary artery diastolic pressure is high, and from this peak velocity the instantaneous pressure difference between the pulmonary artery and right ventricle can be calculated. In patients with normal mean pulmonary artery pressures, the peak velocity of regurgitation is seen at the beginning of diastole and diminishes early. The persistence of a high velocity of regurgitant flow throughout diastole with minimal decline in the velocity profile confirms the existence of a high gradient between the pulmonary artery and the right ventricle at end-diastole. This is indicative of an elevated mean pulmonary artery pressure and irreversible pulmonary vascular disease. In some cases, the pulmonary regurgitation wave-form may have an high early peak followed by an early decrease in maximal velocity, but with a significant calculated pressure difference between the PA and RV even at end-diastole. For such patients, it would not be possible to predict the degree of reversible pulmonary hypertension or the severity of pulmonary vascular disease using Doppler alone. The inability to quantitate pulmonary vascular resistance or the degree of reversible pulmonary hypertension constitutes one of the major limitations of Doppler ultrasound in the assessment of lesions associated with a large volume of left to right shunting.

Doppler Color Flow Mapping

Doppler color flow mapping (CFM) provides unique information about these complex defects. Standard praecordial and subcostal imaging views should be used, as described above, to obtain the CFM information. The interatrial shunt across the primum defect (which is usually non-restrictive), will be seen as an area of laminar red flow crossing the ASD from left to right (Fig. 10-7). Many patients have associated secundum ASDs and will also demonstrate a similar flow abnormality higher in the septum in the region of the foramen ovale. Attempts have been made to correlate shunt size with the width of the jet, and the area of the right atrium occupied by it, but these are very rough estimates, and are only applicable in the absence of significant right atrioventricular valve regurgitation or a left ventricle to right atrium shunt [20]. Additionally, in primum atrial septal defects the color map will indicate that the shunted blood crosses the right atrioventricular valve immediately after passing through the septal defect, so it is impossible to quantify the area of the right atrium it may have occupied.

Increased velocities of forward flow across the right and left atrioventricular valves in the presence of a large shunt or severe atrioventricular valve regurgitation will produce aliasing and turbulence within the color map in diastole.

Atrioventricular valve regurgitation can be readily seen as turbulent systolic jets directed from the ventricles into the atria, in the apical or subcostal transducer position (Fig. 10-7). It is usual to find two distinct "mitral" regurgitant jets, one through the central portion of the orifice and the second in the region of the "cleft" between the bridging leaflets. A semi-quantitative measurement of left atrioventricular valve regurgitation can be made, based on the area of the left atrium occupied by the regurgitant jet. However, the extension of the regurgitant jet into the left atrium depends also on the difference in pressure between the ventricle and atrium in systole, and the compliance of both the atrium and pulmonary veins.

Right atrioventricular valve regurgitation can been seen in the apical four-chamber view or the parasternal short axis view at the level of the right atrioventricular valve. The degree of regurgitation cannot be estimated from the extent of flow reversal (seen as red flow in systole), in the hepatic veins or IVC, in the presence of an LV to RA shunt. CFM however, clearly demonstrates the two regurgitant jets into the right atrium, one from the left (LV to RA) and one from the right (RV to RA) ventricle. Such spatial separation of the regurgitant jets allows accurate alignment with each, and measurement of RV systole pressure by using CW Doppler in conjunction with CFM (Fig. 10-8).

CFM will also show restrictive interventricular communications, particularly those in the interspaces between chordae tethering the bridging leaflets to the crest of the interventricular septum and muscular VSDs in the trabecular septum. Such defects may not be seen on cross-sectional imaging alone. High velocity turbulent flow patterns will indicate the restrictive nature of these defects. In a significant proportion of restrictive VSDs, left to right shunting in diastole will also be evident. In the presence of a non-restrictive interventricular communication, the color map will indicate low velocity laminar flow across the defect, in keeping with equal ventricular pressures. Bidirectional shunting may also be evident through large defects with equal ventricular pressures. Under these circumstances, the ability of CFM to detect additional small VSDs is also limited.

CFM therefore allows accurate estimation of right ventricular systolic pressure in the majority of patients. The dominant site of shunting can be determined, and the severity of atrioventricular valve regurgitation can be estimated semi-quantitatively.

Intraoperative Echocardiography

The aim of surgery in atrioventricular septal defects is to close existing atrial and ventricular septal defects and to produce two competent, non-stenotic atrioventricular valves. The amount of valve cusp tissue available to reconstruct competent atrioventricular valves needs to be assessed at operation, as this cannot be estimated from preoperative cross-sectional imaging alone. Intraoperative epicardial cross-sectional imaging however allows better assessment of atrioventricular valve morphology and chordal attachments. Whether trifoliate repair of the left atrioventricular valve or approximation of the bridging leaflets needs to be performed can be decided from CFM evidence of the presence and degree of regurgitation through the "cleft" between the bridging leaflets.

The quality of the repair and ventricular function can be assessed immediately, and CFM will show the presence of residual shunts or atrioventricular valve regurgitation. Left ventricular outflow obstruction, which may manifest after corrective surgery, can also be determined immediately [21]. In theory therefore, intraoperative echocardiography introduces the possibilty of immediate revision of the surgery in the event of significant residual defects. The degree of residual left atrioventricular valve regurgitation following repair of the atrioventricular valves, as assessed by CFM should provide guidelines for the necessity of valve replacement.

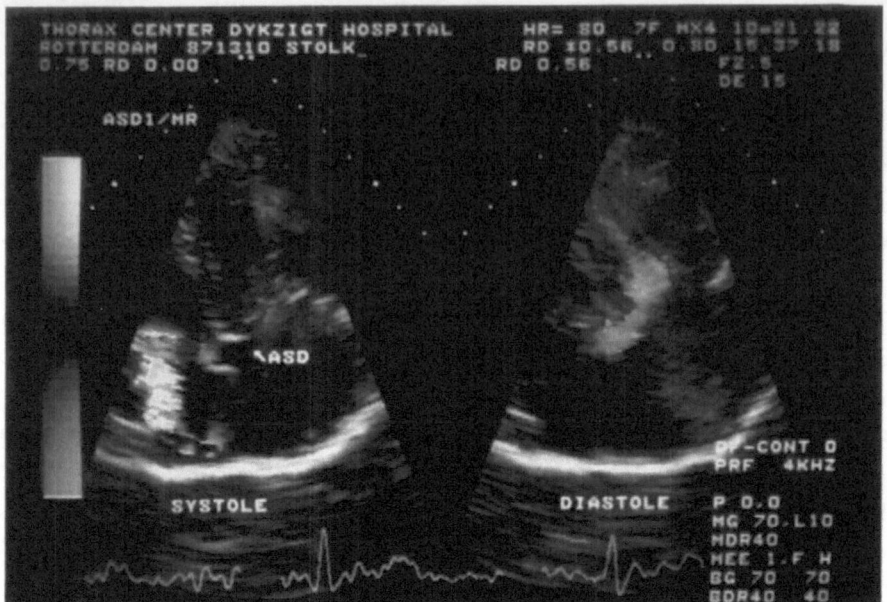

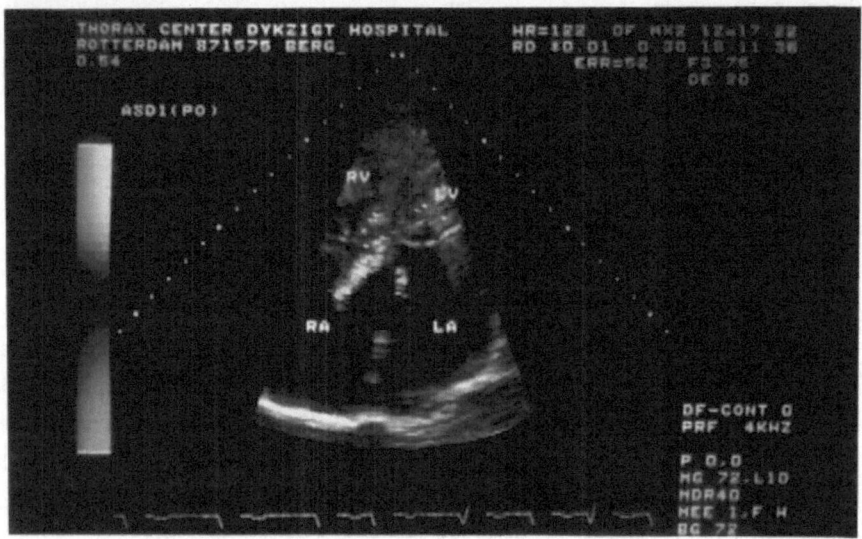

Fig. 10-7. *Partial atrioventricular septal defect: apical four-chamber view. Doppler CFM: a) The diastolic frame shows left to right shunting across the primum atrial septal defect. The uniform red color is indicative of laminar flow through a non-restrictive defect. b) The systolic frame shows high velocity left atrioventricular valve regurgitation, seen as aliased flow away from the transducer. ASD=atrial septal defect. Other abbreviations as before.*

Fig. 10-8. *Partial AV septal defect: Doppler CFM from the apical four-chamber view showing RV to RA and LV to RA shunting in systole. The spatial separation of the two regurgitant jets can be difficult without CFM. Failure to recognize the existence of the LV to RA shunt can result in gross overestimation of the RV systolic pressure by CW Doppler, if this shunt is mistaken for "tricuspid" regurgitation and the peak velocity of flow used to estimate the right ventricular systolic pressure. Abbreviations as before.*

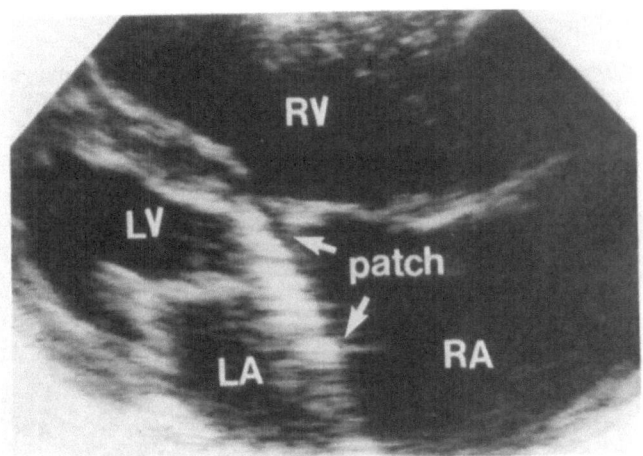

Fig. 10-9. Cross-sectional echocardiogram of a partial atrioventricular septal defect (four-chamber) view, following patch closure of the atrial septal defect. The atrial septum appears intact on imaging. Abbreviations as before.

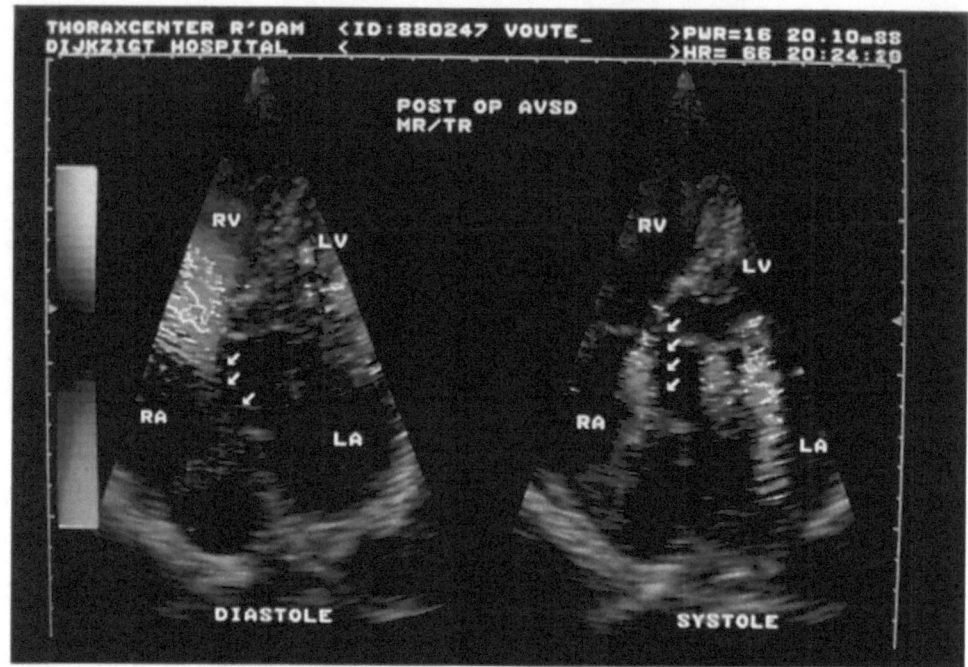

Fig. 10-10. Post operative Doppler CFM from the patient in figure 9. The apical four-chamber view shows residual right and left atrioventricular valve regurgitation. CFM clearly demonstrates two separate regurgitant jets through the left atrioventricular valve: one through the central portion of the orifice and a second jet through the "cleft" (see text). The arrows show the location of the atrial patch.

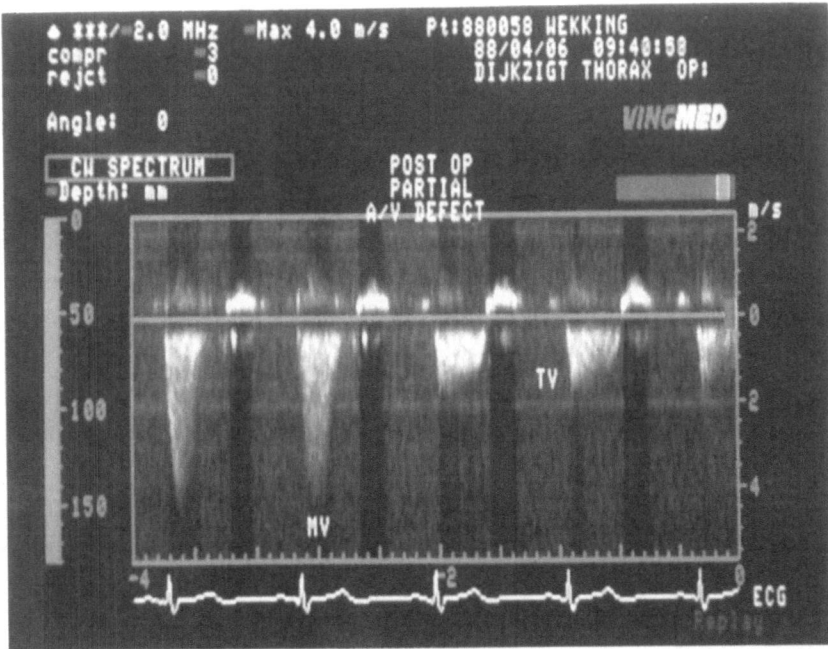

Fig. 10-11. Post operative CW Doppler velocity profiles of right and left atrioventricular valve regurgitation. The RV systolic pressure has been calculated from the peak velocity of right atrioventricular valve regurgitation, and is within the normal range. MV=mitral (left AV) valve; TV=tricuspid (right AV) valve.

Post Operative Follow-up

It is common to find some degree of residual left and right atrioventricular valve regurgitation after corrective surgery for partial or complete atrioventricular septal defects. The long-term significance of the left atrioventricular valve regurgitation needs to be established, but assessment should be possible by serial follow-up examination using cross-sectional and Doppler echocardiography. Right heart pressures can be monitored serially from residual right atrioventricular regurgitation, by CFM-guided measurement of regurgitant velocities using continuous wave Doppler (Figs.10&11).

Summary

Cross-sectional and Doppler echocardiography (PW, CW and CFM) provide accurate morphologic and hemodynamic information in these complex defects to allow surgical repair in the majority of infants or young children to be undertaken without prior catheterization. They also facilitate evaluation of the quality of surgical repair and are of great value in long term, non-invasive follow-up.

References

1) Piccoli GP, Gerlis LM, Wilkinson JL, Loszadi K, Macartney FJ, Anderson RH. Morphology and classification of atrioventricular defects. Br. Heart J 1979; 42:621-32.

2) Wakai CS, Edwards JE. Development and pathologic considerations in persistent common atrioventricular canal. Proceedings of the staff meetings of the Mayo Clinic 1956; 31:487-500.

3) Rastelli GC, Kirklin JW, Titus JL. Anatomic observations on complete form of persistent common atrioventricular canal with special reference to atrioventricular valves. Mayo Clin Proc 1966; 41:296-308.

4) Smallhorn JF, Tommasini G, Anderson RH, Macartney FJ. Assessment of atrioventricular septal defects by two-dimensional echocardiography. Br Heart J 1982; 47:109-21.

5) Sutherland Gr, Godman MJ, Smallhorn JF, Guiterras P, Anderson RH, Hunter S. Ventricular septal defects. Two-dimensional echocardiographic and morphological correlations. Br Heart J 1982; 47:316-28.

6) Ebels T, Meijboom EJ, Anderson RH, van Leeuwen JMS, Lenstra D, Eijgelaar A, Bossina KK, van der Heide JNH. Anatomic and functional "obstruction" of the outflow tract in atrioventricular septal defects with separate valve orifices ("ostium primum atrial septal defect"): an echocardiographic study. Am J Cardiol 1984; 54:843-7.

7) Mortera C, Rissech M, Payola M, Miro C, Perich R. Cross sectional subcostal echocardiography: atrioventricular septal defects and the short axis cut. Br Heart J. 1987; 58:267-73.

8) Smallhorn JF, de Laval M, Stark J, et al. Isolated mitral cleft. Two-dimensional

echocardiographic assessment and differentiation from "clefts" associated with atrioventricular septal defects. Br. Heart J. 1982; 48:109-16.

9) Lipshultz SE, Sanders SP, Mayer JE, Colan SD, Lock JE. Are routine preoperative cardiac catheterisation and angiography necessary before repair of ostium primum atrial septal defect? J Am Cardiol 1988; 11:373-8.

10) Miyatake K, Okamoto M, Kinoshita N, Olta M, Kozuka T, Sakakibara H, Nimura Y. Evaluation of tricuspid regurgitation by pulsed Doppler and two-dimensional echocardiography. Circulation 1982;66:777-84.

11) Abbasi AS, Allen MW, De Christofaro D, Ungar J. Detection and estimation of the degree of mitral regurgitation by range-gated pulsed Doppler echocardiography. Circulation 1980;61:143-7.

12) Stevenson JG, Kawabori I, Dooley T, Guntheroth WG. Diagnosis of ventricular septal defects by pulsed Doppler echocardiography - sensitivity, specificity and limitations. Circulation 1978; 58:322-6.

13) Hatle L, Rokseth R. Noninvasive diagnosis and assessment of ventricular septal defect by Doppler ultrasound. Acta Med Scand 1981; 645:47-56.

14) Sanders SP, Yeager S, Williams RG. Measurement of systemic and pulmonary blood flow and QP/QS ratio using Doppler and two-dimensional echocardiography. Am J Cardiol 1983; 51:952-6.

15) Barron JV, Sahn DJ, Valdes-Cruz LM, Lima CO, Goldberg SJ, Grenadier E, Allen HD. Clinical utility of two-dimensional Doppler echocardiography techniques for estimating pulmonary to systemic flow ratios in children with left to right shunting atrial septal defect, ventricular septal defect or patent ductus ateriosus. J Am Coll Cardiol. 1984; 3: 169-78.

16) Stevenson JG, Kawabori I. Noninvasive determination of pulmonic to systemic flow ratio by pulsed Doppler echo. Circulation 1982; (Suppl II): 232.

17) Greenfield JC, Griggs DM. The relation between pressure and diameter in main pulmonary artery of man. J Appl Physiol. 1983; 18:557-9.

18) Fisher DC, Sahn DJ, Friedman MJ, et al. The mitral valve orifice method for noninvasive two-dimensional determinations of cardiac output by echo Doppler. Circulation 1983; 67:873-7.

19) Miyatake K, Okamoto M, Kinoshita N, Matsuhisa M, Nagata S, Beppu S, Park YD, Sakakibara H, Nimura Y. Pulmonary regurgitation studied with the ultrasonic pulsed Doppler technique. Circulation 1982; 65:969-76.

20) Kyo S, Omoto R, Takamoto S, Takanawa E. Clinical significance of colour flow mapping real-time two-dimensional Doppler echocardiography (2-D Doppler) in congenital heart diasease. Circulation 1984; 70(Suppl II):37.

21) Taylor NC, Somerville J. Fixed subaortic stenosis after repair of ostium primum defects. Br Heart J. 1981; 45:689-97.

CHAPTER XI

THE DOPPLER EVALUATION OF PATENT DUCTUS ARTERIOSUS

James V. Chapman

Patent Ductus Arteriosus

In normal fetal circulation, the aorta and the pulmonary artery are connected at the level of the pulmonary artery bifurcation and the aorta just distal to the left subclavian artery by the ductus arteriosus. It closes in response to increased oxygen in the blood flow through the ductus shortly after birth. This functional closure of the ductus is followed by an anatomic closure in the first two to three weeks of life, however it may remain patent, in which case there is a shunting of blood flow from the aorta to the pulmonary artery. This shunting may also be from the pulmonary artery to the aorta if there is a severe pulmonary hypertension.

Patent ductus arteriosus may occur as an isolated lesion or may coexist in the setting of a complex lesion such as ventricular septal defect, coarctation, and atrioventricular canal defect. In fact there is a group of lesions, including hypoplastic left heart syndrome and preductal coarctation, which are dependent on the patency of the ductus for systemic perfusion.

The patient with a small isolated patent ductus arteriosus may present without symptoms. In a large patent ductus arteriosus heart failure can be noted as early as the second month but usually before the sixth month of life. The size of the patent ductus arteriosus is generally larger, and therefore leads more rapidly to heart failure, the more prematurely an infant is born. In the adult patient heart failure, rupture, aneurysm, and aortic dissection can occur. There is an increased risk of bacterial endocarditis in all patients with patent ductus arteriosus. The presence of a patent ductus arteriosus after six weeks of age is abnormal and generally requires surgical closure. The timing of the surgery is based on the child's hemodynamic status and physical condition, but is usually performed in early childhood. The surgical correction of patent ductus arteriosus carries a low risk and morbidity in the child and adolescent, however surgical intervention is more difficult in older adult patients as the ductus becomes friable.

The closure of the patent ductus arteriosus can occur over a period of hours, days, or spontaneously. The consequences of patent ductus arteriosus are primarily hemodynamic and Doppler ultrasound permits this parameter to be observed noninvasively. The presence of ductal flow can be ascertained using either pulsed, continuous wave, or color flow mapping Doppler. Pulsed Doppler may be applied to measure volumetric flows and the Qp/Qs ratio. Continuous wave Doppler can be used to derive various measurements such as pulmonary artery pressure, which reflects the effects of the shunt on pulmonary resistance. The color flow mapping technique can be used to semi-quantify the severity of the patent ductus arteriosus. In the setting of complex lesions dependent on the patent ductus arteriosus for adequate systemic perfusion, the ductal patency can be monitored by Doppler, and if it closes spontaneously, the ductal status can be followed after administration of prostaglandin E_1 to ascertain that patency has been re-established.

Imaging in Patent Ductus Arteriosus

The muscular tube which comprises the duct can sometimes be imaged by two dimensional echocardiography. There are two primary approaches which can be used for imaging. The long axis view of the bifurcation of the pulmonary artery can be imaged in most patients from a left parasternal transducer position (LV short axis view), at the level of the second or third intercostal space. The duct can be tortuous and difficult to follow from the pulmonary artery to the aorta. The presence of a small duct can be quite difficult to diagnose by imaging alone with a high degree of confidence due to echo drop out, suboptimal resolution, etc. [1].

The ductus can also be visualized from the suprasternal notch position in some patients. The long axis of the descending aorta and the short axis of the pulmonary artery are visualized. The ductus will usually be noted to arise at the level of the descending aorta at a level slightly distal to the left subclavian artery. The major limitations with imaging are: 1) The resolution required to visualize the duct is difficult to achieve in the practical setting 2) The tortuous characteristic of the duct makes it difficult to follow and 3) The possibility of artifacts such as shadowing and echo drop out. But most importantly, the bidimensional and TM imaging modes yield no direct observation of hemodynamic events.

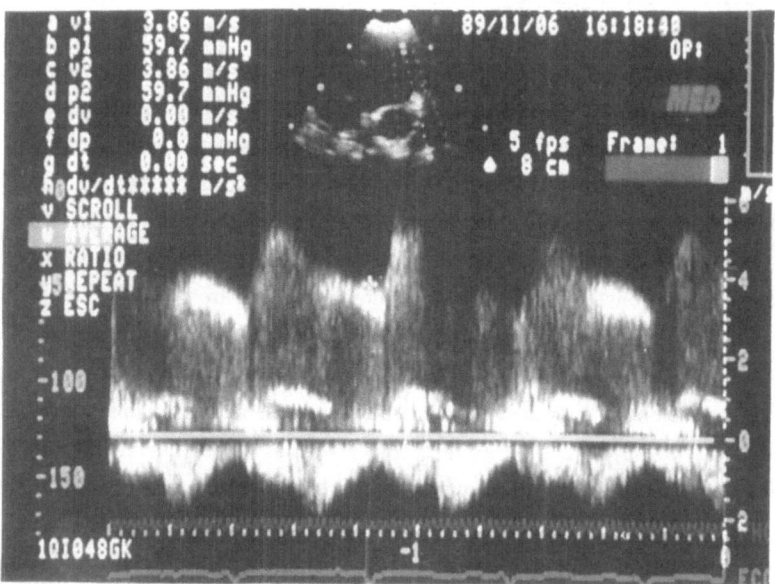

Fig. 11-1. The ductus can sometimes be directly visualized from parasternal short axis view at the base of the heart. In the study the tunnel like duct is seen arising from descending aorta and connecting to the pulmonary artery, the HPRF sample volume is positioned in the duct to measure a shunt flow of 5 m/s.

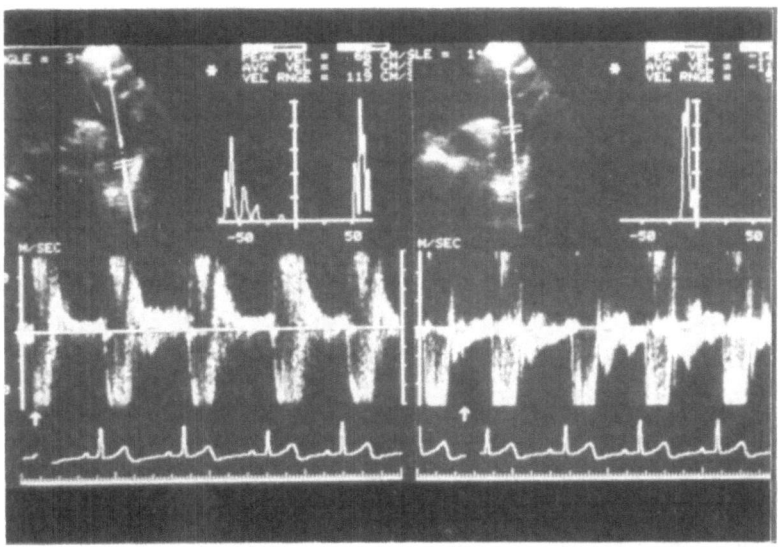

Fig. 11-2. The PD sample volume is positioned in the descending aorta in this study. When the sample volume is distal to the duct, the diastolic flow into the pulmonary artery is towards the transducer. When positioned proximal to the duct, the diastolic flow is away from the probe.

Pulsed Doppler Applications

Pulsed Doppler can be used to study patent ductus arteriosus flow in various ways [2,3,4,5]. The presence of a ductus is demonstrated by positioning the sample volume in the main pulmonary artery and obtaining a continuous systolic and diastolic flow, which is severely aliased in most situations. The flow often adheres to the lateral wall of the main pulmonary artery and can be difficult to localize. Increasing the size of the sample volume may help in these instances.

From the suprasternal notch, one can image the descending aorta as previously described (Fig.11-2). The sample volume is positioned in the aorta proximal to the ductus, and a diastolic flow away from the transducer will be noted. As the position is moved more distally the diastolic flow velocity increases and, as the sample volume is positioned diastal to the ductus the diastolic flow will reverse direction. This diastolic flow is unlike the flow reversal seen in the setting of aortic regurgitation in that the diastolic flow in regurgitation is towards the transducer the whole length of the descending aorta, and it is not influenced by sample volume position.

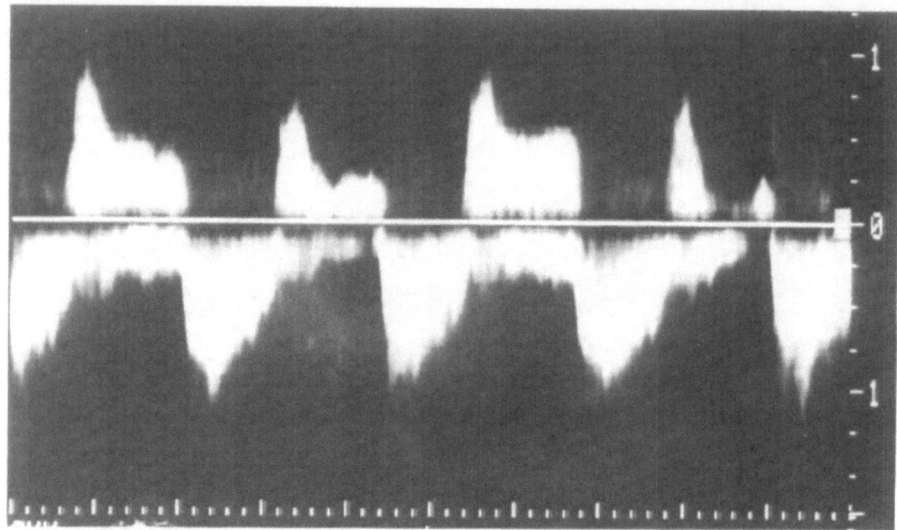

Fig. 11-3. This HPRF Doppler recording is from a child with a PDA and pulmonary hypertension. The left to right shunt is seen in diastole (positive flow) and the flow velocity is low (< 1m/s) indicating a severe pulmonary hypertension is present. The systolic pulmonary artery flow trace demonstrates that the acceleration time is decreased, an other frequent finding in the setting of pulmonary hypertension.

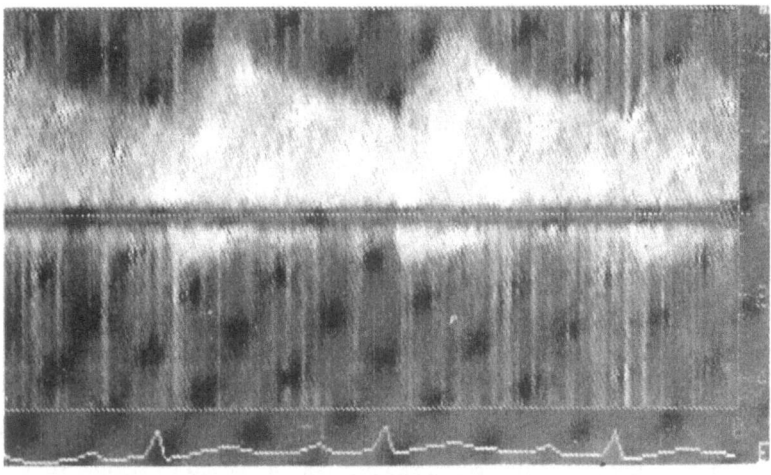

Fig. 11-4. Using CW Doppler to study ductal flow, a continuous stystolic/diastolic flow is recorded. The peak velocity is over 4.25 m/s, indicating that the pulmonary artery pressure is not elevated.

Continuous Wave Applications

The continuous wave Doppler recording of patent ductus arteriosus flow is a wide bandwidth signal with a peak velocity of 4 to 5 m/s (unless pulmonary hypertension is present) and the audio signal has a characteristic grainy sound [6]. The best alignment to flow is obtained from the left parasternal window in most cases. The velocity of the patent ductus arteriosus flow is directly related to the pulmonary artery pressure. The lower the pulmonary pressue the greater the pressure difference, and therefore the higher the velocity. If conversely, the pulmonary artery pressure is increased, the pressure difference is decreased as is the velocity of flow.

The diastolic pulmonary artery pressure can be calculated from the peak velocity measurements. The peak velocity is measured and the Bernoulli equation used to calculate the gradient between the pulmonary and systemic circulations. Subtracting the Doppler derived gradient from the systolic pressure measured by blood pressure cuff yields the pulmonary artery pressure. In our experience this method is adequate for routine clinical measurements, though the gradient does tend to be underestimated in long segment ducts. However, this underestimation is not so great as to cause error in the stratification of patients into grades of normal pulmonary artery pressure, mildly elevated pressure, moderately elevated pressure, or severe pulmonary hypertension.

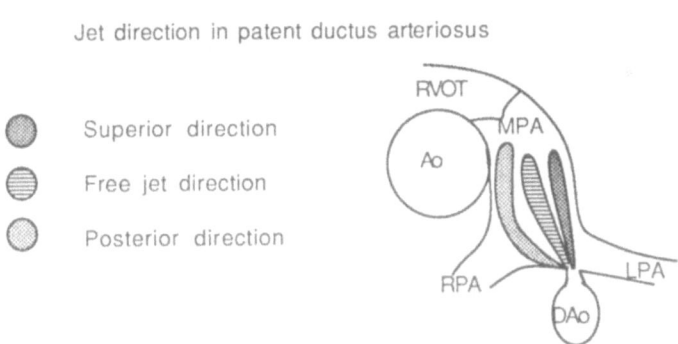

Fig. 11-5. This schematic demonstrates the most commonly encountered jet directions in the setting of patent ductus arteriosus. The superior direction in which the jet adheres to the superior wall of the main pulmonary artery is the most frequently noted jet direction, the posterior jet direction the least frequently encountered.

Color Flow Mapping

The application of color flow mapping permits one to localize the shunt and evaluate the size of the patent ductus arteriosus semi-quantitatively [7,8]. This is the best ultrasonic method for localizing the ductus because the spatial resolution is excellent: the ductal shunt flow may be quite localized, the spatial separation with other flows minimal, and the flow volume small.

The patent ductus arteriosus can usually be interrogated from the parasternal window in adolescents, or the parasternal window and the suprasternal notch in infants and children. From the parasternal short axis view of the left ventricle the long axis of the main pulmonary artery and bifurcation are noted. The short axis of the descending aorta can be seen posterior to the bifurcation, and if the ductus is large enough it may be visualized communicating between the aorta and pulmonary artery. This orientation of the duct makes interrogation by color flow mapping a relatively simple application in most patients. In the presence of ductal shunting, the flow, which is encoded in shades of red by color flow mapping, is most frequently seen to adhere to the superior wall of the main pulmonary artery. However, less frequently the jet can be directed towards the posterior wall, or a free jet can occur. It has been suggested that the direction of the jet relates to the degree of constriction present. The greater the degree of constriction the more inferiorly the jet is directed. In a left to right shunt a high velocity continuous flow with a systolic peak will be demonstrated. The greater the left to right heart pressure gradient, the higher the ductal flow velocity. This high velocity flow leads to aliasing of the sampled signal, which along with the disturbed characteristic of the ductal flow accounts for the very wide bandwidth signal being obtained. The color coding used to represent this flow is therefore a combination of red, blue, and green, as previously discussed for disturbed flow delineation.

In the setting of pulmonary hypertension, the gradient between the aorta and pulmonary artery is small and the patent ductus arteriosus flow velocity low. As aliasing is not present in this situation the flow bolus may be encoded in solid red. In significantly increased pulmonary vascular resistance the ductal flow may shunt right to left, in which case the patent ductus arteriosus flow will be encoded in blue and will be directed from the pulmonary artery to the descending aorta.

Various methods of flow mapping have been proposed to quantify patent ductus arteriosus severity. There are many inherent problems in attempting to flow map a ductal flow, which compromises the utility of the technique. All of the problems associated with flow mapping regurgitant lesions i.e. gain and reject dependency, pulse repetition frequency and transducer frequency dependency, etc. are encountered. In addition, the influence of the systolic right ventricular outflow as a competing flow and the strong influence of intracardiac pressure dynamics on flow volume must be considered. However, if the continuous wave Doppler is used to ascertain that a high velocity flow exists across the patent ductus arteriosus the following statement can be made ; a small jet area indicates a small patent ductus arteriosus and a large jet indicates a large patent ductus arteriosus. It is when the duct is very large or the left to right heart pressure difference is small for another reason, such as primary hypertension, that this method becomes unreliable. Visualization of the flow diameter at the level of the connection is a more reliable indicator of severity because the shunt diameter at this level is not greatly affected by the volumetric flow rate and velocity of flow, as is the area of the shunt flow. Ludomirsky and coworkers have found that even a small ductus diameter ($\approx$ 1 mm) can be hemodynamically significant in very premature neonates. It is therefore necessary to set up the instrument to optimize the color flow mapping spatial resolution. Any beam averaging or smoothing should be minimized, and the color flow mapping modes sample volume length reduced to a minimum length, reduction of color flow mapping angle (the image angle is not so important, and can be left wide enough to permit one to obtain adequate structural information) so that a higher pulse packet is obtained for improved signal quality. Also, a higher frame rate is obtained in conjunction with this improved signal quality resulting in the best tradeoff between temporal, spatial, and frequency resolution.

Post-Operative Follow-up

In the post-operative examination of the repair of the ductus one may use pulsed, continuous wave and color flow mapping Doppler in the same way as in the native lesion to examine for the presence of residual leakage. But as leakage can be quite small and localized the color flow mapping mode is better suited for this application. The continuous wave Doppler can be used to measure the pulmonary artery pressure as previously described (chapter VII).

The Doppler methods described for native patent ductus arteriosus are also useful for evaluation and follow-up of patients after palliative surgical maneuvers such as Blalock-Taussig procedure, insertion of a Waterson shunt, or aortopulmonary windows. All Doppler modalities can be used to demonstrate patency of the shunt, but once again, the color flow mapping mode is best suited for this application due to the high degree of spatial resolution obtained. The possible complications in the setting of these procedures include residual ventricular septal defects, right ventricular outflow tract obstruction, and right ventricular failure. All of these potential problem areas can be evaluated by Doppler. One can localize the site of a residual ventricular septal defect if present, using pulsed or continuous wave Doppler. The right ventricular systolic pressure can be monitored by continuous wave techniques, and the ventricular function can be evaluated based on pulsed Doppler measurements of stroke volume. In palliative procedures, the Doppler methods can also be applied to demonstrate the hemodynamic status after final repair of the lesion and re-establishment of a normal flow circuit.

Conclusion

It has been demonstrated that Doppler yields useful information in the setting of a patent ductus arteriosus and articopulmonary shunts. The patency can be demonstrated in a qualitative manner, and some idea of the size of the shunt derived using color flow mapping Doppler. Pulsed Doppler can be used to quantitatively measure the Qp/Qs ratio in some cases, and continuous wave Doppler can be used to measure intracardiac pressures. In fact the pressure measurement is probably the most useful quantitative information obtained by Doppler in the setting of patent ductus arteriosus. The current surgical practice of correcting patent ductus in childhood make quantitative measurement of shunt size less important, as the following questions can be answered by the Doppler examination. A) Is the duct present ?, B) Is the shunt volume more than trivial ?, C) What is the pulmonary artery pressure, and is it increased ?, D) are there associated lesions present.?

We have demonstrated that Doppler is an ideal method for the follow-up evaluation of patients with a patent ductus arteriosus closure, and for monitoring patency in those situations in which pulmonary flow is maintained via a shunt.

Color Plate 11-1. These CFM studies were all obtained in patients with a patent foreman ovale. In a PDA in the setting of pulmonary hypertension (A) the degree of aliasing is far less than in a patient with a normal pulmonary artery pressure (B), reflecting the low left to right gradient in the latter. The ductus can be visualized in some individuals from the suprasternal notch position (C).

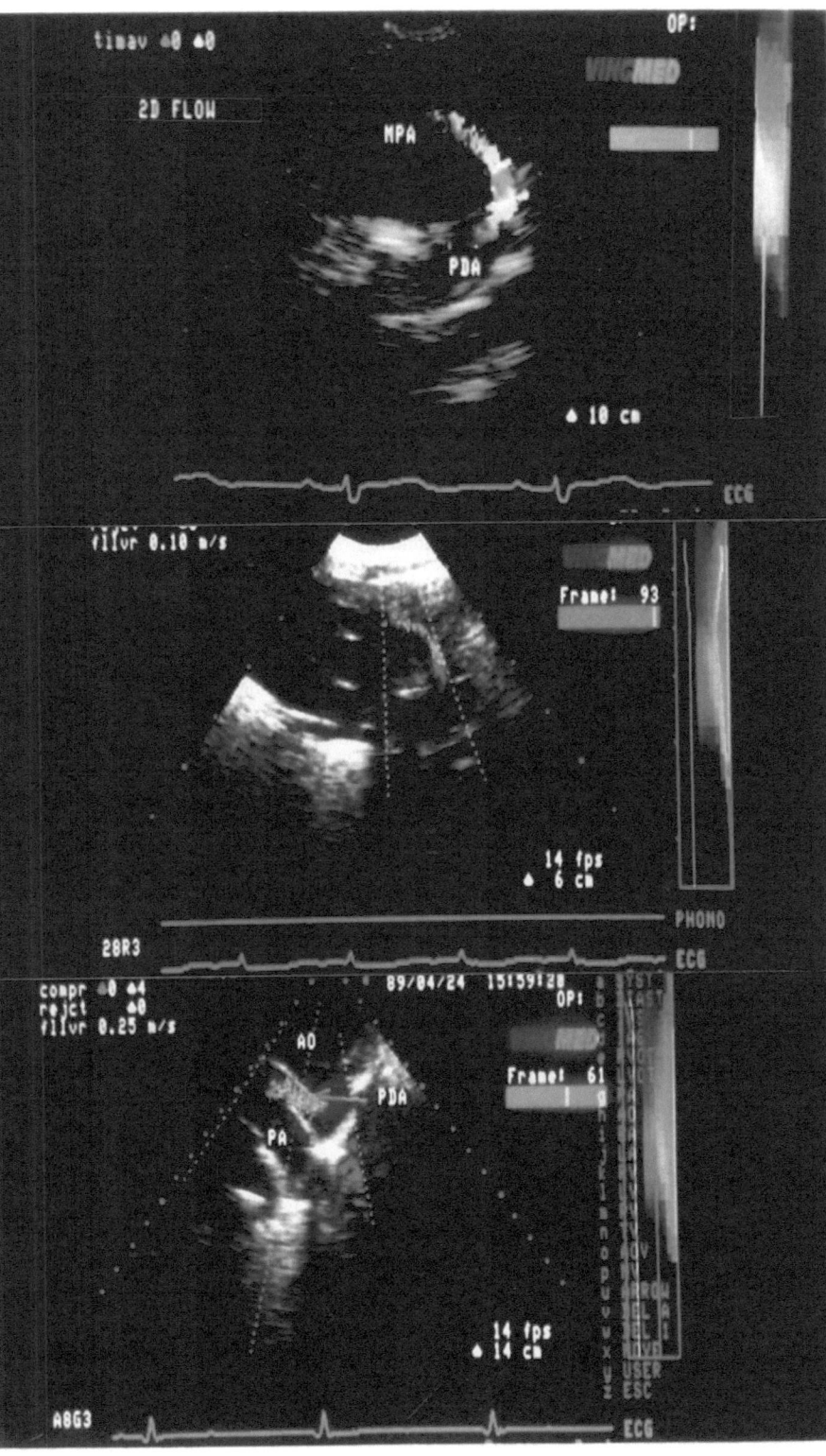

References

1) Daniels O, Hopman JCW, Stelinga, et al. Doppler flow characteristics in the main pulmonary artery and the LA/Ao ratio before and after ductal closure in healthy newborns. Pediatr Cardiol 1982; 3 : 99-104.

2) Allen HD, Sahn DJ, Lange L, Goldberg S. Noninvasive assessment of surgical systemic to pulmonary artery shunts by range-gated pulsed Doppler echocardiography. J Pediatrics 94;395-491, 1979.

3) Cacciapuoti T, Varrichio M, D'Avino M, et al. Noninvasive evaluation of left to right shunts by pulsed Doppler echocardiography. Int J Card 13:1; 57-67, 1986.

4) Stevenson JG, Kawabori I, Dooley TK, et al. Pulsed Doppler echocardiographic detection of pulmonary hypertension in patent ductus arteriosus, Circulation 60:355, 1979.

5) Stevenson JG, Kawabori I, Guneroth WG. Pulsed Doppler echocardiographic evaluation of the cyanotic newborn: Identification of the pulmonary artery in transposition of the great arteries. Am J Cardiol 46; 849, 1980.

6) Hatle L, Angelsen BAJ. Doppler Ultrasound in Cardiology: Physical Principles and Clinical Applications (2nd ed), Lea & Febiger, Philadelphia, 1985.

7) Chapman JV, Sgalambro A. Basic Concepts in Doppler Echocardiography pp 155-165, Martinus Nijhoff Publishers, Doredrecht, 1987.

8) Swenssen RE, Valdes-Cruz, Sahn DJ, et al. Real time Doppler color flow mapping for detection of patent ductus arteriosus. J Am Coll Cardiol 1986; 8: 1059-65.

CHAPTER XII

DOPPLER FINDINGS IN HYPOPLASTIC LEFT HEART SYNDROME

George R. Sutherland
Naryswamy Sreeram

Introduction

Hypoplastic left heart syndrome is characterised by underdevelopment of the morphologic left ventricle to varying degree, accompanied by atresia or stenosis of its inlet and outlet valves. Although hypoplasia of the left ventricle can exist in association with univentricular atrioventricular connection, discordant atrioventricular and/or ventriculoarterial connection or complete atrioventricular septal defect, this section will deal with the commonest morphologic pattern of hypoplastic left heart syndrome, i.e. with severe hypoplasia of the left ventricle and atresia of the mitral and aortic valves in the setting of usual atrial arrangement and concordant atrioventricular and ventriculoarterial connections.

The cross-sectional echocardiographic features of the disorder are well recognised:[1]. In most patients the left ventricle is incapable of supporting the systemic circulation, which therefore occurs via the right ventricle and patent duct. As a consequence of aortic atresia, the coronary arteries are also perfused in a retrograde manner through the duct. The syndrome normally manifests itself in the first week of the neonatal period; constriction of the patent duct during this period rapidly brings about poor systemic perfusion and myocardial ischemia.

Pulsed Doppler Echocardiography

Neonates with hypoplastic left heart syndrome usually present with heart failure and poor systemic perfusion, with the onset of ductal constriction. Any assessment of the hemodynamics, particularly semi-quantitative volumetric estimates or calculation of gradients across site/s of obstruction have to take into account the cardiac output at the time of examination. It is now common practice in several centres to administer E type prostaglandins to maintain patency of the duct, and thereby attempt to "normalise" cardiac output, while assessing the neonate with a view to potential palliative surgery. In the forthcoming discussion of the value of pulsed Doppler echocardiographic assessment of hypoplastic left heart syndrome, it is assumed that such measures to restore adequate systemic and coronary perfusion have been instituted.

Mitral Valve, Aortic Valve and Atrial Septum

A confident diagnosis of hypoplastic left heart syndrome can usually be made on cross-sectional echocardiography alone, given the appropriate clinical setting[1]. Pulsed Doppler techniques, when used in conjunction with imaging, allow better hemodynamic assessment of the lesion[2]. In the severe form of the defect, the left ventricle is extremely underdeveloped, and this is associated with atresia of the mitral and aortic valves. Pulsed Doppler interrogation of the mitral and aortic valves from standard precordial imaging planes will confirm the absence of flow across these structures, or within the left ventricle. The left atrium is usually smaller than normal, but the atrial septum may bulge towards the right, due to a restrictive interatrial communication. With atresia of the mitral valve, an interatrial communication (usually a patent oval foramen) is mandatory, to allow the pulmonary venous return to reach the systemic circulation. From the subcostal transducer position, interrogation of the atrial septum will identify the interatrial communication. The flow across the atrial septum will be from left to right, and occurs throughout the cardiac cycle. The peak velocities that can be recorded will depend on the degree to which the interatrial communication is restrictive; in the majority (with restrictive hemodynamics), flow tends to be turbulent and of high velocity.

Tricuspid and Pulmonary Valves

The tricuspid valve annulus is usually larger than normal. Pulsed Doppler interrogation of the tricuspid valve will show an increased velocity of inflow across the valve in diastole, in the presence of a large left to right shunt at atrial level, reflecting an unobstructed interatrial communication allowing free drainage of the pulmonary venous return into the right arium. Tricuspid regurgitation is present in the majority of neonates. Assessment of the degree of regurgitation is particularly important in these patients with the introduction of palliative surgery for the syndrome, and eventually establishing a Fontan type of circulation using the right ventricle as the systemic ventricle. Pulsed Doppler "mapping" techniques both within the right atrium and caval veins, as have been described in previous sections, may be used for this purpose.

Pulsed Doppler assessment of the pulmonary valve and main pulmonary artery may also reveal an increased peak velocity of flow in systole in neonates with a high pulmonary blood flow. Retrograde flow in diastole may also be recorded in some patients, as shunting through the patent duc may be from left to right in diastole.

Ascending Aorta, Aortic Arch and Duct.

Interrogation of the ascending aorta from the suprasternal or apical transducer positions will demonstrate the characteristic pattern of retrograde flow within this structure. This helps to distinguish the syndrome from severe congenital aortic stenosis with underdevelopment of the left ventricle and mitral valve, in which condition ascending aortic flow will be prograde, albeit restricted. As the systemic circulation, and coronary perfusion, is dependent on persistent patency of the arterial duct, it may be predicted that flow within the duct will be from right to left for the major part of the cardiac cycle. The duct when patent is usually a very prominent structure that can be imaged in the majority of patients with hypoplastic left heart syndrome. Placement of the pulsed Doppler sample volume within the duct (using the suprasernal or high left parasternal transducer positions), will confirm the dynamics of flow within the duct. Although the major portion of flow will represent right to left shunting (pulmonary artery to descending aorta and retrograde perfusion of the ascending aorta), it is not uncommon to also detect a smaller component of left to right ductal shunting in diastole, due to the differences in systemic and pulmonary vascular resistance[2]. Constriction of the duct may be assessed from the higher peak velocities of flow through the duct, though this is best done with continuous wave Doppler.

An important associated anomaly is coarctation of the aorta, the incidence of which varies from 20 to 80% in patients with hypoplastic left heart syndrome[2,3]. Both preductal and juxtaductal coarctation occur with equal frequency. Careful cross-sectional imaging from the suprasternal notch will usually identify the narrowed site, but better assessment of the precise site of coarctation may be made with pulsed Doppler interrogation of the aortic arch. It must be remembered that assessment of the site and degree of narrowing of the aorta will be dependent on the cardiac output at the time of examination. If the duct is severely constricted, with significant reduction of systemic perfusion in a sick neonate, it may not be possible to identify the severity of coexisting coarctation. Normalisation of the cardiac output by administration of E type prostaglandins may therefore be required as an initial step in assessing coarctation. However, the presence of a widely patent duct also introduces problems in assessing aortic arch anatomy from cross-sectional imaging alone. It is common to see some degree of kinking of the aortic isthmus a the site of ductal insertion. Careful pulsed Doppler assessment of the entire arch may be helpful in identifying localised areas of narrowing, from the acceleration of flow at the site of narrowing. Where very high velocities are encountered, continuous wave Doppler may be used to measure the peak velocities of flow at the suspected site of coarctation, although problems may arise in differentiating the high velocity of flow at the coarctation site from flow through a constricted duct. In summary, pulsed Doppler allied with cross-sectional imaging provides important information about the flow characteristics across the atrial septum (restrictive or unrestrictive), within the ascending aorta (retrograde flow), and through the patent duct (right to left shunting for the major part of the cardiac cycle).

Continuous Wave Doppler

Continuous wave Doppler echocardiography has little to add to pulsed Doppler techniques in the assessment of the hypoplastic left heart syndrome prior to considering palliative surgery. It may help in recording the peak velocities of flow in systole and diastole across a constricted duct. Ductal constriction of significant degree can however, be readily recognised from the clinical picture (poor peripheral pulses and cyanosis) and from pulsed Doppler recordings within the ascending and descending aorta. Although continuous wave Doppler has been reported to be helpful in the assessment of the severity of coarctation in the neonate and young infant, it can be misleading particularly in the presence of a coexisting patent duct[4,5]. When the duct is widely patent, and supplies the distal aorta (beyond the site of coarctation, high velocities of flow at the coarctation site may not be recorded. Alternately, when high velocities of flow are recorded by CW Doppler from the suprasternal notch, this may reflect increased velocity of flow through a constricted duct[5]. Serious limitations therefore exist in the ability to precisely determine the severity of coexisting coarctation in neonates with hypoplastic left heart syndrome.

Continuous wave Doppler assessment however, becomes imporant in assessing the quality of initial palliative surgery, as it enables estimation of the degree of obstruction to systemic blood flow, and the pulmonary artery systolic pressure (see below).

Color Flow Mapping

Left Ventricle, Mitral Valve and Aortic Valve

Color flow mapping (CFM), aids in the rapid recognition of the anomalies associated with the hypoplastic left heart syndrome. Once the morphologic left ventricle is identified, it is a relatively easy matter to recognise the presence or absence of flow within the ventricular cavity. Associated mitral and aortic atresia can also be readily seen from absence of flow through these structures on the color flow map. The precise site of interatrial shunting, and the nature of the communication (restrictive versus unrestrictive) can also be seen from the flow characteristics (velocity and variance modes on CFM) of the atrial septal defect. Pulsed Doppler interrogation of the atrial septum, to record the peak velocities of flow across the ASD, may be guided from such knowledge of the precise site of the shunt, and its direction within the right atrium.

Tricuspid Valve and Pulmonary Valve

The peak velocities of inflow across the tricuspid valve may be higher than normal, and this is identified by aliasing on the color flow map. The presence of tricuspid regurgitation can be readily recognised by CFM. CFM techniques for semi-quantification of atrioventricular valve regurgitation, based on the area occupied by the regurgitant jet relative to the area of the arium, have been discussed previously, and are applicable to the assessment of tricuspid regurgitation in patients with hypoplastic left heart syndrome, assuming that the cardiac output is near normal. From the subcostal transducer location, it will also be possible to recognise flow reversal in systole within the inferior vena cava and right atrium in patients with significant tricuspid regurgitation.

Higher than normal velocities of flow across the pulmonary valve are also easily recognised with CFM, as also the presence of pulmonary regurgitation. The assessment of pulmonary regurgitation has important implications in planning staged repair of the hypoplastic left heart syndrome. Eventually, with the currently used techniques of palliation/repair, the aim of surgery is to utilise the morphologic right ventricle as the systemic ventricle, with the pulmonary valve being the "systemic" arterial valve[4,5]. CFM criteria for volumetric assessment of pulmonary or aortic regurgitation are less well categorised than for AV valve regurgitation; this is an area in which the value of Doppler ultrasound (pulsed Doppler or CFM) remains to be established.

Ascending Aorta, Aortic Arch and Duct

The color flow map of the ascending aorta will readily demonstrate retrograde perfusion of this segment vis the duct. As discussed in the section on pulsed Doppler echocardiography, this finding, together with the absence of flow out of the left ventricle, will distinguish hypoplastic left heart syndrome from severe aortic valve stenosis. The duct can be easily recognised by CFM, and the pattern of flow within it categorised. It will be seen that the predominant direction of shunting is from right to left within the duct, with a smaller component of left to right shunting in diastole. Associated defects such as coarctation of the aorta, or rarely interruption of the aortic arch may also be recognised more easily when CFM allied to imaging is used.

Conclusion

Precise morphologic diagnosis of the hypoplastic left heart syndrome, and assessment of the haemodynamics of the lesion have become particularly important with the advent of successful techniques for palliation, and subsequent "physiologic" correction of this hitherto fatal lesion. The objectives of initial palliation are to establish unobstructed systemic and coronary blood flow, to normalise pulmonary blood flow, pulmonary artery pressure and pulmonary vascular resistance, and to relieve pulmonary venous obstruction. The feasibility of palliation (RV function and volume, presence and degree of tricuspid regurgitation), and the precise measures required (e.g. atrial septectomy to relieve pulmonary venous obstruction) can be readily assessed from cross-sectional imaging allied with pulsed Doppler and color flow mapping. For the reasons discussed previously, assessment of the presence and severity of preductal or juxtaductal coarctation can be difficult, even with the combined use of imaging, spectral Doppler and CFM.

Noninvasive assessment of palliative surgical measures for hypoplastic left heart syndrome. Noninvasive imaging techniques may however, have an even more important role in the morphologic and hemodynamic evaluation of the quality of palliative surgical procedures, and in deciding on the timing, and nature of subsequent repair with a Fontan type of procedure. Thus, using a combination of the techniques and methods described previously, it will be possible assess right ventricular function, to determine whether the interatrial communication following septostomy or septectomy is adequate; the presence and degree of residual or newly developed obstruction to systemic blood flow may be estimated from imaging, and from continuous wave Doppler measurement of the peak velocities of flow across the connection between the main pulmonary artery and the aorta; the pulmonary artery systolic pressure can be esimated from the pressure drop across the aorto-pulmonary shunt derived from the peak systolic velocity of flow through the shunt. The severity of tricuspid regurgitation may be assessed semi-quantitatively using the methods described above. Pulmonary regurgitation may also be readily detected using pulsed Doppler or color flow mapping, although there are significant problems in volumetric assessment.

Noninvasive imaging and Doppler techniques (pulsed wave, continuous wave and color flow mapping) may therefore obviae the need for cardiac catheterisation prior to planning palliative surgery or subsequent "physiologic" correction in selected patients with hypoplastic left heart syndrome.

References

1) Lange LW, Sahn DJ, Allen HD, Ovitt TW, Goldberg SJ. Cross-sectional echocardiography in hypoplastic left ventricle: echocardiographic-angiographic-anatomic correlations. Pediar Cardiol 1980; 1: 287-99.

2) Bash SE, Huhta JC, Vick GW, Gutgesell HP, Ott DA. Hypoplastic left heart syndrome: is echocardiography accurate enough to guide surgical palliation? J Am Coll Cardiol 1986; 7: 610-6.

3) Moulton AL, Anderson RH, Zuberbuhler JR. Hypoplastic left heart - anatomic variations with surgical palliation in view (abstr). 1985; World Congress of Paediatric Cardiology.

4) Robinson PJ, Wyse RK, Deanfield JE, Franklin R, Macartney FJ. Continuous wave Doppler velocimetry as an adjunct to cross-sectional echocardiography in the diagnosis of critical left heart obstruction in neonates. Br Heart J 1984; 52: 552-6.

5) Wilson N, Sutherland GR, Gibbs JL, Dickinson DF, Keeton BR. Limitations of Doppler ultrasound in the diagnosis of neonatal coarctation of the aorta. Int J Cardiol 1989; 23: 87-9.

6) Norwood WI, Kirklin JK, Sanders SP. Hypoplastic lef heart syndrome: experience with palliative surgery. Am J Cardiol 1980; 45: 87-91.

7) Lang P, Norwood WI. Hemodynamic assessment after palliative surgery for hypoplastic left heartsyndrome. Circulation 1983; 68: 104-8.

CHAPTER XIII

DOPPLER ECHOCARDIOGRAPHY EVALUATION OF TOTAL ANOMALOUS PULMONARY VENOUS DRAINAGE

George R. Sutherland
Naryswamy Sreeram

Introduction

Total anomalous pulmonary venous drainage (TAPVD) is an uncommon disorder, accounting for approximately 2% of congenital cardiac malformations[1]. It is characterised by pulmonary veins that do not drain into the anatomic left atrium. Patients usually present in the neonatal period or early infancy. The clinical manifestations depend on whether the pulmonary venous drainage is obstructed or unobstructed, and can vary from a picture of severe cyanotic congenital heart disease (obstructed venous drainage) to acyanotic right sided cardiac failure (unobstructed drainage and volume overload of the right ventricle). In the neonate, it may also mimic various respiratory disorders.

The cross-sectional echocardiographic appearances of TAPVD vary with the site of pulmonary venous drainage. Three basic patterns of drainage are commonly recognised: 1) supracardiac: where the veins drain into a common chamber that connects via an ascending vein either to the left innominate vein and thence to the superior vena cava (SVC), or directly into the right sided SVC; 2) cardiac: where the common pulmonary venous confluence or individual pulmonary veins drain into the coronary sinus, or less often directly into the right atrium; 3) infracardiac: where the pulmonary venous confluence connects via a descending vein to the inferior vena cava or hepatic veins below the diaphragm. Rarely, there may be a combination of these drainage sites ("mixed" drainage), and this is usually more difficult to recognise.

Cross-sectional echocardiography is the diagnostic technique of choice in the assessment of the sites of pulmonary venous drainage[2,3]. Normally in neonates and infants, from an apical or subcostal four-chamber view, at least two pulmonary veins can be seen to enter the right atrium (right upper and left lower). Failure to clearly identify these structures should lead one to suspect anomalous pulmonary venous drainage, if the clinical picture is compatible with the diagnosis. Using a combination of suprasternal, precordial and subcostal planes of section, it is possible in the majority to make an unequivocal diagnosis of TAPVD, and to categorise the precise site/s of drainage of the pulmonary veins.

Several indirect indices of anomalous pulmonary venous drainage may also be recognised on cross-sectional echocardiography. These include the presence of a small left atrium and a dilated right atrium and ventricle, especially if there is an associated restrictive interatrial communication; the left innominate or the coronary sinus may appear dilated if either of these structures are the site/s of pulmonary venous drainage.

Pulsed Doppler Echocardiography

Pulsed Doppler echocardiography is a valuable adjunct to cross-sectional echocardiography in the diagnosis of TAPVD[4,5,6,7]. Although it may be possible to make the diagnosis with PW Doppler in combination with M-mode echocardiography, the ability to directly visualise both normal and abnormal venous connection/s, and then to interrogate flow at each of these sights represents a significant advance on M mode echocardiography.

Supracardiac TAPVD

The commonest pattern of supracardiac TAPVD is where the pulmonary veins reach a common confluence, above and behind the left atrium. From this confluence, an ascending vein drains into the left innominate vein, thus returning the pulmonary venous blood into the right atrium via the superior vena cava. Typical patterns of flow may be recorded in each of these structures. The specific flow patterns vary depending on the presence or absence of obstruction within the ascending vein. With the transducer in the suprasternal notch, and with the PW Doppler sample volume located in the ascending vein itself, a characteristic phasic venous flow towards the transducer will be recorded with unobstructed drainage[7]. The direction of flow readily distinguishes the ascending vein from other venous structures such as a persistent left superior vena cava, in which the flow will be away from the transducer (towards the heart). The phasic flow towards the transducer reflects pressure dynamics within the right atrium, into which the pulmonary venous blood eventually drains. There may also be some variation in peak velocities with respiration. In all such cases, higher velocities of flow than normal can be recorded also within the left innominate vein, and followed into the right SVC.

The increased volume of flow through the tricuspid valve is reflected in increased velocities of diastolic flow across the valve, on pulsed Doppler sampling. For the same reason, higher velocities of flow with spectral dispersion can also be recorded in systole within the main pulmonary artery and its central branches, from the precordial or suprasternal transducer positions. Careful imaging of the interatrial septum from the subcostal or precordial scanning planes will identify the obligatory interatrial communication. Pulsed Doppler interrogation of the atrial septum will reveal a continuous pattern of right to left shunting across the septum, with the peak velocity of flow being recorded in diastole.

Where the pulmonary venous confluence drains directly into the superior vena cava, cross-sectional imaging will usually identify the connecting vein. Pulsed Doppler sampling of this vein can then be performed; the pattern of flow in the absence of obstruction to pulmonary venous drainage is as described previously; systolic and diastolic peaks can be recorded, and flow is usually of low velocity and laminar. As expected, higher than normal velocities of flow will also be recorded within the SVC. The intracardiac flow patterns are not dissimilar to those described previously.

Obstruction to pulmonary venous return, either within the ascending veins, or stenosis of individual pulmonary veins alters the flow patterns significantly. PW Doppler interrogation of the ascending vein then reveals a continuous pattern of flow, with mild variations during respiration.

This pattern of nonphasic flow suggests that pulmonary venous return is no longer inversely related to atrial pressure dynamics, and strongly suggests obstructed pulmonary venous return. With sequential sampling within the ascending vein, high velocity turbulent flow can be recorded distal to the point of obstruction.[5,7].

Flow within individual pulmonary veins also shows a nonphasic pattern in the presence of obstruction to pulmonary venous return.

TAPVD with Drainage to the Coronary Sinus or Right Atrium

This is the commonest pattern of drainage of the anomalous pulmonary veins directly to the heart. The venous confluence is located posterior to the left atrium, and connects with the coronary sinus via a bridging vein. Occasionally individual pulmonary veins enter the coronary sinus directly. The coronary sinus is usually enlarged, and projects into the back of the left atrium at the atrioventricular groove. Once the venous confluence has been imaged, pulsed Doppler sampling combined with cross-sectional imaging will enable the delineation of the site of drainage of the connecting vein. In the presence of high pulmonary blood flow, higher than normal velocities of flow can be recorded within the coronary sinus.

Where the drainage site of the pulmonary veins is directly into the right atrium, the pulmonary venous channel can be seen behind the left atrium, and followed into its drainage site within the right atrium. Again PW Doppler sampling within this venous channel will enable recording of the direction and peak velocity of flow. The patterns of flow both within the common venous channel and individual pulmonary veins differ depending on the presence or absence of obstruction to pulmonary venous return, as described previously.

Infradiaphragmatic TAPVD

It is in the detection of infradiaphragmatic TAPVD that pulsed Doppler echocardiography is most valuable[6]. The site of drainage of the descending vein from the pulmonary venous confluence is into either the inferior vena cava, or the portal circulation. Subcostal scanning in a sagittal plane will identify the inferior vena cava and the aorta in their long axis. A third channel (the descending vein), can also be imaged in its long axis in the majority of infants with infradiaphragmatic TAPVD. This channel can usually be followed from its origin behind and below the left atrium, and thence in its course through the diaphragm. Occasionally, compression of this vein below the diaphragm by the liver may cause difficulties in imaging its infradiaphragmatic course. Pulsed Doppler sampling in the three vascular structures that can be identified below the diaphragm will demonstrate characteristic flow patterns through each. Flow through the aorta will be phasic, occurring in systole. IVC flow will be directed towards the heart (away from the transducer in the subcostal position). It will show variation with the phases of respiration, with peaks occurring in systole and diastole. Nearer the right atrium (just below the diaphragm) a flow reversal associated with atrial systole can also be recorded. Flow within the third vascular structure (the descending vein) will be away from the heart (towards the subcostal transducer)[6]. It is usually continuous, turbulent flow and of high velocity, reflecting obstruction within the descending vein, as is usually the case. The direction, velocity and turbulent nature of flow will distinguish this structure from the IVC, or any other infradiaphragmatic vein, in all of which flow will be towards the heart. The infradiaphragmatic type of TAPVD is commonly associated with stenosis or obstruction of the descending vein, and consequently PW Doppler sampling of individual pulmonary veins will also show a nonphasic pattern of flow, with some respiratory variation in the peak velocities recorded.

Flow Characteristics within Individual Pulmonary Veins

The recorded pattern of flow within individual pulmonary veins will vary depending on the presence or absence of distal obstruction, or stenosis within the pulmonary vein itself. With unobstructed forms of TAPVD, flow will be phasic, and laminar. The recorded peak velocities will vary with the phases of respiration. Distal obstruction is reflected by a pattern of nonphasic flow within the pulmonary vein. Stenosis of the pulmonary vein itself produces a pattern of high velocity, nonphasic turbulent flow within the vein, distal to the point of obstruction. Although TAPVD may exist in association with other complex malformations, some of which can result in diminished pulmonary blood flow, the patterns of flow within the pulmonary veins are similar, and depend only on the presence or absence of obstruction[7].

Doppler Color Flow Mapping

Color flow mapping (CFM) enables easier identification of the pulmonary venous confluence and the precise site of communication of the confluence with the systemic venous return[8]. For the common type of supracardiac TAPVD (ascending vein connecting pulmonary veins to the left innominate vein), suprasternal echocardiography with CFM will identify flow coming towards the transducer within the ascending vein. The direction of flow distinguishes this vein from other venous flows (all other venous flows are directed towards the heart, and therefore away from the transducer). Higher velocities than normal, as depicted by aliasing on the color flow map, may be recorded not only within the ascending vein, but also within the innominate vein. Higher velocities of flow across the tricuspid and pulmonary valves will be shown as aliased flow on CFM. Transatrial flow will clearly be demonstrated as occurring from right to left; if the interatrial communication is restrictive, this will be seen as turbulent flow occurring throughout the cardiac cycle. Additional sites of drainage (to SVC, right atrium, or coronary sinus) can also be convincingly demonstrated by CFM once the pulmonary venous confluence has been identified on imaging. Obstruction to venous return at any point will be represented as a mosaic pattern in the color flow map, distal to the point of obstruction.

Distinction of TAPVD from Cor Triatriatum

Where imaging demonstrates apparent partitioning of the left atrium into two chambers (as may happen with TAPVD to the coronary sinus, and consequent protrusion of the coronary sinus into the left atrium), CFM will enable easy distinction of this appearance from cor triatriatum, by demonstrating the absence of flow between the two "partitioned areas" of the left atrium. This apparent partitioning of the left atrium has been recognised by M mode echocardiography[4] in patients suspected of having TAPVD; but the definite diagnosis or exclusion of either TAPVD or cor triatriatum is facilitated by CFM (or pulsed Doppler) interrogation of flow within the two chambers. The absence of a communication between the two chambers (as demonstrated by an absence of flow from one into the other) will rule out the diagnosis of cor triatriatum. In addition, in cor triatriatum, normal pulmonary venous drainage into the posterior and superior chamber can usually be demonstrated by apical or suprasternal cross-sectional echocardiography.

Infradiaphragmatic TAPVD

Color flow mapping is also of value in conjunction with cross-sectional imaging, both in demonstrating the descending vein and the pattern of flow within it[8]. The descending vein can usually be followed from its origin through the diaphragm, from the parasternal and subcostal imaging planes. Sagittal subcostal views will demonstrate the inferior vena cava to the right, the aorta to the left, and the descending vein which usually passes anterior to these two structures (thereby distinguishing it from the azygos vein that normally lies behind these structures). It is however, in demonstrating the direction and pattern of flow through each of these vessels that CFM is most useful. Flow within the aorta will be seen in red (towards the subcostal transducer); it will be phasic, occurring in systole. Flow within the IVC will be coded blue (away from the transducer and towards the heart). Within the descending vein itself, continuous turbulent flow away from the heart will be seen. This pattern of flow reliably distinguishes the descending vein from all other infradiaphragmatic vascular structures.

Conclusion

Cross-sectional imaging is the investigative technique of choice in the assessment of normal and abnormal patterns of pulmonary venous connections. From a combination of suprasternal, precordial and subcostal scan planes, it should be possible in the majority of patients with TAPVD both to make a correct diagnosis of the abnormality, and to define the precise site/s of drainage of the pulmonary veins. Both pulsed wave Doppler and color flow mapping enhance the diagnosis of TAPVD, by enabling flow within the connecting vein (ascending or descending), the innominate vein, the inferior vena cava and across the atrial septum to be characterised. Obstruction to flow, either within the common venous channel or within individual pulmonary veins can be reliably recognised from the recorded patterns of flow which show characteristic variations; the precise site of obstruction may also be demonstrated in some patients. Multiple sites of drainage of the pulmonary veins ("mixed TAPVD") is sometimes difficult to diagnose by noninvasive means. A combination of cross-sectional imaging and color flow mapping should however make it possible to identify individual pulmonary veins and their sites of drainage within the heart or to other extracardiac vascular structures in the majority of patients, and most patients with "uncomplicated" TAPVD can, in our experience be referred for surgery on the basis noninvasive investigation alone.

References

1) Fyler DC, Buckley LP, Hellebrand WE, Cohn HE. Report of the New England Infant Cardiac Program. Pediatrics 1980; 65 (Suppl): 376-461.

2 Sahn DJ, Allen HD, Lange LW, Goldberg SJ. Cross-sectional echocardiographic diagnosis of the sites of total anomalous pulmonary venous drainage. Circulation 1979; 60: 1317-25.

3) Smallhorn JF, Sutherland GR, Tommasini G, Hunter S, Anderson RH, Macartney FJ. Assessment of total anomalous pulmonary venous connection by two-dimensional echocardiography. Br Heart J 1981; 46: 613-23.

4) Stevenson JG, Kawabori I, Guntheroth WG. Pulsed Doppler echocardiographic detection of total anomalous pulmonary venous return: resolution of left atrial line. Am J Cardiol 1979; 44: 1155-8.

5) Skovranek J, Tuma S, Urbancova D, Samanek M. Range-gated pulsed Doppler echocardiographic diagnosis of supracardiac total anomalous pulmonary venous drainage. Circulation 1980; 61: 841-7.

6) Cooper MJ, Teitel D, Silverman NH, Enderlein MA. Study of the infradiaphragmatic total anomalous pulmonary venous connection with cross-sectional and pulsed Doppler echocardiography. Circulation 1984; 70: 412-6.

7) Smallhorn JF, Freedom RM. Pulsed Doppler echocardiography in the preoperative evaluation of total anomalous pulmonary venous connection. J Am Coll Cardiol 1986; 8: 1413-20.

8) Vitarelli A, Scapato A, Sanguigni V, Caminiti MC. Evaluation of total anomalous pulmonary venous drainage with cross-sectional color flow Doppler echocardiography. Eur Heart J 1986; 7: 190-5.

THE EVALUATION OF COMPLEX SHUNT LESIONS

Howard M. McAlpine

George R. Sutherland

Introduction

Complex intracardiac shunting, whether congenital or acquired often presents a difficult diagnostic challenge. The physical signs may be confusing or misleading, particularly in patients who have multiple sites where intracardiac shunting is occurring, and an accurate diagnosis cannot always be established despite cardiac catheterisation.

Noninvasive ultrasound studies have revolutionised the investigation of complex shunting in both congenital and acquired heart disease. Cross-sectional imaging can visualise most significant anatomical defects, although small defects may go undetected, and "echo dropout" can lead to erroneous false positive diagnoses. The diagnostic accuracy of cardiac ultrasound is markedly increased by Doppler studies, which can locate the site of small defects by identifying the blood flow disturbance associated with shunting. Nonetheless, interrogation of the cardiac chambers and great vessels by pulsed wave Doppler with the care that is necessary to exclude small or multiple sites of shunting is a time consuming process, and considerable operator experience is necessary in order that accurate results can be obtained. Furthermore, the spatial directions of the jets associated with high velocity restrictive shunts are difficult to predict and can be missed. In addition, both pulsed and continous wave Doppler may fail to detect non restrictive defects where flow is low velocity and laminar.

The advent of color flow mapping has greatly increased the ease and speed with which normal and abnormal intracardiac flow patterns can be identified. This modality is also more sensitive than conventional Doppler techniques for determining the presence of complex intracardiac shunts. Moreover, color flow mapping is the only noninvasive means of reliably identifying multiple sites of shunting occuring within the same cardiac chamber. Complex or rapidly changing flow patterns can be confusing on the color flow image, and the direction and timing of a shunt is often more readily appreciated by obtaining a color M-mode through the region of interest. When a shunt has been located, further hemodynamic information can be obtained by determining its velocity profile using pulsed and continuous wave Doppler. Color flow mapping can facilitate optimal alignment of the Doppler beam to the site of maximum shunt flow allowing accurate measurement of its peak velocity, and the direction and timing of flow can also be confirmed. The characteristic hemodynamic features of a shunt determined in this way assists in identifying its site of origin. Table 1 summarises the hemodynamic characteristics of most of the complex shunts encountered in relation to the cardiac chambers involved. Some of the more common sites of complex intra and extracardiac shunting are described in greater detail below.

CFM IN COMPLEX INTRACARDIAC SHUNTING		Diastolic		
		High velocity		**Low velocity**
Systolic	**High velocity** (> 2 m/sec) i) ii) iii) iv) v)	VSD/AR Coronary sinus fistulae Coronary artery fistulae Ao/RA fistulae Ao/LA fistulae	i) ii) iii) iv)	Congenital VSD Post infarct VSD LV Pseudo aneurysm LV/RA fistulae
	Low velocity (< 2 m/sec) i) ii)	Restrictive ASD Cor Triatriatum	i) ii) iii) iv)	ASD PAPVD Coronary sinus LV Pseudo aneurysm

Table 14-1 . CFM in Complex Intracardiac Shunting

Ruptured Sinus of Valsalva

A sinus of Valsalva aneurysm is a relatively uncommon congenital abnormality which usually occurs as an isolated anomaly, but may be associated with ventricular septal defects, aortic valve abnormalities and other congenital lesions. Most sinus of Valsalva aneurysms remain clinically silent and only present in adult life if rupture occurs. The resultant loud too and fro murmur may be confused with that associated with a patent arterial duct, a coronary artery fistula, severe aortic regurgitation, or the combination of ventricular septal defect and aortic incompetence. The right sinus of Valsalva is most often involved. This structure can rupture into the right ventricular outflow tract or right atrium. Occasionally a ruptured aneurysm may cause dissection of the interventricular septum or enter the left ventricle [1-4]. Rupture into two cardiac chambers is also possible if aneurysms involve more than one coronary sinus.

Discontinuity of echos at the apex of the aneurysm on 2-D imaging supports the diagnosis of rupture, although echo dropout may cause diagnostic difficulties. Pulsed wave Doppler is unlikely to miss the turbulent flow in systole and diastole when rupture is into the atria or right ventricle if a careful search is made, and color flow mapping facilitates localisation of the shunt (Fig.14-1). Continuous wave Doppler demonstrates high velocity systolic and diastolic shunting due to the high pressure gradient which exists between the aorta and the right heart chambers throughout the cardiac cycle. Occasionally, the aneurysm ruptures into the left ventricular outflow tract and may be mistaken for aortic regurgitation by pulsed wave Doppler. Indeed, aortic incompetence may coexist with a sinus of Valsalva rupture and neither pulsed nor continuous wave Doppler is able to reliably differentiate between these two jets. In contrast, color flow mapping readily demonstrates that the turbulent flow originates from the aneurysm rupture rather than through the valve orifice.

The rare condition of aorto-left ventricular tunnel should be considered in any neonate or infant with features suggesting sinus of valsalva rupture or severe aortic incompetence. Most cases are only diagnosed at surgery or autopsy, and angiography is difficult to interpret due to the associated severe aortic incompetence. Cross-sectional imaging can visualise the mouth of the tunnel above the sinus of Valsala and Doppler will confirm high velocity systolic and diastolic flow in the tunnel and left ventricular outflow tract [5-7].

Coronary Artery Lesions

(a) Anomalous Origin of the Coronary Arteries:

Anomalous origin of either the left or right coronary artery from the pulmonary artery usually causes significant left to right shunting in infancy or childhood and is associated with the development of severe ischemic cardiomyopathy and heart failure [8]. A minority are identified as teenagers when they present with symptoms of myocardial ischemic or are noted to have a murmur suggesting mitral incompetence. An accurate, early diagnosis is essential if left ventricular function is to be preserved. When anomalous origin of the left coronary artery is the only abnormality, the diagnosis will usually be clinically apparent. Nonetheless, the associated systolic murmur may be misinterpreted when mitral incompetence is present or overlooked when forming part of other complex congenital cardiac disorders. Moreover, aortic root angiography can give rise to appearances suggesting normal coronary artery connections, or may fail to accurately show the location of the connection to the pulmonary artery [9].

Anomalous origin of the left coronary artery is more common than involvement of the right system, and in either instance, visualisation of the connection with the pulmonary artery by cross-sectional imaging is extremely difficult. Dilatation of the right coronary artery, if present, is suggestive but not diagnostic of anomalous origin of the left coronary system, and could also occur with a right coronary artery fistula. Furthermore, the left coronary artery may appear to connect normally with the aortic root due to false "dropout" of echos between the aortic wall and the left coronary artery.

Pulsed and continuous wave Doppler can detect the turbulent diastolic shunt flow in the pulmonary artery, but this is of limited diagnostic value unless abnormal coronary artery connections are suspected, and tracing the origin of the shunt flow may not be possible [10]. Color flow mapping resolves these difficulties, and reliably shows the reversal of flow in the coronary artery, and the mosaic turbulent jet arising from the coronary ostium into the pulmonary artery [9,11,12]. In some instances, identification of the abnormal coronary flow on the color flow map may be the only clue as to the correct diagnosis. The site of connection to the pulmonary artery is usually but not invariably at a point just distal to the pulmonary valve and precise localisation of the coronary orifice with color flow mapping assists the surgeon to find it at operation.

(b) Coronary Artery Fistulas:

A coronary artery fistula is an abnormal communication between a coronary artery and any cardiac chamber, a pulmonary artery, or great vein. The majority are congenital in origin, but rarely may result from penetrating injuries, cardiac surgery or myocardial infarction [13-16]. More than 90% involve the right coronary artery with drainage into the right atrium, coronary sinus, or right ventricle [17]. A continuous murmur may arouse suspicion of a coronary artery fistula in otherwise asymptomatic children, and as shunting may become more severe in later life, coupled with the risk of endocarditis, elective closure is the preferred mode of management [13].

Recent reports document the ability of cross-sectional imaging and pulsed Doppler to detect coronary artery fistulas, but identification of the origin, course and site of drainage necessary for surgical intervention is not always possible [18-20]. The timing and velocity of the flow jet will depend on the magnitude of the shunt as well the site of drainage, and localisation of a small shunt can be extremely difficult with pulsed Doppler alone. In contrast, color flow mapping is a highly sensitive technique for detecting even small coronary artery fistulas, and has the additional advantage of being able to demonstrate that in some instances, multiple fistulous connections are present [11,21]. During surgical repair, intraoperative color flow mapping provides the surgeon with the opportunity to assess whether all such fistulous connections have been sucessfully ligated.

In adults, small clinically silent coronary artery fistulas are detected in approximately 1% of routine coronary angiograms [22]. The true incidence of these unimportant filamentous coronary connections is unknown, but it is likely that they will be increasingly detected as incidental findings by the more sensitive technique of color flow mapping.

Connections Between the Aorta and Pulmonary Artery

(1) Patent Ductus Arteriosus:

An isolated patent ductus arteriosus does not usually escape clinical detection, but when present with other complex cardiac disorders may be more difficult to diagnose. Identification of ductal patency is important in congenital heart disease, particularly when cyanosis is present, and the direction of flow within it should be established. Visualisation of the ductus arteriosus by cross-sectional imaging has been widely reported [23-26], but is of limited value in assessing patency of a small ductus. If the pulmonary arterial pressure is normal, there is continuous high velocity shunting from the ductus, directed along the anterolateral wall of the pulmonary artery towards the pulmonary valve. In systole, the ductal flow mixes with the antegrade pulmonary flow, and if pulsed doppler sampling is not in close proximity to the ductus, only normal systolic pulmonary flow may be recorded. In diastole, the retrograde ductal jet may reach as far as the pulmonary valve, before reversing direction and returning along the contralateral wall of the pulmonary artery. The retrograde flow jet can be traced back towards the bifurcation of the pulmonary artery and into the mouth of the patent ductus with pulsed wave Doppler. The peak velocity of the ductal shunt measured with continuous wave Doppler allows the pulmonary arterial pressure to be calculated [27]. Left to right shunting from the aorta also causes diastolic flow reversal in the descending aorta distal to the ductal diverticulum, and the extent of flow reversal provides a measure of the shunt magnitude.

When the ductus is small, the narrow retrograde diastolic jet in the pulmonary artery is easily missed, although it is usually possible to record the continuous diastolic antegrade flow along the opposite wall of the pulmonary artery. Thus it is important with pulsed Doppler to make multiple measurements across the width of the pulmonary artery in order that the characteristic flow patterns can be determined.

The diagnostic certainty of ductal patency is strengthened by color flow mapping which makes the task of identifying the mosaic retrograde diastolic jet very much easier, and it can be traced back to the mouth of a constricted ductus [28,29]. Additional problems are encountered using pulsed Doppler alone in the presence of pulmonary hypertension, when retrograde pulmonary artery diastolic ductal flow is of low velocity and may be difficult to separate from pulmonary incompetence, or non specific flow reversals in a dilated pulmonary artery. Color flow mapping differentiates between these different flow patterns, and may be the only means of identifying right to left shunting when pulmonary hypertension is severe [28]. The ease and speed with which the ductus arteriosus can be identified by color flow mapping is of particular benefit when keeping examination time short in critically ill infants.

(2) Aortopulmonary Window:

An aortopulmonary window is a direct communication between the ascending aorta and the main pulmonary artery due to incomplete division of the aorto-pulmonary septum. Functionally this may be similar to a patent ductus arteriosus, and results in similar clinical signs. The size and position of an aortopulmonary window is variable, and although cross-sectional imaging can visualise the defect, the accuracy of this technique is unknown. A ventricular septal defect or patent ductus arteriosus can coexist with aortopulmonary window, and as echo dropout on the aorto-pulmonary setum is often passed as normal, this potentially serious defect may be overlooked. Pulsed Doppler will show turbulent systolic and diastolic flow in the pulmonary artery, and color flow mapping confirms the presence of the defect by displaying continuous flow across the region of echo dropout in the aorto-pulmonary septum [30]. If the shunt is large, retrograde diastolic flow can also be recorded in the ascending aorta but unlike patent ductus arteriosus, the retrograde flow is proximal rather than distal to the ductal diverticulum.

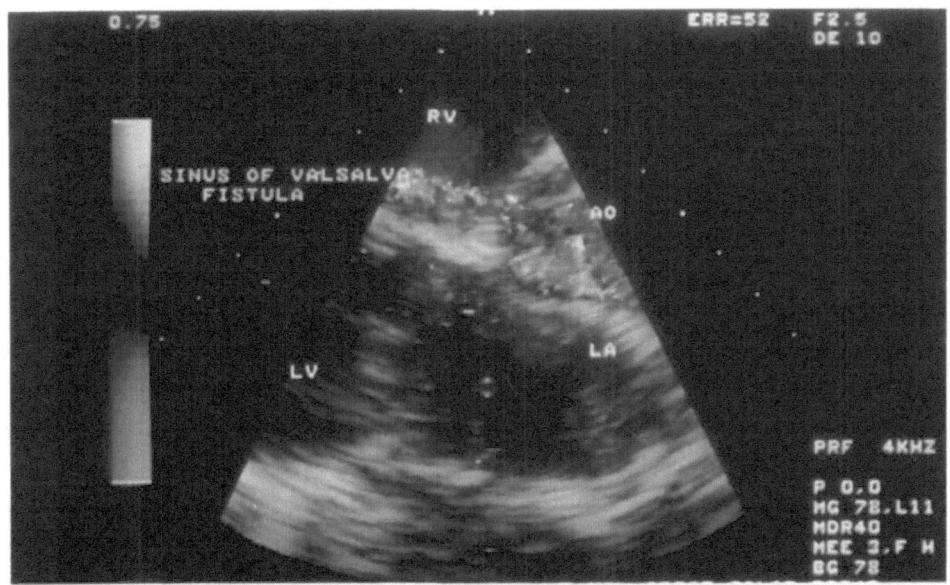

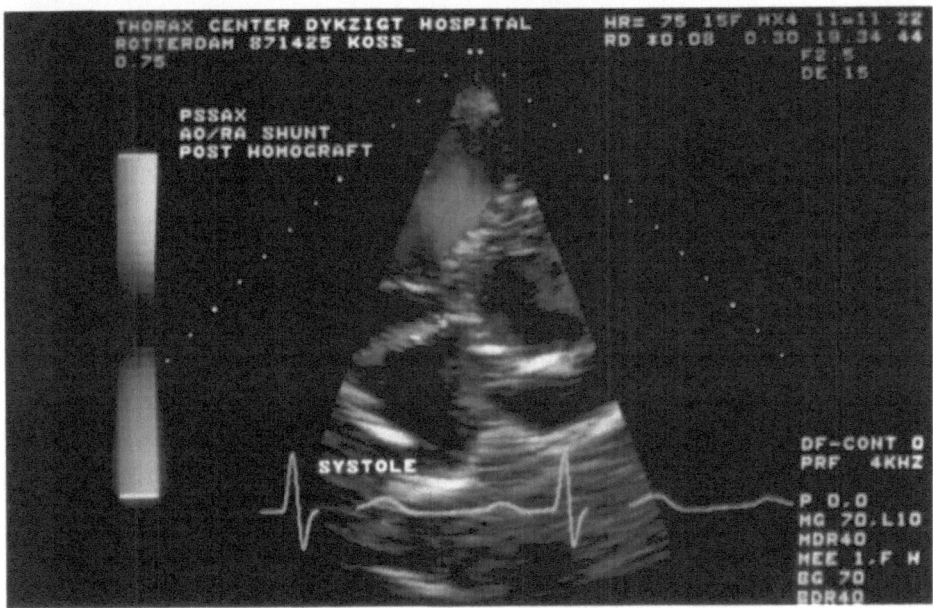

Figure 14-1. Parasternal long-axis view recorded during systole in a patient with a ruptured right sinus of Valsalva aneurysm. Color flow mapping shows a mosaic turbulent jet passing from the aortic wall into the right ventricle.

Figure 14-2. Parasternal short-axis view in a patient with a homograft aortic valve replacement. color flow mapping frozen in systole shows a shunt to the right atrium. High velocity flow was recorded throughout the cardiac cycle consistent with an aorto-right atrial communication.

(3) Aorto-pulmonary Shunts:

An aorto-pulmonary shunt is frequently carried out as a palliative procedure in patients with congenital cyanotic heart disease. These cyanotic infants may also have a patent arterial duct, and as both of these shunts cause continuous murmurs, the clinical distinction between them may be impossible. Over the years several methods have been devised for channeling aortic flow to the pulmonary circulation. The earliest shunts involved the creation of a direct aorto-pulmonary communication as in the Potts or Waterston shunts. More recently, an indirect shunt to the right pulmonary artery via the subclavian artery has been favoured as in the Blalock Taussig shunt, or by using an interposition graft between the aorta and the pulmonary artery. From a high right parasternal or suprasternal approach, the communication with the right pulmonary artery can often be visualised, and Doppler sampling within the shunt demonstrates high velocity continuous turbulent flow directed towards the pulmonary artery [31]. Pulsed Doppler sampling in the right pulmonary artery will show turbulent systolic and diastolic flow with a right Blalock-Taussig shunt, but similar appearances can arise from a large ductal shunt. Color flow mapping is helpful in locating the Blalock-Taussig shunt by the appearance of continuous mosaic colors of turbulent flow within its lumen. In comparison, as viewed from the suprasternal approach, flow in the ascending aortic flow is towards the transducer encoded in red, and the laminar flow in the superior vena cava encoded blue. A left Blalock–Taussig shunt can be located in a similar fashion, by imaging the transferse and descending aorta, and searching for a communication with the left pulmonary artery using color flow mapping and pulsed Doppler sampling.

Endocarditis Related Shunts

(1) Valve Lesions:

The visualisation of vegetations on valves by cross-sectional echocardiography provides important confirmatory evidence of infection in patients with suspected endocarditis. Valvar incompetence is common, and can be confirmed by pulsed and continuous wave Doppler. Color flow mapping aids quantification of the valvar incomptence, and may occasionally disclose that the regurgitant flow arises from a perforation in a valve leaflet rather than, or in addition to regurgitation through the valve orifice [32,33]. When a bioprosthetic valve becomes incompetent, the presence of a periprosthetic jet can be determined by color flow mapping, whereas neither pulsed Doppler nor conventional angiography can distinguish paravalvar regurgitation from an eccentric regurgitant jet caused by a peripheral tear in the valve cusp [34,35].

(2) Aortic Root Communications:

An aortic root abscess is a serious complication of infective endocarditis and is associated with an increased mortality. Visualisation of an abscess cavity is usually extremely difficult by praecordial cross-sectional imaging, although its presence is suggested by excessive thickening of the aortic wall. Transesophageal echocardiography provides much more detailed imaging of the medial, lateral and posterior aspects of the aortic root than praecordial echocardiography, and is now the technique of choice for identifying abscess cavities. Imaging from the oesophagus has the additional advantage of overcoming the problem of echo masking of the posterior aspect of the aortic root when a mechanical prostheses is in situ.

Extension of the abscess cavity from the aorta into the perivalvar tissue may ultimately lead to penetration of the atria or the right ventricle [36]. As in the case of sinus of Valsalva rupture discussed earlier, color flow mapping provides an excellent means of identifying the direction of abscess rupture (Fig. 14-2). Subsequent interrogation of the flow jet by continuous wave Doppler will identify the high velocity systolic and diastolic flow pattern consistent with an aortic communication.

(3) Left Ventricular Outflow Tract Communications:

Occasionally, an abscess cavity involves the left ventricular outflow tract and communicates with the left atrium or right ventricle (Fig.14-3). The defect may be visualised on cross-sectional imaging, and Doppler will show turbulent systolic flow in the region of the defect [37]. In the case of a left atrial communication, the flow jet must be distinguished from an eccentric regurgitant jet through the mitral orifice or a peripheral leaflet perforation, and this is most easily accomplished by color flow mapping.

(4) Left ventriculo-right atrial communications:

A left ventricular to right atrial communication due to a defect in the atrioventricular septum is rarely congenital in origin, and is more commonly associated with either aortic valve replacement or aortic valve endocarditis (Fig. 14-4). The shunt is usually small and not recognised until cardiac catheterisation. Opacification of the right atrium after left ventriculography is diagnostic, although small defects may go undetected. Pulsed wave Doppler shows turbulent systolic flow entering the right atrium in the region of the defect, and must be distinguished from tricuspid regurgitation which may also be present. When two flow jets entering the right atrium are in close proximity or cross, it is possible that one may be overestimated or the other missed entirely by pulsed Doppler. Color flow imaging can guide pulsed Doppler sampling for velocity measurement to sites where the flow jets do not intermingle, and may also help to determine the origin of the shunt. Blood flow in the left ventricle accelerates as it approaches the communication with the right atrium causing a localised area of aliasing on the color map. Thus, by scanning the left ventricular outflow tract and the atrioventricular septum, the appearance of a convergence zone of aliased high velocity flow on the wall of the left ventricle identifies the origin of the shunt.

Congenital communications between the left ventricle and the right atrium can be divided into those that occur above or below the level of the attachment of the tricuspid valve. In the infravalvar form, the septal leaflet of the tricuspid valve is often cleft or perforated and may be closely adherent to the margins of a perimembranous ventricular septal defect. Thus the shunt occurs indirectly, passing through the cleft in the tricuspid valve, and this can be confirmed by color flow mapping.

In addition to a cleft in the mitral or tricuspid valve, more extensive anatomical abnormalities of the atrioventricular connections including a straddling tricuspid valve or a common atrioventricular valve may be associated with atrioventicular canal defects. Valvar regurgitation is common, and color flow mapping is the most appropriate technique for identifying whether single or multiple regurgitant jets are present (Fig. 14-5).

Conclusion

In conclusion, this chapter has dealt with several uncommon but important causes of left to right shunting. Although dealt with separately here, it should be appreciated that in congenital heart disease, several sites of shunting may coexist . The complete ultrasound examination should include a careful search for unsuspected communications, and screening is optimally carried out by a combination of cross-sectional imaging and color flow mapping. If abnormal flow is recorded, pulsed and continuous wave Doppler provide complimentary information relating to the characteristic waveform and velocity of individual shunts and allows calculation of shunt magnitude. Growing experience with color flow mapping is showing that it not only facilitates alignment of spectral Doppler beams, but it is also the quickest and most accurate technique for identifying complex intra and extracardiac shunts. In some circumstances, such as with small coronary artery fistulas, color flow mapping may be the only means of detecting these abnormalities.

Those not familiar with the spectral waveforms from pulsed and continuous wave Doppler find color flow maps easier to understand, and abnormal jets can be appreciated at a glance. This is particularly useful when time is short during intraoperative studies or when dealing with very ill children. In the future it seems likely that color flow mapping will progressively reduce the need to resort to invasive proceedures to establish diagnoses, and surgeons will become more confident in accepting echocardiographic findings. From initial beginnings when it was viewed simply as an appealing way to demonstrate intracardiac flow, color flow mapping is now firmly established as a powerful diagnostic tool.

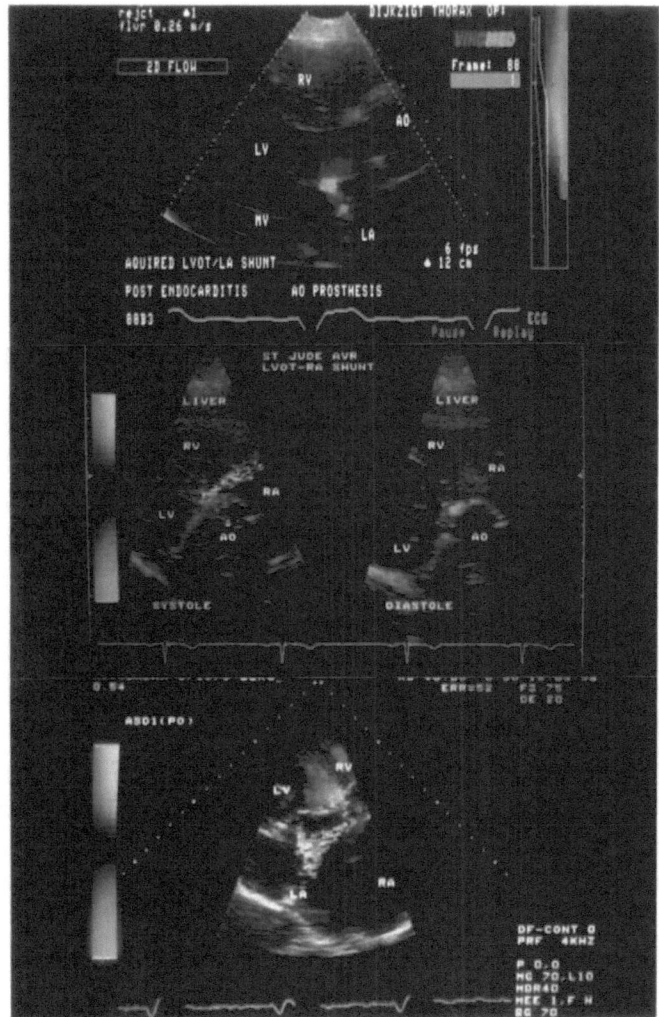

Figure 14-3. Parasternal long-axis view in a patient treated for endocarditis of the prosthetic aortic valve. Color flow mapping shows a mosaic jet from the left ventricular outflow tract to the left atrium in systole in keeping with penetration by an abscess cavity.

Figure 14-4. Subcostal cross-sectional imaging following a St Jude aortic valve replacement. Color flow mapping shows a turbulent systolic jet passing from the left ventricular outflow tract to the right atrium. A small low velocity, non turbulent jet is seen within the communication during diastole.

Figure 14-5. Color flow mapping in the four-chamber view demonstrating a central orifice jet of regurgitation through a common atrioventricular valve and a second reurgitant jet through a cleft.

References

1. Cheng CW, Lin FC, Fang BR, Kuo CT, Lee YS and Chang CH. Doppler and two-dimensional echocardiographic features of sinus of Valsalva aneurysm. Am Heart J 1988;116:1283-1288

2. Terdjman N, Bourdarias JP, Farcot JC, Gueret P, Dudourg O, Ferrier A and Hanania G. Aneurysms of sinus of Valsalva: two dimensional echocardiographic diagnosis and recognition of rupture into the right heart cavities. J Am Coll Cardiol 1984;3:1227-1235.

3. Chen WWC and Tai YT. Dissection of the interventricular septum by aneurysm of sinus of Valsalva. Br Heart J 1983;50:293-295.

4. Chow LC, Dittrich HC, Dembitsky WP and Nicod PH. Accurate localisation of ruptured sinus of Valsalva aneurysm by real-time Doppler flow imaging. Chest 1988;94:462-465.

5. Norwicki ER, Aberdeen E, Friedma S and Rashkind WJ. Congenital left aortic sinus-left ventricular fistula and review of aortocardiac fistulas. Am Thorac Surg 1977;23:378-388.

6. Perry JC, Nanda NC, Hicks DG and Harris JP. Two dimensional echocardiographic identification of aortico-left ventricular tunnel. Am J Cardiol 1983;52:913-4.

7. Bash SE, Huhta JC, Nihill MR, Vargo TA and Hallman GL. Aortico-left ventricular tunnel with ventricular septal defect: two dimensional/Doppler echocardiographic diagnosis. J Am Coll Cardiol 1985;5:757-760.

8. Wesselhoeft H, Fawcett JS and Johnson AL. Anomalous origin of the left coronary artery from the pulmonary trunk. Its clinical spectrum, pathology, and pathophysiology, based on a review of 140 cases, with seven further cases. Circ 1968;38:403-425.

9. Houston AB, Pollock JCS, Doig WB, Gnanapragasam J, Jamieson M, Lilley S and Murtagh EP. Anomalous origin of the left coronary artery from the pulmonary trunk: Elucidation with colour Doppler flow mapping. Br Heart J 1990;63:50-54.

10. King DH, Danford DA, Huhta JC and Gutgesell HP. Non-invasive detection of anomalous origin of the left main coronary artery from the pulmonary trunk by pulsed Doppler echocardiography. Am J Cardiol 1985;55:608-609.

11. Saunders SP, Parness IA and Colan SD. Recognition of abnormal connections of coronary arteries with the aid of Doppler color flow mapping. J Am Coll Cardiol 1989;13:922-926.

12. Swensson RE, Murillo-Olivas A, Elias W, Bender R, Daily PO, and Sahn DJ. Non-invasive Doppler color flow mapping for detection of anomalous origin of the left coronary artery from the pulmonary artery and for evaluation of surgical repair. J Am Coll Cardiol 1988;11:659-661.

13. Liberthson RR, Sagar K, Berkoben JP, Weintraub RM and Levine FH. Congenital coronary arteriovenous fistula. Report of 13 patients, review of the literature and delineation of management. Circ. 1979;59:849-853.

14. Liberthson RR, Barron K, Harthorne JW, Dinsmore RE, and Daggett WM. Traumatic coronary arterial fistula. A case report and review of the literature. Am Heart J 1973;86:817-821.

15. Lee RT, Mudge GH and Colucci WS. Coronary artery fistula after mitral valve replacement. Am Heart J. 1988;115:1128-1130.

16. Yu R, Sharma B and Franciosa JA. Acquired coronary artery fistula to the left ventricle after acute myocardial infarction. Am J Cardiol 1986;58:557-558.

17. Eagle KA, Haber E, De Santis RW, and Austen WG, Eds. The Practise of Cardiology. Second Edition 1988 pp630-636. Little, Brown and Company, Boston/Toronto.

18. Chen CC, Hwang B, Hsiung MC, Chiang BN, Meng Lc, Wang DJ and Wang SP. Recognition of coronary arterial fistula by Doppler 2-dimensional echocardiography. Am J Cardiol 1984;53:392-394.

19. Miyatake K, Okamoto M, Kinoshita N, Fusejima K, Sakakibara H and Nimura Y. Doppler echocardiographic features of coronary arteriovenous fistula. Br Heart J 1984;51:508-518.

20. Reeder GS, Tajik AJ and Smith HC. Visualisation of coronary fistula by two-dimensional echocardiography. Mayo Clin Proc 1980;55:185-189.

21. Velmis H, Schmidt KG, Silverman NH, and Turley K. Diagnosis of coronary artery fistula by two dimensional echocardiography, pulsed Doppler ultrasound and color flow imaging. J Am Coll Cardiol 1989;14:968-976.

22. Lefevre T and Bernard A. Left coronaro-ventricular microfistula. Arch Mal Coeur 1988;81:285-292.

23. Sahn DJ and Allen HD. Real-time cross-sectional echocardiographic imaging and measurement of the patent ductus arteriosus in infants and children. Circ 1978;58:343-354.

24. Smallhorn JF, Huhta JC, Anderson RH and Macartney FJ. Suprasternal cross-sectional echocardiography in assessment of patent ductus arteriosus. Br Heart J 1982;48:321-330.

25. Huhta JC, Gutgesell HP, Latson LA and Huffines FD. Two-dimensional echocardiographic assessment of the aorta in infants and children with congenital heart disease. Circ 1984;70:417-424.

26. Perez JE, Nordlicht SM and Geltman EM. Patent ductus arteriosus in adults: diagnosis by suprasterna and parasternal pulsed Doppler echocardiography. Am J Cardiol 1984;53:1473-1475.

27. Musewe NN, Smallhorn JF, Benson LN, Burrows PE and Freedom RM. Validation of Doppler-derived pulmonary arterial pressure in patients with ductus arteriosus under different haemodynamic states. Circ 1987;76:1081-1091.

28. Swensson RE, Valdes-Cruz LM, Sahn DJ, Sherman FS, Chung KJ, Scagnelli S and Hagen-Ansert S. Real-time Doppler color flow mapping for detection of patent ductus arteriosus. L Am Coll Cardiol 1986;8:1105-1112.

29. Liao PK, Su WJ and Hung JS. Doppler echocardiographic flow characteristics of isolated patent ductus arteriosus: better delineation by Doppler color flow mapping. J Am Coll Cardiol 1988;12:1285-1291.

30. Alboliras ET, Chin AJ, Barber G, Helton JG and Pigott JD. Detection of aortopulmonary window by pulsed and color Doppler echocardiography. Am Heart J 1988;115:900-902.

31. Stevenson JG, Kawabori I and Bailey WW. Noninvasive evaluation of Blalock-Taussig shunts: determination of patency and differentiation from patent ductus arteriosus by Doppler echocardiography. Am Heart J 1983;106:1121-1132.

32. Miyatake K, Yamamoto K, Park YD, Izumi S, Yamagishi M, Sukakibara H and Nimura Y. Diagnosis of mitral valve perforation by real time two-dimensional Doppler flow imaging technique. J Am Coll Cardiol

1986;8:1235-1239.

33. Decroly P, Vandenbossche JL and Englert M. Anterior mitral valve aneurysm perforation secondary to aortic valve endocarditis detected by Doppler colour flow mapping. Eur Heart J 1989;10:186-189.

34. Kapur KK, Fan P, Nanda NC, Yoganathan AP and Goyal RG. Doppler color flow mapping in the evaluation of prosthetic mitral and aortic valve function. J Am Coll Cardiol 1989;13:1561-1571.

35. Alam M, Rosman HS, Lakier JB, Kemp S, Khada F, Hautamaki K, Magilligan DJ and Stein PD. Doppler and echocardiographic features of normal and dysfunctioning bioprostheic valves. J Am Coll Cardiol 1987;10:851-858.

36. Arnett EN and Roberts WC. Clinicopathological analysis of 22 necropsy patients with comparison of observations in 74 necropsy patients with active infective endocarditis involving natural left-sided cardiac valves. Am J Cardiol 1976;38:281-291.

37. Fisher EA, Estioko MR, Stern EH and Goldman ME. Left ventricular to left atrial communication secondary to a para aortic abscess: color flow Doppler documentation. J Am Coll Cardiol 1987;10:222-224.

38. Sutherland GR, Balaji S, Monro JL. Potential value of intraoperative Doppler colour flow mapping in operations for complex intracardiac shunting. Br Heart J 1989;62:467-469.

CHAPTER XV

TETRALOGY OF FALLOT, PULMONARY ATRESIA AND TRUNCUS ARTERIOSUS

George R. Sutherland

Tetralogy of Fallot

Morphologic considerations.

This common condition is characterised by three coexisting morphologic abnormalities; 1) a large unrestrictive ventricular septal defect which is sub aortic in position; 2) override of the aorta above the defect with aortic displacement toward the right ventricle and; 3) obstruction of the right ventricular outflow tract. Tetralogy of Fallot normally presents as an isolated lesion but may be associated with other complex morphologic abnormalities (such as a complete atrioventricular defect) in a small number of cases.[1,2]

Each of the three coexisting abnormalities can vary considerably in its morphology.The sub-aortic ventricular septal defect is most commonly of the perimembranous outlet type (Fig.15-1) but can be solely located in the muscular outtlet septum. The defect is normally large and non-restrictive (i.e, the peak systolic pressure in the ventricles are equal). However where there has been a posterior extension of the perimembranous outlet defect into the inlet septum rare cases have been reported of the defect becoming progressively more restrictive as a result of ingrowth of tissue around the defect margins from the tricuspid valve septal leaflet.This fibrous tissue ingrowth forms a tricuspid pseudoaneurysm around the defect margins. More commonly additional multiple ventricular septal defects may coexist with the additional defects usually occurring in the apical or central trabecular septum.

The degree of aortic displacement varies considerably within the spectrum of Tetralogy of Fallot. At one end of the spectrum override may be minimal and the morphologic diagnosis of a combination of an isolated perimembranous outlet ventricular septal defect with associated infundibular or valvar pulmonary stenosis may be more correct. At the other end of the spectrum Tetralogy shades imperceptibly into the spectrum of hearts whose morphology is defined as Double Outlet Right Ventricle. While little change normally occurs in either the morphology of the ventricular septal defect or in the degree of aortic override during the natural history of patients with Tetralogy it is the changes in the morphology of the right heart outlet obstructive lesions which determines the clinical course. Four main outlet lesions may be present 1) infundibular (muscular) pulmonary stenosis, 2) pulmonary valve stenosis (with or without valve hypoplasia), 3) supra-pulmonary stenosis and 4) branch pulmonary artery stenosis. All four forms can be progressive lesions. Each of the four obstructive lesions may occur in isolation but in virtually every case of Tetralogy at least two are present.

Cross-sectional Imaging.

Within the spectrum of complex heart lesions Tetralogy of Fallot is one of the easiest of cross-sectional imaging diagnoses to make as b~ th the large sub-arterial ventricular septal defect and the presence of aortic override are readily appreciated as soon as the left ventricular long axis plane is scanned. However, these cross-sectional imaging features are also common to hearts with Tetralogy, Double Outlet Right Ventricle, Pulmonary Atresia with Ventricular Septal Defect and Truncus Arteriosus. Thus the differentiation of Tetralogy from the other three entities depends on the definition of both the right ventricular outflow tract anatomy and the morphology of the vessels supplying the lungs.

In normal patients an imaging scan of the right ventricular outflow tract and pulmonary arteries carried out from a series of middle to high left parasternal positions will allow the direct visualisation of the pulmonary valve ring and valve leaflets, the main pulmonary artery and the proximal portions of its right and left main branches. In the normal patient little is seen of the infundibulum of the right ventricle when imaging from the precordial approach. However, in small infants and some young children the whole of the right ventricle (inlet and outlet muscular infundibulum) can be scanned in a sagittal plane with the transducer placed in the subcostal position. This unique view of the right ventricular infundibulum cannot normally be obtained in older children and adults.[3]

To distinguish Tetralogy for the other lesions with similar intracardiac morphology (Pulmonary Atresia with Ventricular Septal Defect; Truncus Arteriosus) a complete scan of the right ventricular infundibulum, valve, main and branch pulmonary arteries should be carried out[4]. In virtually every case of Tetralogy, short-axis precordial cross-sectional imaging will demonstrate the presence of a normally positioned and patent right ventricular outflow tract and pulmonary valve ring. Where the pulmonary valve ring is significantly hypoplastic, the degree of hypoplasia be readily appreciated on the cross-sectional image. Where the pulmonary valve leaflets are conclusively seen to open then pulmonary atresia at valve level can effectively be excluded. However, imaging alone can give no information on the severity of either the infundibular or valve stenosis. The main and branch pulmonary arteries will normally be seen to be confluent and to be in continuity with the pulmonary valve. Cross-sectional imaging however is a poor technique for use in the evaluation of possible main or branch pulmonary artery stenosis. Furthermore it cannot define the relative severity of any stenosis thus imaged. However the identification of a patent pulmonary valve on the cross-sectional imaging examination will distinguish Tetralogy from Truncus and Pulmonary Atresia with Ventricular Septal Defect (in the case of the latter abnormality, ambiguity in the differentiation from Tetralogy will exists only where the pulmonary atresia is caused by an imperforate membrane at valve level. In such cases it may be impossible to distinguish this entity from severe pulmonary stenosis without the demonstration of obstructed trans-valve flow by continuous wave Doppler).

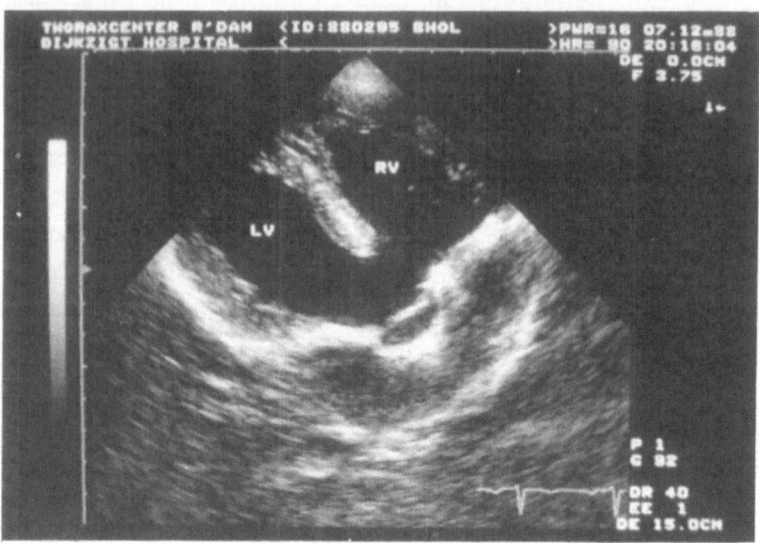

Figure 15-1. A precordial apical four chamber view demonstrating a large perimembranous outlet ventricular septal defect in a patient with Tetralogy of Fallot. Note the large aorta which overrides the defect. The aortic valve is seen to form the upper margin of the defect.

The Role of Doppler in the Evaluation of Tetralogy of Fallot.

a. In the Initial diagnosis - Evaluation of the right ventricular outflow tract.

The majority of infants born with Tetralogy of Fallot are clinically acyanotic during the first few weeks or months of life. It is only with the development of increasing sub pulmonary or pulmonary valve obstruction that significant right to left shunting across the non-restrictive ventricular septal defect occurs. Continuous wave Doppler examination in the neonate is of value in detecting the abnormal high velocity waveform over the right ventricular outflow tract which is indicative of obstruction. This waveform may be one of two types 1) fixed obstructive (Fig 2) (associated with valve stenosis) or 2) dynamic obstructive (Fig 3) (associated with dynamic infundibular stenosis due to smooth muscle contraction). Indeed, using an appropriate transducer position from which the interrogating Doppler beam transects both obstructive lesions (where both are present) in a sequential manner then both systolic waveforms, dynamic and fixed, can be recorded simultaneously one within the other (Figs 2 + 4). The highest peak velocity of the combined waveforms thus recorded will usually represent the maximal instantaneous pressue drop across the whole right ventricular outflow tract. Thus the two components to the lesion can effectively be considered as a single combined lesion and should not be analysed as two serial lesions.

When studying a neonate with Tetralogy it is usual to record both the dynamic and a fixed obstructive waveforms. However some neonates may have only a dynamic obstructive waveform indicative of isolated infundibular stenosis. It is our experience that such infants are particularly prove to developing hypercyanotic attacks during the first few weeks or months of life. In two cases we have carried out a continuous wave Doppler study during such a hypercyanotic spell and its subsequent treatment. Both studies demonstrated the same sequence of events to occur within the right ventricular outflow tract. With the onset of hypercyanotic symptoms, the time from the onset of the dynamic obstruction to the peak pressure gradient became progressively later in systole with no related increase in its peak velocity. With disappearance of the systolic murmur on clinical examination the signal strength of the dynamic waveform became progressively less until in one case it became absent altogether. With appropriate therapy in both cases the dynamic waveform rapidly returned to baseline level.

In both the neonate and infant, prior to surgical correction, no pulmonary incompetence waveform is normally recorded by continuous wave Doppler examination. However, in the few patients with Tetralogy and Absent Pulmonary Valve Syndrome severe pulmonary incompetence will be present from birth. In this condition no true pulmonary valve is formed but ridges of valve tissue are often present in the right ventricular outflow tract. These can give rise to outflow tract obstruction which is usually moderate and which on continuous wave Doppler examination is associated with a fixed obstruction waveform. It is this combination of obstruction to forward flow and severe pulmonary incompetence which gives rise to the "sawing" murmur so characteristic of the neonate with this rare lesion.

The Ventricular Septal Defect.

The majority of neonates and infants with Tetralogy remain acyanotic during the first few months of life. Indeed, many will have only left to right shunting at ventricular level. It is only with the development of increasing right ventricular outflow tract obstruction that significant bi-directional shunting occurs over the ventricular septal defect and the infant becomes clinically cyanotic. Indeed in some cases so large is the initial left to right shunt that turbulent flow may be observed within both the defect itself and in the adjacent portion of the right ventricular cavity. Both pulsed Doppler and color M-mode examinations of the flow characteristics within the defect will define the precise duration and direction of flow. Continuous wave Doppler may record a peak jet velocity of up to 2.5 metre/sec where there is a large left to right shunt but normally the peak velocity of flow within the defect is < 1.5 metre/sec. Apart from in those patients with very large left to right shunts (previously described) color flow mapping will demonstrate flow within the defect to be laminar (Fig 5). As in all patients where equal peak systolic ventricular pressures are associated with multiple ventricular septal defects then color flow mapping may be of limited value in defining other defects within the trabecular septum. This is equally true of patients who have Tetralogy of Fallot. A detailed search for distal defects should always be made but it should be appreciated that if such defects exist they will often be missed even in the most experienced hands.

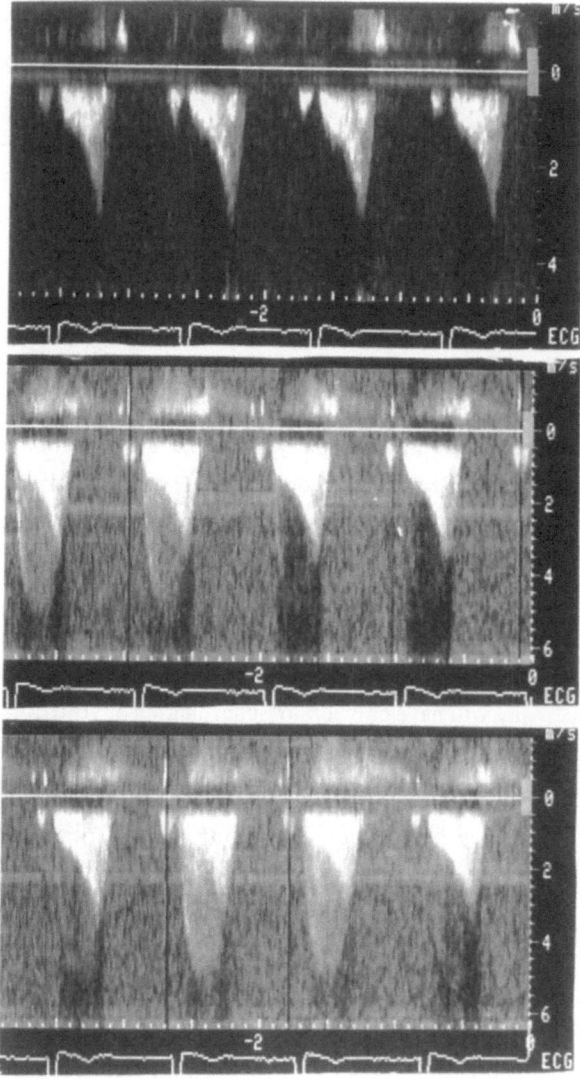

Figure 15-2. A continuous wave Doppler recording of the velocity profiles within the right ventricular outflow tract from a patient with Tetralogy of Fallot in whom the obstruction was predominately at valve level. Both fixed and dynamic obstructive are seen. Upper panel: this demonstrates an isolated dynamic obstruction waveform obtained from a low left parasternal transducer position with the transducer angled towards the mid-to-upper portion of the right ventricular outflow tract. Mid panel: with subsequent transducer angulation superiorly towards the pulmonary valve, two waveforms are recorded, one within the envelope of the other. The fixed obstructive waveform is well seen in the first two beats and is the waveform with the higher peak velocity which rises more rapidly to a peak. The dynamic waveform is seen within the velocity envelope of the fixed obstruction and is seen to rise to a late velocity peak. Lower panel: With further transducer angulation towards the pulmonary valve the dynamic waveform may be lost and only the fixed waveform recorded. This sequence of recordings can be made in almost every case of Tetralogy of Fallot.

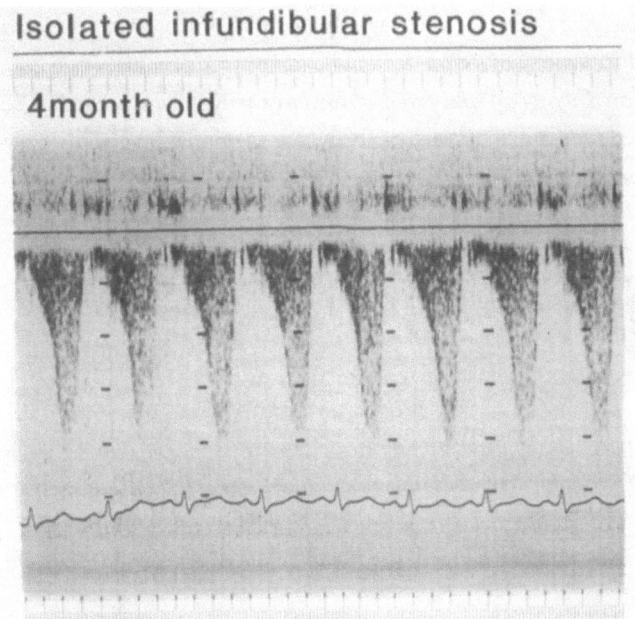

Fig 15-3. An isolated dynamic obstructive waveform recorded by continuous wave Doppler from an infant with Tetralogy of Fallot. It is unusual to have no co-existing fixed obstruction in this condition but this may occur in neonates and infants.

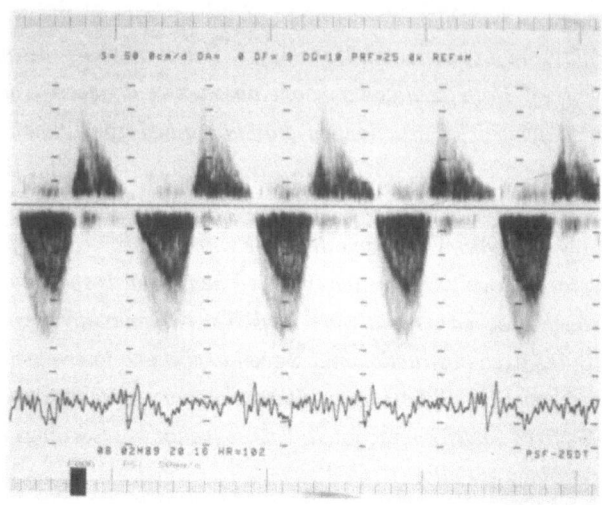

Fig 15-4. A post operative continuous wave Doppler study of right ventricular outflow tract flow in a patient with Tetralogy of Fallot. Residual mild obstruction persists within the outflow tract with both residual dynamic and fixed obstructive waveforms recorded. Note also the diastolic waveform of pulmonary incompetence which is almost invariably present in cases where a trans-annular patch has been placed at surgery.

Fig 5. A color flow map recorded from an unoperated patient with Tetralogy of Fallot. The heart is viewed in the left ventricular long-axis plane. Note the large non-restrictive ventricular septal defect with the aorta over-riding the defect. Color flow mapping demonstrates laminar systolic flow from left to right across the defect. This is indicative of equal peak systolic ventricular pressures.

Fig 6. An apical four-chamber view from a post operative patient with Tetralogy of Fallot. The color flow map demonstrates a systolic turbulent jet crossing the upper end of the septal defect patch from left to right ventricle. This confirms the presence of a residual ventricular septal defect.

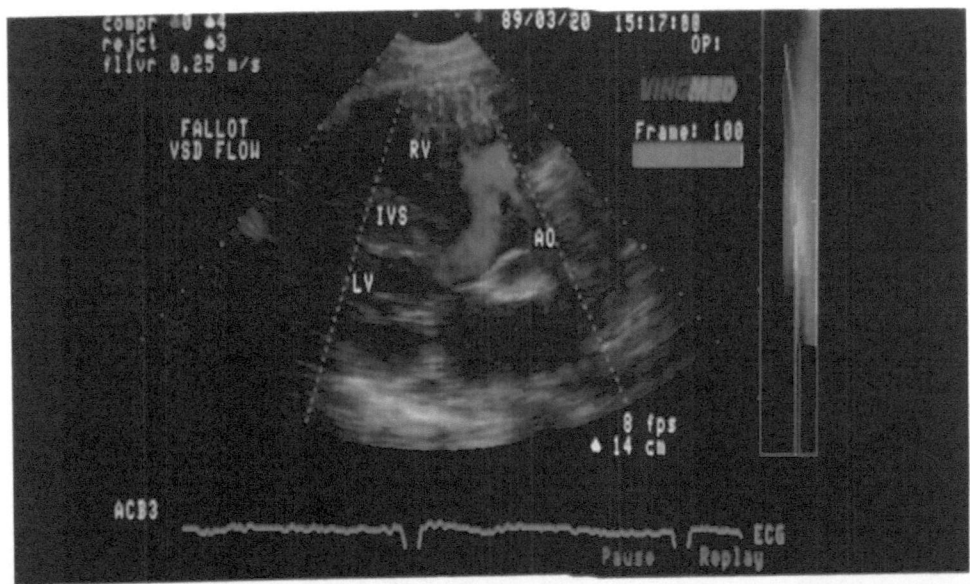

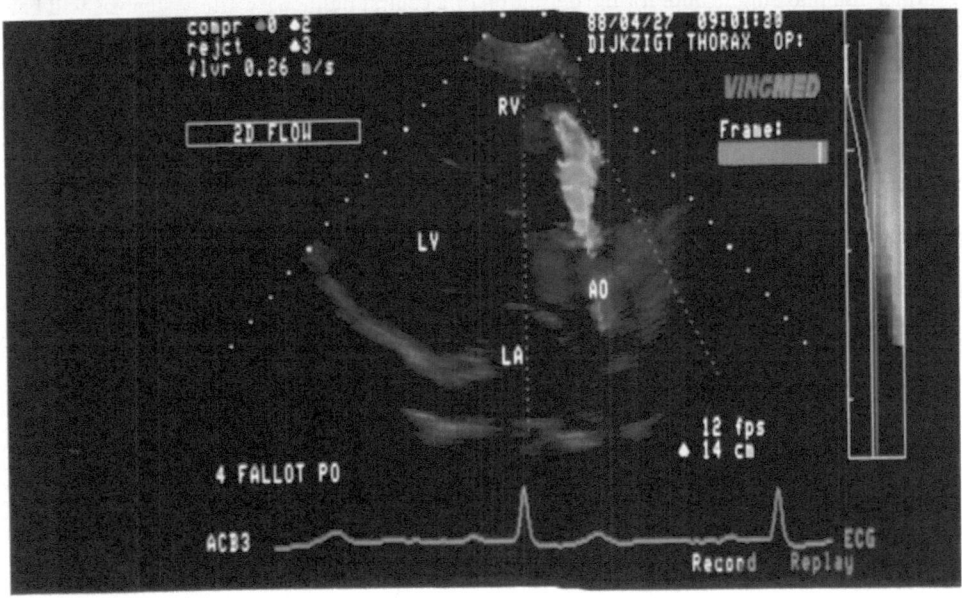

The Definition of the Pulmonary Arteries

Frequently cross-sectional imaging of pulmonary artery morphology is difficult in Tetralogy of Fallot. This may be due to hyperinflation of the lungs, a chest deformity or prior cardiac surgery. Neither the right ventricular outflow tract, pulmonary valve and valve ring nor the main and branch pulmonary arteries may be adequately visualised. Color flow mapping is frequently of additional value in defining these entities. This is because within the ultrasound machine the Doppler information which is processed to make up the color flow maps is acquired and analysed separately from the imaging information and is only overlain on the cross-sectional image as a final step in the production of the combined image. Thus, because of its inherent sensitivity, color flow mapping information can demonstrate areas of flow within structures within a cross-sectional image when no discernable structure can be seen. Furthermore the color flow mapping information can demonstrate where flow is laminar, aliased or turbulent and thus can give much indirect information evidence on cardiac morphology.

Areas of obstructed flow, denoted by systolic turbulence on the color flow map, will normally be visualised within the right ventricular outflow tract and over the pulmonary valve in patients with Tetralogy who have obstructions at these levels. The turbulent flow caused by the valvar stenosis normally extends far out into the branch pulmonary arteries. In this situation any further obstructions within the central pulmonary arteries will normally be masked (imaging alone is a very insensitive technique for defining main or branch pulmonary artery narrowings). A further complicating feature for the definition of a central pulmonary artery stenosis will be the concomitant presence of turbulent duct or aorto-pulmonary shunt flow into the pulmonary arteries. The widespread intra-pulmonary turbulence caused by either of these entities can similarly mask a central pulmonary artery stenosis

In Summary, the combination of information derived from cross-sectional imaging, spectral Doppler and color flow mapping should always allow the diagnosis of patients with Tetralogy of Fallot to be made. However, less than optimal information may be obtained on the number of ventricular septal defects, the precise morphology of the infundibular stenosis and the morphology of the central or distal pulmonary arteries. In addition, coronary artery anomalies cannot be excluded. Angiography remains an essential adjunct prior to surgical repair of this abnormality.

Ultrasound in the Evaluation of the Repair of Tetralogy of Fallot

The various Doppler modalities when appropriately integrated can provide a very accurate assessment of the results of the repair of Tetralogy of Fallot. Cross-sectional imaging alone is of limited value in the evaluation of this patient group as it can neither reliably identify a residual septal defect nor does it provide information of value in excluding residual right ventricular outflow tract obstruction. As such residual defects are virtually always partially restrictive color flow mapping is a very sensitive technique in detecting any residual interventricular shunting either associated with patch dehiscence (Fig 6) or with the presence of an unsuspected additional defect in a distal site. Continuous wave Doppler interrogation can normally derive the peak velocity of systolic flow across the defect and thus allow an accurate estimation of right ventricular peak systolic pressure to be made (Fig 7). Continuous wave Doppler can also determine accurately the systolic and diastolic velocity profiles of flow over right ventricular outflow tract (Fig 8). Any residual outflow tract obstruction can be excluded. The presence of pulmonary incompetence is normally easily identified and much can be deduced about its severity from the pulmonary incompetence waveform. In general, the lower the peak velocity in diastole and the shorter the time taken to equalise pulmonary artery and right ventricular diastolic pressures, the greater the degree of pulmonary incompetence. Pulsed Doppler should be used to better define the diastolic waveform. Athough residual obstruction (either dynamic or fixed) within the outflow tract can be accurately measured problems arise when attempting to exclude or evaluate any branch pulmonary artery stenosis. This is because such lesions are seldom well visualised by cross-sectional imaging and are normally lie at right angles to the interrogating Doppler beam (Fig 9). Color flow mapping is both a sensitive and specific technique for identifying such lesions within the central pulmonary arteries. Even where imaging fails to demonstrate any structure discernable as the pulmonary arteries color flow mapping can demonstrate areas of turbulence within the sector image indicative of obstruction within the central pulmonary arteries (Figs 10 + 11). Severe obstruction between the main pulmonary artery and either left or right pulmonary artery will normally be associated with systolic antegrade turbulence across the obstruction with holo-diastolic turbulent flow back across the obstruction into the main pulmonary artery. More distal obstructive lesions within the pulmonary arterial bed cannot be excluded by ultrasound examination and their exclusion requires either angiographic or magnetic resonance imaging exclusion.

Ultrasound Evaluation of Pulmonary Atresia with VSD

The methodology used in the evaluation of the intracardiac morphology associated with this condition should be essentially the same as that previously described in the section on Tetralogy of Fallot. The most common abnormality of right ventricular outflow tract morphology in this condition is absence of the connexion between the right ventricle and the pulmonary arteries. The right ventricular outflow tract is either absent or miniscule. The morphology of the lung blood supply is extremely variable in this condition and may be very complex.The main pulmonary artery may be absent or very short and hypoplastic. The right and left pulmonary arteries may both be present and of normal size but may or may not be confluent. In Complex Pulmonary Atresia lung blood supply is effected primarily by collateral vessels which take origin from the descending aorta. These may or may not connect with a true intrapericardial central pulmonary arterial system. If this latter entity is present it is usually extremely hypoplastic. If the above description suggests that the complexity of the pumonary vessel morphology which may be present would preclude accurate ultrasound evaluation this is not quite correct. Some useful information can be obtained in this patient group by carefully conducted ultrasound studies. This is especially true of the evaluation of neonates presenting with this condition in whom both medical and surgical management decisions can frequently be made based on only ultrasound information [5].

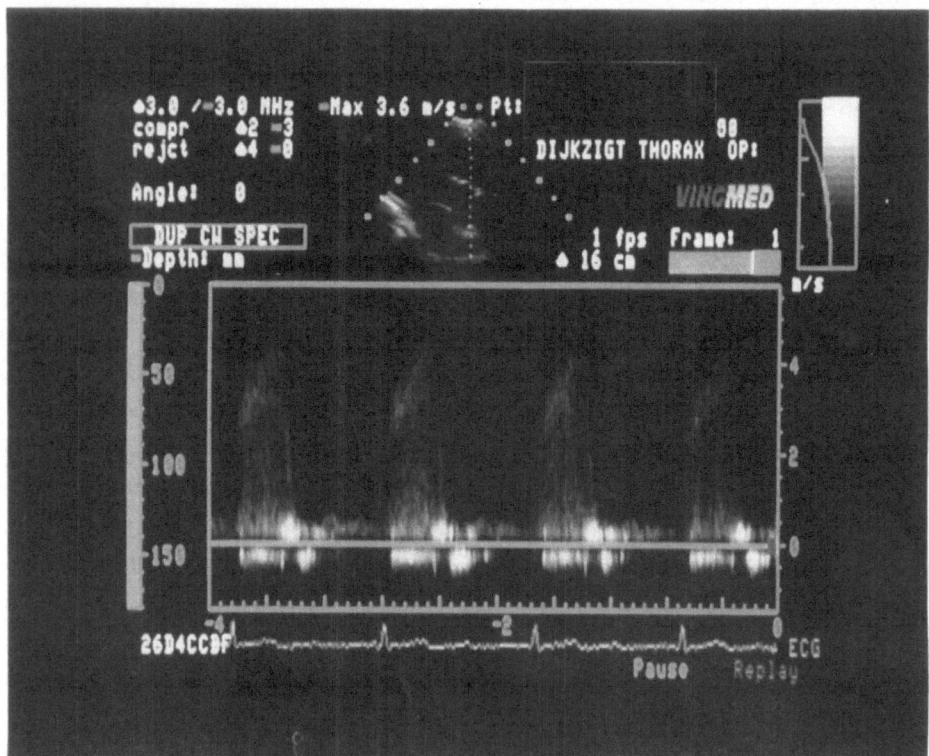

Fig 15-7. The continuous wave Doppler recording from a patient with Tetralogy of Fallot who has a small post operative residual ventricular septal defect. These defects are best detected with the transducer placed in a mid left parasternal position. In this case the peak systolic jet velocity was 4.3 metres/sec. indicating that the trans-septal pressure gradient was high and that right ventricular peak systolic pressure was near normal.

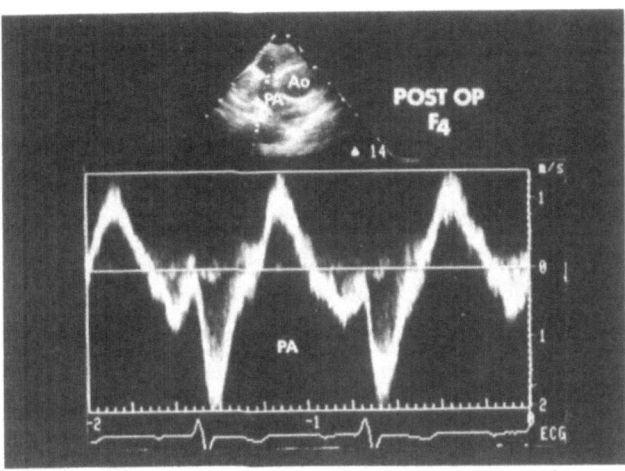

Fig 15-8. A High Pulsed Repetition Frequency recording of flow across the right ventricular outflow tract in a patient who has severe pulmonary incompetence following repair of Tetralogy of Fallot. Note the abnormal late diastolic forward flow in the pulmonary artery indicative of an abnormally high end diastolic pressure being generated in the non-compliant right ventricle following atrial systole. The peak velocity of forward flow over the outflow tract is also increased because of the large volume of systolic forward flow related to the severe pulmonary incompetence. The diastolic retrograde waveform is characteristic of severe pulmonary incompetence.

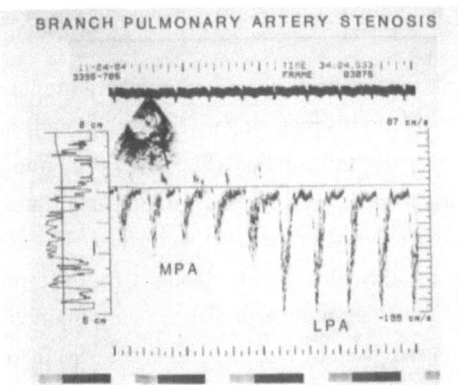

Fig 15-9. A pulsed doppler scan from main to left pulmonary artery demonstrating an increase in peak systolic velocity across a known vessel stenosis. Note that the insonnating beam is at 90 degrees to the flow and thus little can be deduced about the severity of the lesion.

It is perfectly possible in neonates and infants to both demonstrate atresia of the right ventricular outflow tract and determine whether the intrapericardial main pulmonary artery is present or not. Continuous wave Doppler will fail to identify a high velocity systolic jet within the right ventricular outflow tract. Pulsed Doppler interrogation will demonstrate low velocity continuous flow in the central pulmonary arteries where the arterial duct is non-restrictive (Fig 12). Where the duct is restrictive, Pulsed Doppler will demonstrate aliased continuous flow and Continuous Wave Doppler should be used to determine the peak velocity of flow and hence determine the degree of duct restriction. Color flow mapping (either with or without the use of color M-mode registration to confirm the continuous nature of the flow) will demonstrate confluent flow within the main, right and left pulmonary arteries if these are in continuity and are unobstructed. In neonates with unobstructed arterial ducts color flow mapping will demonstrate laminar flow throughout the central pulmonary vessels. However, where the duct is restrictive flow will be uniformly turbulent within the proximal pulmonary arteries. In this situation the localised area of turbulent flow which normally acts as the marker for a stenosis within the proximal pulmonary arteries will be masked by the generalised turbulence caused by the duct flow. However, where laminar flow across the arterial duct is present then the localised turbulence associated with an isolated stenosis will normally be defined.

The combination of cross-sectional imaging and color flow mapping can consistently define the presence of normally positioned, confluent and adequate-sized intrapericardial central pulmonary arteries. Imaging from the suprasternal position will normally confirm that the source of pulmonary blood flow is a single arterial duct. In such cases our experience has shown that aorto-pulmonary shunting can be safely carried out based only on the ultrasound information.

Problems arise for a complete ultrasound examination where the lung blood supply is not unifocal in origin. It is impossible to distinguish between a single arterial duct or a collateral based on either imaging or Doppler information (Fig 13). Furthermore, it is impossible to ascertain with any degree of accuracy either the number of collaterals present or their individual morphologies. Indeed the collateral vessels are often so tortuous in their course that a single vessel may be transected by the ultrasound beam two or three times in the one echocardiographic plane and thus may be interpreted as being multiple vessels. In addition, collateral stenoses cannot be interrogated by Doppler and thus no useful noninvasive evaluation of the arterial pressure in the distal lung vessels can be made. Of the ultrasound techniques available only transesophageal imaging can reliably identify the presence of intra-pericardial hypoplastic central pulmonary arteries which are supplied from collateral vessels arising from the descending aorta.

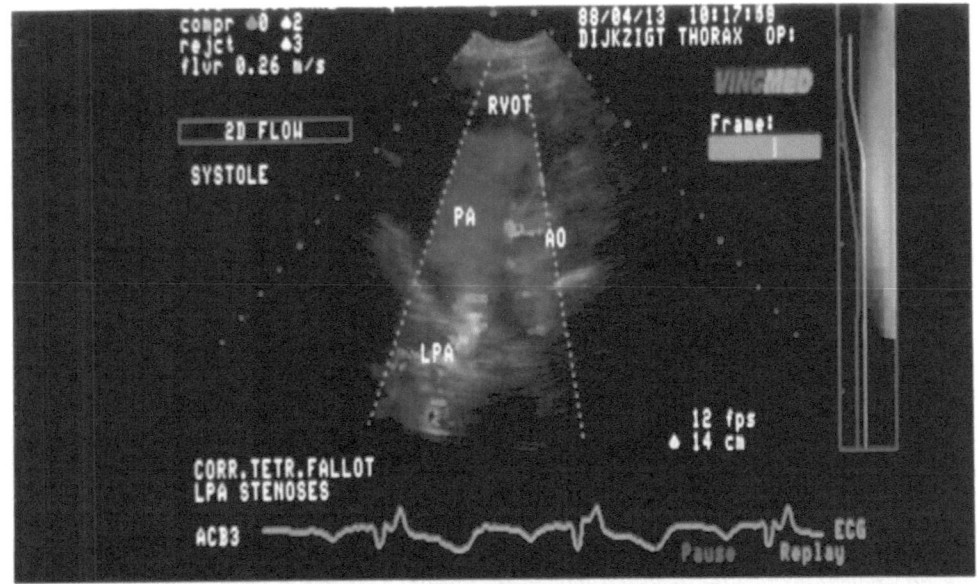

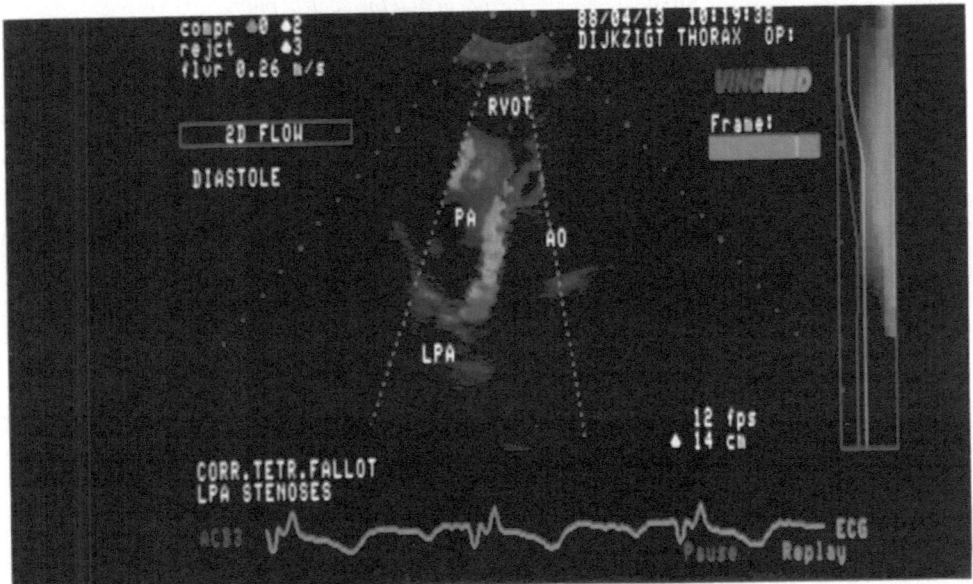

Fig 15-10. A color flow map recorded with the transducer in a high left parasternal position from a patient who has had Tetralogy of Fallot repaired. An area of systolic turbulent flow is present at the bifurcation of the main and left pulmonary artery. This appearance is diagnostic of a stenosis at this site.

Fig 15-11. A diastolic frame from the color flow map demonstrated in Fig 10. In this image a diastolic turbulent jet is seen to exit from the left pulmonary artery into the main pulmonary artery. This appearance is always associated with a significant obstruction within the central pulmonary arteries.

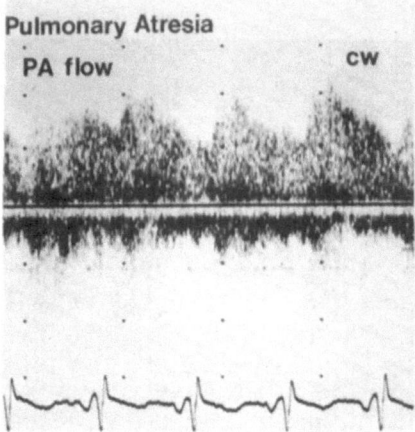

Fig 12 . *A continuous wave Doppler recording of flow within the central pulmonary arteries in a neonate with pulmonary atresia with ventricular septal defect. Note the continuous nature of the flow indicating that the focus of supply is the aorta. The low peak velocity of flow indicates that there is little pressure gradient between the aorta and the central pulmonary vessels.*

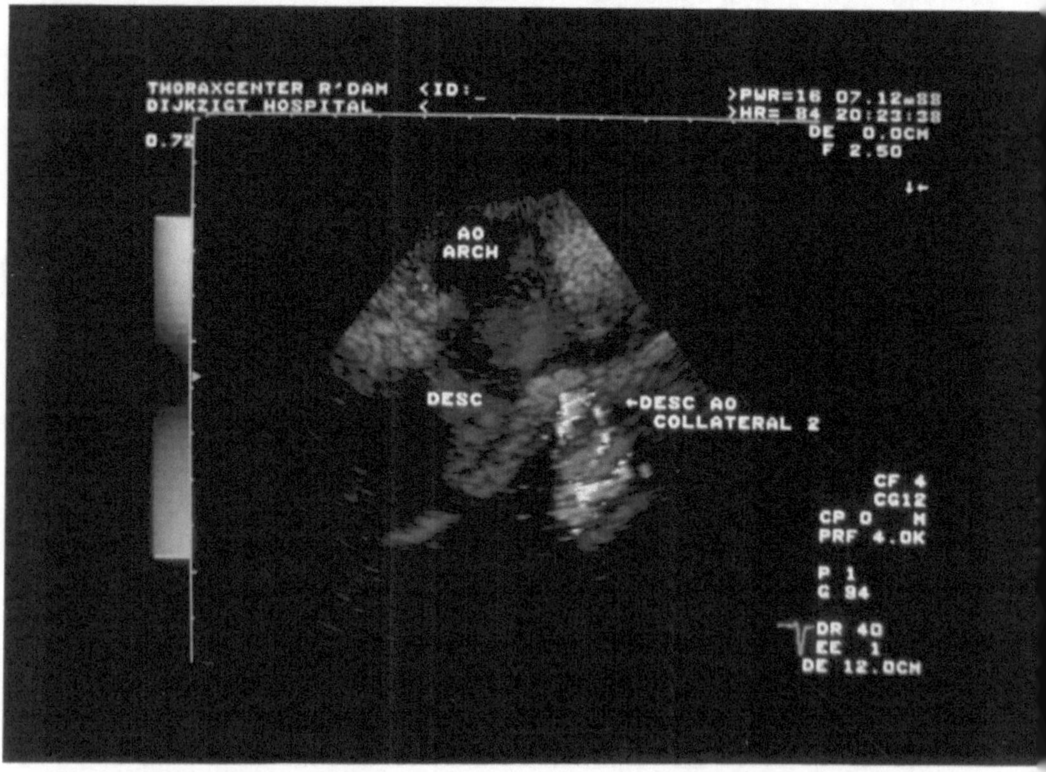

Fig 13 . *A suprasternal color flow map from a patient with pulmonary atresia with ventricular septal defect in whom the pulmonary blood supply was derived from aorto-pulmonary collateral vessels. This image demonstrates turbulent flow in a para-aortic position which represents flow in one of the two large descending aortic collaterals which were present in this patient.*

Truncus Arteriosus

Again the intracardiac morphology in this lesion is essentially similar to that encountered in both Tetralogy of Fallot and Pulmonary Atresia with a Ventricular Septal Defect. The ventricular septal defect is non-restrictive and bidirectional low velocity laminar flow should be identified within the defect both on Pulsed Doppler and color flow mapping studies. Truncal valve incompetence is almost an invariable finding in this lesion and its severity can be evaluated using the combination of continuous wave Doppler and color flow mapping. Such an evaluation, although only semi-quantitative in its assessment of the degree of incompetence, should provide essentially the same information as angiography. Color flow mapping is also of value when attempting to define the morphology of the vessels which take origin from the single arterial trunk and which supply the lungs. These may be difficult to visualise using cross-sectional imaging alone. Rarely the situation is encountered in which one pulmonary artery arises from the ascending aorta and the other is supplied from a descending aortic collateral or an arterial duct. This is normally a cross-sectional imaging diagnosis but again color flow mapping will help to confirm the morphology. The flow in the central pulmonary vessels in this condition is normally turbulent because of the extremely high lung blood flow. Thus, in the presence of wide-spread turbulence, any central stenoses within the pulmonary arteries may be missed on color flow mapping examination. Where the orifice of the common trunk is stenotic either high pulsed repetition frequency or continuous wave Doppler can be used to determine the systolic gradient. Care must be taken when using Doppler to evaluate any suspected truncal valve stenosis. Both the pre-and post-valve peak flow velocities should be measured and incorporated into the modified Bernoullie equation to allow accurate gradient estimation.(If the post valve peak systolic velocity alone is used to derive the peak instantaneous gradient too high a pressure drop will be calculated because of the high forward flow across the truncal valve in those cases with coexisting truncal valve regurgitation).

References

1. Anderson RH, Macartney FJ, Shinebourne EA, Tynan M. Pulmonary atresia with ventricular septal defect. In: Anderson RH, Macartney FJ, Shinebourne EA, Tynan M, eds. Paediatric Cardiology. Edinburgh: Churchill Livingstone, 1987:799-827.

2. Somerville J, Saravalli O, Ross D. Complex pulmonary atresia with congenital systemic collaterals: classification and management. Arch Mal Coeur 1978;71:322-328.

3. Silove ED, de Giovanni JV, Shiu MF, Myint Myint YI. Diagnosis of right ventricular outflow obstruction in infants by cross-sectional echocardiography. Br Heart J 1983;50; 416-420.

4. Sanders SP, Bierman FZ, Williams RG. Conotruncal malformations: diagnosis in infancy using sub-xiphoid 2-dimensional echocardiography. Am J Cardiol 1982;50:1361-7.

5. Smyllie JH, Sutherland GR, Keeton BR. The value of colour flow mapping in determining pulmonary blood supply in infants with pulmonary atresia with ventricular septal defect.

CHAPTER XVI

THE USE OF INTRAOPERATIVE ULTRASOUND IN CONGENITAL HEART DISEASE

George R. Sutherland

Oliver F.W. Stümper

Introduction

The first report in the literature on the use of intraoperative echocardiography appeared in 1972 and dealt with the M-mode echocardiographic assessment of mitral valve operations [1]. In the following years there were several further reports concerning the usefulness of this technique in a variety of intraoperative applications: 1. for monitoring left ventricular function [2,3], 2. for the demonstration of outflow tract stenosis in Tetralogy of Fallot [4] and 3. in the evaluation of hypertrophic subaortic stenosis [5]. As the M-mode technique could only provide insight into the dimensions and motion of cardiac structures, it was rapidly replaced by cross-sectional imaging, which allowed detailed morphologic information to be acquired. The clinical applications of epicardial cross-sectional imaging for monitoring ventricular function [6,7,8], and for precise demonstration of the anatomy of cardiac valves, cardiac tumors, and coronary artery disease have all been reported [9,10,11].

In 1985 a large series of patients who underwent cardiac surgery for congenital heart disease were studied by intraoperative epicardial cross-sectional imaging [12]. The study reported a yield of additional new information in ten percent of the patients, provided by the pre-bypass studies, which either refined or altered the surgical approach. Further post-bypass studies revealed information that contributed to surgical management in nine percent of the patients. With continuing improvements in angiography and refinements in preoperative cardiac ultrasound the preoperative diagnosis nowadays might be thought to be seldom incomplete after combined investigations. However this is not the case. Our own recent experience in some 230 complete intraoperative studies in congenital heart disease has demonstrated a continuing yield of new important morphologic or hemodynamic information of value to surgical management in approximately one fifth of the patients. These in general were not new or unsuspected major morphologic malformations, but were important new insights which were relevant to surgical decision making.

The major disadvantage of using cross-sectional imaging alone in the early intraoperative studies was that it could not provide any direct hemodynamic information, thus considerably limiting any complete assessment of surgical repair. Only the adjunct of intraoperative contrast echocardiography allowed some insight into hemodynamic results. The initial intraoperative use of contrast echocardiography was in the evaluation of both valve incompetence and intracardiac shunts by the injection of echogenic contrast medium, such as agitated patient's blood or saline solution, into an appropriate cardiac chamber. Valvular incompetence or intracardiac shunting was assumed to be absent in cases where no contrast "leakage" could be detected into the "upstream" chamber [13]. Such contrast echo studies performed immediately post-repair proved to be of some value for the evaluation of reconstructive valve repair [14,15] and for the exclusion of significant residual shunts after surgical closure of ventricular septal defects [16]. However, with increasing clinical experience the major inherent limitations of this technique became obvious. The contrast information obtained turned out to depend on a multitude of factors, such as type, amount, site, velocity and exact timing of injectate, thus largely reducing the reproducibility of these investigations. Furthermore, contrast echocardiography could neither define the precise site and numbers of regurgitant jets or residual shunts, nor could it provide any information concerning flow characteristics, such as flow velocity and turbulence. On the basis of these limitations contrast echocardiography proved to be of only limited value for the intraoperative assessment of repair of complex forms of congenital heart disease.

Since the introduction of Doppler ultrasound and, in particular, color flow mapping there is now renewed interest in intraoperative echocardiography for assessment of surgical repair of congenital heart disease. This has been caused by the unique inherent properties of color flow mapping, which can provide the equivalent of intraoperative angiography. By using this technique in combination with high resolution cross-sectional imaging it should, in theory, be possible for the surgeon to assess both the underlying morphologic and hemodynamic features of almost any congenital heart lesion. In the intraoperative setting it is only the combination of both ultrasound modalities which achieves optimal results.

Though increasing experience with intraoperative ultrasound in patients undergoing cardiac surgery both for acquired valvular heart disease and coronary artery disease has recently been reported [17], experience with the complete range of intraoperative ultrasound in congenital heart disease is still limited. Initial reports on its use in a small series of children undergoing surgery for congenital malformations have been published both by Takamoto [18] and Hagler [19]. These studies indentified a high incidence of minor residual lesions, such as small residual VSDs and minor degrees of valvular regurgitations, which might have otherwise gone undetected. Subsequent correlation of these intraoperative findings with the findings obtained by postoperative studies demonstrated the high sensitivity of immediate post-bypass epicardial ultrasound studies in detecting residual hemodynamic abnormalities.

Thus, the potential role of this new technique should be to provide the surgeon with detailed information regarding the hemodynamic results achieved by his repair, as well as clearly demonstrating the post repair morphology. Following repair he must first rule out any significant lesions which may require immediate further repair during a second period of bypass, and second, he must identify those patients with minor residual lesions which influence the immediate post operative management and long term results. Used in this way intraoperative Doppler ultrasound could be a valuable means of further reducing perioperative hospital mortality in this group of patients, in which early mortality is still largely related to the existence of significant residual lesions. With increasing experience the practice of intraoperative ultrasound might also influence surgical technique [20]. However, current experience is still too limited to allow confirmation of these statements.

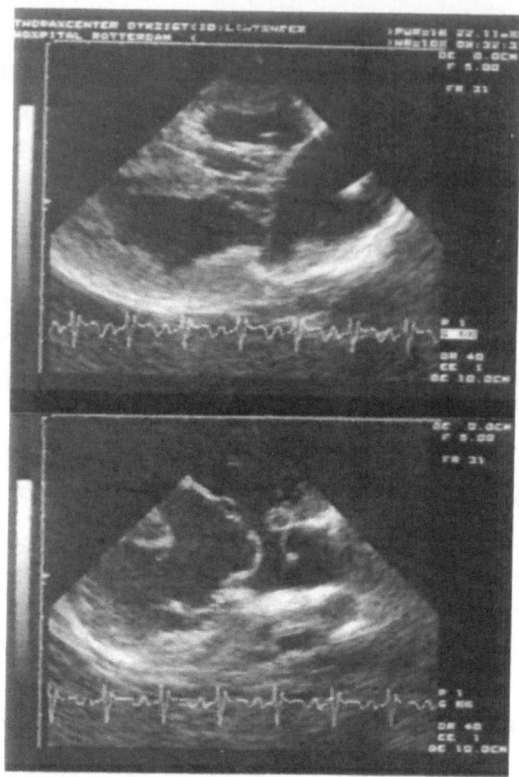

Figure 16-1. a: Modified epicardial four-chamber view of the common valve in a patient with complete atrioventricular septal defect. Note the close packed chordae inserting into the crest of the interventricular septum and the large atrial component of the defect. b: Rotation of the probe allows the assessment of the left ventricular outflow tract and the outlet portion of the interventricular septum. In this diastolic frame the exact morphology of the superior bridging leaflet is visualized. (LV = left ventricle).

Clinical Practice of Intraoperative Ultrasound

Intraoperative echocardiographic studies in surgery for congenital heart disease yield the maximal value when they are performed, interpreted and discussed in close cooperation between the responsible cardiac surgeon and the attending pediatric cardiologist. The information obtained by ultrasound investigations in the operative setting is in most cases too complex to allow exact on-line evaluation even in the most experienced hands. Immediate slow motion or frame by frame analysis of video recordings is required to interpret both pre- and post-repair ultrasound studies. The evaluation of the studies, including the estimation of the hemodynamic results has to take into account 1. the preoperative diagnosis, 2. the repair performed, 3. the hemodynamic situation immediately post bypass, 4. the most likely short and long term history of any residual lesion and

5. the feasibility versus the risks of immediate further repair.

The rapidly changing hemodynamic situation immediately after weaning from cardiopulmonary - bypass may prevent exact and reproducible Doppler quantification. Decision making must at all times during the post-bypass study rely on a semi-quantitative approach, which has to be influenced by previous experience gained with this technique.

There are two main ultrasound approaches to the intraoperative assessment of cardiac surgery in congenital heart disease; the epicardial and the transesophageal approaches. The merits and drawbacks of both techniques will now be considered in turn.

Epicardial Studies

The epicardial approach is the standard ultrasound technique in surgery for congenital heart disease. By using a series of modified four chamber, short and long axis scans a complete picture of the underlying malformation and the hemodynamic abnormalities can be obtained in most patients. This direct epicardial high resolution (i.e. high frequency) cross-sectional imaging always allows a more detailed insight into the precise morphology of the lesion than does the praecordial approach. Frequently, in our experience, this increase in the resolution of morphology contributes to alteration or refinements in the surgical management.

All intraoperative epicardial studies should consist of two separate parts: i) the pre-bypass study following thoracotomy and pericardotomy, prior to cannulation for cardio pulmonary bypass, and ii) the post-bypass study before closure of the chest. Prior to commencement of the post-bypass study all cannulae should be removed, as in small children the large diameter of the cannulation tubes, relative to the diameters of the great vessels are likely to produce unpredictable flow patterns and thus preventing exact evaluation. Furthermore, care should be taken not to perform the post-bypass study until the blood pressure and the preload return to near normal. The findings of each study have then to be correlated with one another. A pre-bypass study is mandatory in every case as it serves as the reference basis for interpretation of the post-bypass findings. It is also essential as the hemodynamic situation with the chest open and the patient under anaesthesia and on mechanical ventilation may be considerably changed from the preoperative situation.

<u>Technique</u> The ultrasound transducers and wires are packed in sterile plastic bags after a small amount of sterile ultrasound gel has been applied to the head of the transducer in order to improve ultrasound coupling (initial experience with gas sterilization frequently caused damage to the transducers and has largely been abandoned). Sterility is effectively secured using the above measures. Warm saline solution is then poured into the pericardial sac, in order to reduce the mechanical irritation of the heart by the transducer, which can cause episodes of arrhythmias. It also improves contact of the transducer with the epicardial surface. In addition, when using a high frequency short focus transducer it serves as a stand-off interface which can be used to improve near field resolution. Occasional isolated or coupled premature ventricular beats caused by

epicardial scanning are sometimes observed. The rarely encountered short runs of premature beats are self-terminating after removal of the transducer from the epicardium, and in our experience have never required cardioversion.

The pre- and post-bypass studies should be performed according to a predetermined standardized scheme. Firstly, high resolution cross-sectional imaging is carried out to demonstrate the anatomy of the underlying malformation. Secondly, color flow mapping of the entire heart is recorded. Thirdly, pulsed- and continuous wave Doppler recordings are made where appropriate. The scan positions used for epicardial scanning should be comparable, as far as possible, to those used for precordial imaging in order to facilitate interpretation. However, the relatively small size of thoracotomy relative to the large transducer dimensions limits this approach. Thus a variety of new scan positions have to be used to allow complete assessment of the hemodynamic situation after surgical repair. The echocardiographer and surgeon must familiarize themselves with these new cross-sections. Epicardial scanning in infants and small children is virtually impossible from the apex of the heart and the lateral walls, due to current transducer design. This limits the epicardial approach for complete investigations especially after any extensive use of ultrasound opaque prosthetic material in the repair. Prosthethic materials, such as Dacron or Gore-Tex, cast vast ultrasound shadows, that produce large areas of flow masking in the color flow maps. Further limitations and artifacts frequently encountered during the intraoperative studies are caused by electrical interference from the surrounding apparatus. Diathermy routinely has to be switched off during the studies, as the associated electrical interference makes color flow mapping virtually impossible. Sometimes even diathermy used in the adjacent room prevents Doppler evaluation.

The current limitations in the phased array transducer is that the design prevents a complete intraoperative investigation being carried out with only one probe. At present standard precordial transducers must be used. For cross-sectional imaging in small children a small 5 MHz, 48 - 64 element probe routinely gives best image resolution. Color flow mapping and pulsed wave Doppler investigations are performed with standard 3.75 MHz probes using phased array technology. Emphasis during color Doppler studies should concentrate on the demonstration of flow abnormalities of systemic and pulmonary venous return, flow characteristics across both the atrioventricular and arterial valves within the ventricular outflow tracts. As well as these, the integrity of both the atrial and ventricular septal structures should be routinely assessed. Pulsed wave Doppler is of importance for evaluation of any residual gradients across the cardiac valves and ventricular outflow tracts. Exact evaluation of valvular and subvalvular stenosis and pressure gradients across the interventricular septum require continuous wave Doppler investigations, which are routinely performed with a 2.5 MHz duplex probe. Continuous wave Doppler studies with a pencil probe are difficult to perform and to interpret intraoperatively and are in most cases too time consuming. However an attempt should be undertaken as they can give invaluable additional information on residual valvular and subvalvular stenosis or outflow tract gradients.

To avoid having to use multiple bulky standard precordial transducers a new range of pediatric intraoperative transducers must be developed which are designed specifically for this task. Within a single transducer they should combine high resolution imaging with color flow mapping and spectral Doppler. The transducer should be small enough to allow the surgeon to manipulate it with his finger both lateral to and behind the heart. Such a transducer would allow the problems caused by flow masking by anterior prosthetic material to be circumvented by allowing imaging to be directed at flow masked areas from behind the heart. Such a transducer would make the use of the intraoperative transesophageal approach (which is at present used to circumvent this problem) superfluous.

Transesophageal Studies

Due to the large diameter of currently available transesophageal probes this new window to the heart [21,22] is not as yet routinely accessible in children undergoing cardiac surgery. In our experience, in older patients who undergo corrective surgery of congenital heart disease, this technique (used in combination with the epicardial approach) has proved to be of great additional value to epicardial imaging. Their combined use allows a better evaluation of reconstructive procedures of the atrioventricular valves and of surgical repair of left ventricular outflow tract abnormalities. However the transesophageal technique has major limitations. Experience gained with this technique has revealed it to allow only poor demonstration of the right ventricular outflow tract, the branch pulmonary arteries and the anterior and apical portions of the ventricular septum. In addition the large distance between the esophageal transducer and these structures makes their assessment by color flow mapping virtually impossible [23]. In addition, esophageal image quality is inferior to that obtained from the epicardium using the range of currently available transducers . Furthermore, the number of imaging planes obtainable is limited and most esophageal probes do not allow continuous wave Doppler measurements, though there are reports of transesophageal probes with continuous wave Doppler in the literature, which have recently become available. With further miniaturization of the probes, the transesophageal technique may become a valuable adjunct to the epicardial approach in small children undergoing intracardiac repair at atrial and atrioventricular levels and where extensive flow masking occurring behind prosthetic material used in the repair (large VSD patches, conduits, etc.) prevents adequate epicardial imaging and color flow mapping evaluation during the post bypass study. As well as its potential intraoperative use, with the development of miniaturized transducers, transesophageal echocardiography may become the method of choice for prolonged post-operative monitoring in the intensive care unit.

Technique The esophageal probe is introduced in the anaesthetic induction room, after endotracheal intubetion and the patient fully anaesthetized. It is inserted under direct vision into the hypopharynx and then blindly advanced to the lower end of the oesophagus. The probe is left in the oesophagus during the whole operation but has to be switched off while the patient is on bypass, in order to prevent any thermal damage to the oesophagus. With a combination of cross-sectional imaging [25], color flow mapping and pulsed wave Doppler evaluation, a complete assessment of the morphology and the flow characteristics of the underlying malformation should be carried out. Emphasis should be put on evaluation of atrial structures, venous return, atrioventricular valves, the left ventricular outflow tract and ventricular function. The current limitations of single plane transesophageal imaging should be borne in mind.

Post-Operative Studies

The aim of all immediate post-bypass studies is to rule out any hemodynamically significant lesions. Exact Doppler quantification of hemodynamic parameters is of limited value in the intraoperative setting due to the rapid changes of these parameters. Therefore, subsequent post-operative studies should be carried out in the intensive care unit 1) for further exclusion of residual lesions that might have been gone undetected by the post-bypass study, 2) to quantify hemodynamic parameters.

The standard approach for post-operative investigations is transthoracic, but image quality is normally poor due to entrapped air and the presence of suction tubes. These factors together with the impaired signal to noise ratio in the intensive care unit (caused by electrical interference from the surrounding apparatus) may considerably limit color flow analysis.

In the future, transesphageal echocardiography may become the method of choice for routine post-operative studies and prolonged monitoring even in small children. The esophageal approach is easily accessible on the intensive care unit, the image quality and color flow information are constantly far better than these obtained from the precordium.

Assessment of Cardiac Surgery by Epicardial Doppler Ultrasound

Complex congenital malformations of the heart are normally constituted of different specific lesions which occur on various levels of the heart. Cardiac surgery performed on these malformations is in most cases a repair of a series of defects encountered on each of the involved levels. These different levels being the atrial level, the atrioventricular valves, the interventricular septum, the outflow tracts, the arterial valves and the great arteries. Instead of describing the practice of intraoperative epicardial Doppler ultrasound during the various cardiac operations, we prefer to use this level orientated approach, with special reference to complete surgical procedures where this seems appropriate.

Atrial Level

Exact localization of the orifices of all the systematic and pulmonary veins and the coronary sinus is readily demonstrated with cross-sectional epicardial imaging. Individual pulmonary vein drainage is clearly depicted on the color flow maps, and individual flow characteristics can be identified and quantified by means of pulsed wave Doppler sampling. The integrity of the atrial septum can be demonstrated by color flow mapping from the right atrial epicardial surface. The restrictive nature of any present atrial septal defect is readily recognized by depiction of turbulent flow across the defect in the color flow maps. Color flow mapping is a definite advantage, as it can improve the complete understanding of the complex morphology and flow patterns associated with coronary sinus defects, sinus venosus defects, juxtaposed atrial appendages and cor triatriatum, as it clearly demonstrates blood flow direction and the complex flow characteristics within these structures.

Following surgical closure of atrial septal defects color flow mapping investigations can be used to exclude the existence of residual atrial shunting. Significant residual shunting is an infrequent finding, but some minor areas of turbulent flow originating from the sutureline are often encountered in the immediate post bypass study. Such findings, in our experience, are irrelevant in the majority of patients. Their occurrence is independent of surgical technique (direct suture versus patch closure). However, after establishing a Fontan circulation, even small residual ASDs have to be completely excluded by means of color flow mapping, as these defects, associated with the right atrial pressures during the post-operative period, can result in a life-threatening R-L shunting. Recommencement of bypass to effect definitive closure of any such residual atrial septal defect is mandatory. Following a Mustard or Senning procedure for complete transposition of the great arteries baffle obstructions and leaks have to be excluded. As some degree of turbulent flow across the baffle is a common finding, pulsed Doppler evaluation of any potential gradient is of value. However, in practice good alignment to flow direction is difficult to obtain from the epicardial approach. Baffle leaks, which result in predominant L-R shunting, are clearly demonstrated by color flow mapping when appropriate scan positions are chosen to view the entire sutureline of the patch.

Atrioventricular Valves

Pre-bypass epicardial high resolution imaging of the atrioventricular valves and their tensor apparatus should be performed in every patient. This technique, used in combination with color flow mapping, provides a more detailed understanding of the functional morphology of incompetent valves (Fig.16-1a/b). This is of great value for determining the type and extent of any reconstructive valve surgery required. In patients undergoing repair of partial or complete atrioventricular septal defects and Ebstein's malformation of the tricuspid valve, precise planning of the exact localization and the extent of required incisions, resections and plications is facilitated by the ultrasound information obtained.

The high incidence of malformations of the chordae of both atrioventricular valves in patients with double outlet right ventricle, discordant chamber connections and double inlet ventricle [25] stresses the need for systemized investigations of patients with these malformations, as the presence of abnormal chordal insertions may significantly alter the surgical approach. In our experience epicardial cross-sectional imaging is more sensitive than precordial imaging for detection and clear demonstration of both major and minor degrees of straddling.

Following repair, the immediate hemodynamic results of reconstructive valve surgery should be evaluated by color Doppler investigations (Fig.16-2a/b). Color flow mapping is superior to contrast echocardiography for assessment of any residual regurgitations, as contrast findings are frequently too ambiguous to allow accurate evaluation in clinical practice, and do not allow demonstration of the exact site of the regurgitant jet. The grading of residual valvular regurgitation by color flow mapping can only be performed on a semi-quantative basis during intraoperative investigations. A holosystolic broadening jet with maximal length of more than one third of the atrial transverse diameter has to be considered severe regurgitation which suggests further immediate definite repair or valve replacement (Fig.16-3). Feasibility of further reconstructive measures can be demonstrated by cross-sectional high resolution imaging. Flow acceleration across stenotic valves has to be evaluated by a combination of pulsed wave Doppler, with subsequent calculation of the pressure gradients. The existence of residual, or iatrogenic, stenosis of the atrioventricular valves have to be systematically excluded immediately following surgical closure of a cleft in the mitral valve, repair of complete atrioventricular septal defects and after correction of Ebstein's malformation of the tricuspid valve.

Ventricular Level

Following cardio-pulmonary bypass, the need for volume replacement and the need for inotropic support can be readily and continually assessed by cross-sectional imaging while the chest is open. This is one of the most important contributions of intraoperative ultrasound in cardiac surgery. Epicardial short axis scans provide immediate demonstration of ventricular performance, ventricular filling and the detection of dyskinetic areas.

Interventricular Septum

The integrity of the ventricular septum can be easily assessed preoperatively by color flow mapping using a series of foreshortened four-chamber views and long and short axis scans from the right ventricular epicardial surface (Fig.16-4). Surgical closure of any ventricular septal defect should be followed by thorough intraoperative post-bypass color Doppler evaluation, as hemodynamically significant residual defects will exist in about 6-10% of cases [26,28]. These residual defects are either true residual defects at the original site, or additional distal septal defects which were either overlooked, or that have been missed preoperatively by both angiocardiography and Doppler echocardiography. (The failure to detect multiple VSDs preoperatively normally occurs in association with non-restrictive hemodynamics). In addition, apical muscular VSDs frequently have more than one right ventricular orifice in the trabecular septum, which may make complete surgical closure of these defects difficult. Another mechanism, which may cause a significant residual defect is the possibility of immediate patch dehiscence by the pulling through of a couple of stitches along the VSD margin after recommencement of mechanical action of the heart.

The aim of the intraoperative post-bypass study is to exclude any such residual defects. Cross-sectional imaging alone can only detect large residual defects, associated with major areas of patch dehiscence. However, the demonstration of echo drop out around a ventricular septal defect patch is not specific for a residual defect. This may well be caused by image masking by synthetic patch material thus producing a false-positive defect [29]. In addition, confirmation of the integrity of the muscular part of the interventricular septum cannot reliably be performed by cross-sectional imaging alone. Therefore color flow mapping studies which scan the entire inventricular septum are important to exclude residual defects. The specifity and sensitivity of such a color flow mapping technique for detection of multiple VSDs has been reported as being high [30,31], and the exact site and number of defects can be clearly demonstrated. However, major limitations may be encountered using this technique. Equal ventricular peak systolic pressures or very small interventricular pressure gradients (which occur in the presence of large residual defects) result in low velocity laminar flow shunting, which, even with frame by frame analysis, may not be appreciated when interpreting the complex flow maps. An even more important problem in clinical practice is that in the presence of significant residual right ventricular outflow tract stenosis color flow mapping exclusion of a residual perimembraneous or muscular outlet ventricular septal defect is not possible, as the right ventricular outflow tract obstruction procedures systolic turbulence which totally obscures turbulent shunt flow across any residual outlet defect. In this situation an additional contrast echocardiography study, with injection of agitated patients's blood via a left atrial line, and using a scan position which includes the right ventricular outflow tract, is of great help to exclude a significant residual defect [32]. Post-bypass assessment of closure of ventricular septal defects with contrast echocardiography alone is inadequate, as this technique cannot provide all the information required, such as exact site and number of defects. In addition, clinical practice has revealed a high incidence of false-positive contrast findings, due both to concomitant venous injections by the anaesthetist and to the spontaneous appearance of right heart contrast, and false-negative results due to poor imaging or unreliable contrast effect. Problems also arise with color flow mapping as it frequently yields false positive findings concerning the existence of minimal residual shunts, due to misinterpretation of multiple turbulent peri-patch flow abnormalities.

The exact quantification of shunt volume in the post-bypass setting by means of pulsed and continuous wave Doppler evaluation is not feasible, as the hemodynamic situation is rapidlly changing. A semi-quantitative approach based on color flow mapping appearances for grading residual shunts into two categories, mild to moderate and severe, is more suitable and practical for intraoperative use. A broad expanding turbulent jet depicted in the color flow maps, reaching from the interventricular septum far into the cavity or outflow tract of the right ventricle should be considered to represent a significant residual shunt. Further investigations to determine the severity of shunting and the exact site of the residual defect should include the combination of contrast echocardiography and high resolution cross-sectional imaging. The demonstration of a contrast density in the right ventricular cavity which exceeds more than half of the simultaneous density achieved in the left ventricle, following a left atrial injection, is confirmative of a significant residual shunt. The subsequent use of a combination of cross-sectional imaging and color flow mapping should clearly demonstrate the exact site of the residual defect. Some residual shunting, readily demonstrated in the color flow maps, from the sutureline of a patch immediately following bypass is a normal finding [33]. These shunts may appear as multiple early systolic short peri-patch jets on the color flow maps. Flow of these shunts is normally laminar with only minimal turbulence. Contrast studies will exclude significant residual shunting.

In our experience the post-bypass assessment of surgical closed ventricular septal defects is best performed when both techniques, color flow mapping and contrast echocardiography are used in combination [34]. This approach yields the maximal information for definite exclusion of hemodynamically significant residual shunting.

Ventricular Outflow Tracts

During the pre-bypass study both ventricular outflow tracts should be investigated by cross-sectional imaging and color flow mapping for exclusion of turbulent flow patterns due to anatomic stenosis. Intraoperative echocardiography frequently provides better understanding of the relative importance and morphology of coexisting subvalvular and valvular stenosis. Color flow mapping readily indentifies the exact localization of individual stenoses by demonstration of turbulent flow across the relevant area. The pre-bypass epicardial ultrasound study may derive the essential morphologic information for decision making in the surgery of right ventricular outflow tract obstruction. The subsequent results of any surgical procedure can then readily be assessed by combined color and pulsed wave Doppler investigations immediately post-bypass. This method of management may lead to a more conservative approach to the surgery of right ventricular outflow tract obstructions, with a possible reduction in frequency and severity of pulmonary regurgitation [35].

Isolated obstructions of the left ventricular outflow tract in congenital heart disease are most often found in patients with idiopathic hypertrophic subaortic stenosis and discrete fibromuscular obstructions. Epicardial cross-sectional imaging provides excellent information regarding morphology and extent of these lesions, which proves to be a valuable aid for guidance of surgical resection. The combination of intraoperative epicardial and transesophageal echocardiography in these patients can yield even more information. Repair is routinely performed via the aortic valve. Thus post bypass studies are centered on the exclusion of residual significant stenosis, aortic regurgitation and iatrogenic lesions of the mitral valve apparatus.

In patients undergoing surgical repair of malformations which compromise both ventricular outflow tracts, such as double outlet right ventricle, intraoperative epicardial echocardiography can provide more detailed information concerning the spatial relationship of either outflow tract, than can be obtained from the transthoracic approach [36,37]. This allows exact planning for partial resection of stenotic areas, and may guide in the final decision concerning the feasibility of various surgical approaches [38,39], as the likelihood of residual intracardiac and conduit obstructions can be better estimated. Following repair any such obstructions and residual ventricular septal defects have to be excluded by use of a combination of color and pulsed wave Doppler investigations.

The surgical use of an aortic homograft as a valved conduit for correction of outflow tract atresia or severe stenosis is increasingly often performed [40]. Hemodynamic results are potentially endangered by first valvular incompetence of the homograft and second obstruction at either the proximal or distal conduit anastomoses. Valvular incompetence, which might be related to harvesting and sterilization techniques or to gross distortion at the site of the proximal anastomosis, is almost reliably excluded by color Doppler investigations. However, high echodensity of the homograft sometimes limits this approach. Flow obstruction across the proximal and distal anastomoses has to be excluded by color flow mapping and pulsed wave Doppler sampling. Frequently the proximal anastomosis, which is normally incorporated in the right ventricular myocardium, shows some degree of dynamic obstruction, due to systolic narrowing of the anastomosis.

Arterial Valves and Great Arteries

Following surgical relief of an arterial valve stenosis (aortic valve stenosis in particular) the presence of valvular regurgitation has to be excluded by the post bypass study. This can readily be performed by color flow mapping. Prior cross-sectional imaging can help to decide the question whether reconstructive measures are feasible or whether valve replacement is required. Residual gradients across the valves can be evaluated by continuous wave Doppler. In adolescents and adults this can be carried out using the relative large duplex probe, but in small children this is facilitated by the use of a small continuous wave Doppler pencil probe. Intraoperative invasive measurements of pressure gradients across the aortic valve have proved to be of subsequent prognostic value [41].

Patients who undergo definite repair of congenital heart disease after a systemic-pulmonary shunt has been constructed for palliation in the past should be investigated for the existence of peripheral pulmonary artery stenosis, which is a frequently associated finding. Color flow mapping and pulsed wave Doppler studies yield clear information concerning the necessity of patch arterioplasty in these patients. Patency of newly constructed shunts and unobstructed flow across the anastomoses should be documented before closure of the chest.

Color flow mapping of the great arteries should be used for screening for supravalvular stenosis. Areas of turbulent flow have to be evaluated by pulsed or continuous wave Doppler, especially in patients who have undergone the arterial switch procedure.

The presence of a patent ductus arteriosus should be excluded in all patients undergoing surgery for congenital heart disease and subsequent successful ligation should be documented on the color flow maps.

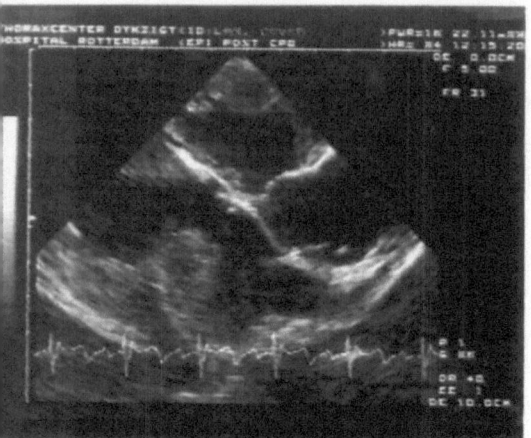
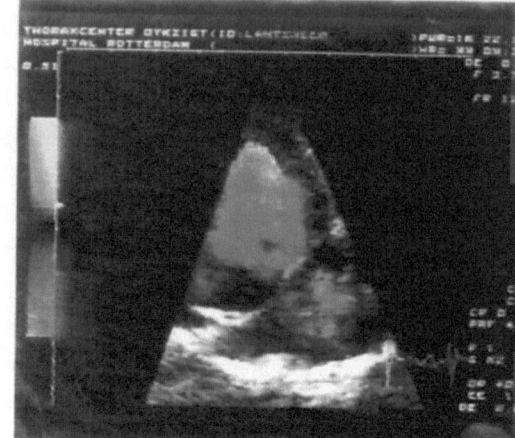
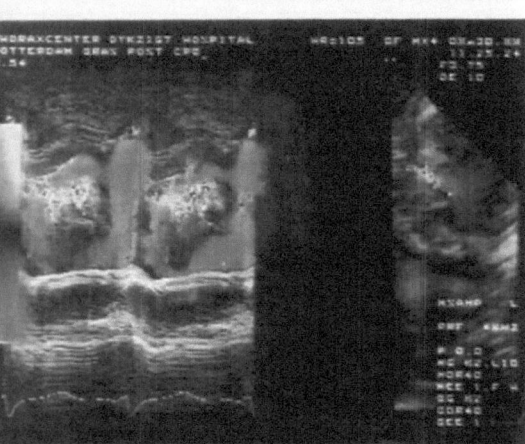
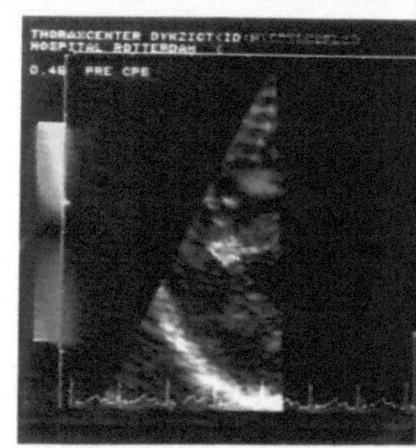
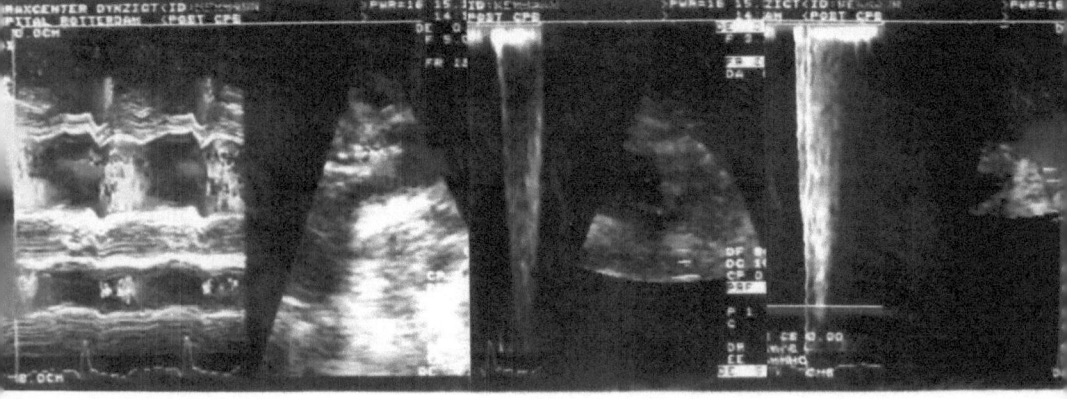

Figure 16-2 . Post bypass study in the same patient as in figure 1.a: the four-chamber view allows exclusion of any gross patch dehisence. The tricuspid valve is readily demonstrated. However ultrasound masking behind the prosthetic patch used for closure of the ventricular defect precludes the assessment of the mitral valve. b: the exclusion of mitral valve regurgitation is therefore better performed when using high left atrial views which are obtained when scanning between the ascending aorta and the pulmonary artery. (LA =left atrium)

Figure 16-3 . Color flow mapping study of the tricuspid valve in a patient after intracardiac repair for double outlet right ventricle. The jet is reaching far into the right atrial cavity (RA) and was graded to be severe. Subsequently this patient underwent a Fontan type procedure during a second period of bypass.

Figure 16-4 . Pre bypass study in a newborn child with transposition of the great arteries. Using short axis epicardial views the color flow mapping studies revealed an additional muscular ventricular septal defect that was not known preoperatively. (LV = left ventricle, RV = right ventricle)

Figure 16-5 . Post bypass epicardial study in an infant following an aterial switch procedure for transposition of the great arteries. a: Color flow mapping study of the aortic valve and the ascending aorta. Turbulent flow patterns are noted at valve level. The corresponding color M-mode clearly documents the holosystolic nature of the turbulence. b: Subsequent pulsed wave Doppler sampling in the ascending aorta revealed a maximal flow velocity of about 2.5 m/s. Immediate revision was not undertaken as the level of obstruction was assumed to be mainly located on valve level. The potential creation of aortic regurgitation was discussed not to outweigh the potential benefit of releaving the obstruction. c: Pulsed wave Doppler sampling in the pulmonary artery (PA) on the level of the anastomosis. The maximal flow velocity was determined to be about 1.9 m/s. However no revision was undertaken.

Doppler Ultrasound During Special Surgical Procedures and Fontan Procedures

Since the introduction of the operation described by Fontan in 1971 [42] for palliation of patients with tricuspid atresia, there have been several operative modifications reported [43]. These modifications have made the Fontan-type procedure also suitable for surgical treatment of various other forms of complex congenital heart disease, such as double inlet ventricle and where the presence of severe straddling atrioventricular valves precludes another approach [44]. After establishing a Fontan circulation the presence of a residual atrial septal defect, or the existence of a (right) ventricular - right atrial shunt through a surgically closed atrioventricular valve will result in rapid deterioration of the patient [45]. The outstanding role of intraoperative Doppler ultrasound following a Fontan procedure is first to exclude with certainty any residual R-L shunt at atrial level, or through a surgically closed right atrio-ventricular valve and second any obstruction of the atrial-pulmonary anastomoses or conduits. This can only be achieved by combined color and pulsed wave Doppler studies immediately post bypass. In case a thorough investigation demonstrates any such finding high resolution cross-sectional imaging should be performed to define the exact site of the residual lesion, in order to guide immediate surgical repair during a second period of bypass.

Senning, Mustard Procedure

Both procedures are performed to correct concordant-discordant hearts by means of construction of an interatrial baffle. The baffle is either constructed by part of the right atrial wall (Senning[46]), which is frequently augmented by a pericardial patch, or by the use of a pericardial or Dacron patch (Mustard [47]). Post repair, the presence of leakage across the patch suture line (which might result in severe bidirectional shunting at atrial level) and the presence of systemic or pulmonary venous obstruction must be excluded. Both color flow mapping and pulsed wave Doppler evaluation of flows into and across the baffle should be performed in every patient. In the presence of a gradient exceeding 3 and 5 mm Hg for systemic venous return and pulmonary venous return respectively further surgery should be contemplated. This also applies for major residual baffle leaks.

Rastelli Procedure

This procedure [48] is used to correct concordant-discordant hearts with a non-restrictive ventricular septal defect and subpulmonary outflow tract obstruction. The role of intraoperative ultrasound during the procedure is multifold. The pre-bypass study has to confirm the initial diagnosis, and to detect any associated lesions. Cross-sectional imaging should concentrate on exact demonstration of the spatial relationships of the ventricular septal defect and the subpulmonary outflow tract. This information is crucial in planning the need for and the exact degree of resection of part of the outlet septum [49] in order to secure unobstructed flow via the ventricular septal defect to the aorta. Furthermore, the existence of straddling atrioventricular valves should be excluded. Following the Rastelli repair the ventricular function should be assessed by a series of short axis scans. Obstructions of the interventricular communication, of both anastomoses of the aortic homograft, and the presence of a residual ventricular septal defect should be excluded by combined color flow mapping and pulsed or continuous wave Doppler investigations.

Arterial Switch Procedure

Following the arterial switch procedure for transposition of the great arteries [50,51] epicardial cross-sectional short axis scans for assessment of ventricular performance are mandatory to detect any dyskinetic or akinetic area. Turbulent flow at the site of the anastomoses of the coronary arteries and the proximal portions of these arteries can be excluded by color flow mapping (Fig.16-5a). In addition, flow velocities across the anastomoses of both great arteries should be carefully evaluated by pulsed wave Doppler sampling (Fig.16-5b/c). Maximal velocities across these anastomoses optimally should not exceed the upper limit in this age group, which is about 1.5 m/s in term children. Stenoses are more frequent at the site of the pulmonary anastomosis [52]. The existence of any other residual lesion, such as a residual ventricular septal defect, should be excluded by a complete post bypass study.

In summary, the use of intraoperative ultrasound as an aid to surgery for congenital heart disease is at present still at an early phase. Many problems have yet to be resolved. It is perhaps the most challenging area for the echocardiographer. On line analysis of the complex information obtained remains difficult even in the most experienced hands. It is a costly technique as an echo machine is tied up in the operating theatre for a long time (3-4 hours), in order to perform two studies which take in total approximately a quarter of an hour. Despite these drawbacks, we conclude that this technique is an important rapidly expanding use of cardiac ultrasound, which is likely to become a standard adjunct to the surgical procedure in both assessing the repair and for monitoring in the immediate post bypass period.

References

1. Johnson ML, Holmes JH, Spangler RD, Paton BC. Usefulness of echocardiography in patients undergoing mitral valve surgery. J Thorac Cardiovasc Surg 1972; 64: 922-934.

2. Spotnitz HM, Troccone NJ, Porter RJ Jr, King DL, Hoffman BF, Malm JR. Simplified measurement of in vivo compliance of the left ventricle. Surg Forum 1976; 27: 283-285.

3. Gaudiani VA, Shemin RJ, Syracuse DC, Henry WL, Conkle DM. Continuous epicardial echocardiographic assessment of postoperative left ventricular function. J Thorac Cardiovasc. Surg 1978; 76: 64-69.

4. Spotnitz HM, Malm JR, King DL, Pooley RW, Bowman FO, Bergman D, Edie RN, Reemsma K, Kongrad E, Hoffman BF. Outflow tract obstruction in tetralogy of Fallot. Intraoperative analysis by echocardiography. NY State J Med 1978; 78: 1100-1103.

5. Syracuse DC, Gaudiani VA, Kash DG, Henri WL, Morrow AG. Intraoperative intracardiac echocardiography during left ventriculomyotomy and myectomy for hypertrophic subaortic stenosis. Circulation 1978; 58: Suppl 1:23-27.

6. Wong CYH, Spotnitz HM. Systolic and diastolic properties of the human left ventricle during valve replacement for chronic mitral regurgitation. Am J Cardiol 1981; 47:40-49.

7. Waggoner AD, Shah AA, Schuessler JS, et al. Effect of cardiac surgery on ventricular septal motion: assessment by intraoperative echocardiography and cross-sectional two-dimensional echocardiography. Am Heart J 1984; 108:1012-8.

8. Beaupre PN, Kremer PF, Cahalan MK, Lurz FW, Schiller NB, Hamilton WK. Intraoperative detection of changes in left ventricular segmental wall motion by transesophageal two-dimensional echocardiography. Am

Heart J 1984; 107:1201-3.

9. Spotnitz HM, Malm JR. Two-dimensional ultrasound and cardiac operations. J Thorac Cardiovasc Surg 1982; 83:43-51.

10. Rosenzweig MS, Nanda NC. Ventricular septal impingement by mitral prosthesis. Detection by two-dimensional echocardiography and its significance (abstr.) Circulation 18=980; 62:Suppl III:20.

11. Sahn DJ, Copeland JG, Temkin LP, Wirt DP, Mammana R, Glenn W. Anatomic-ultrasound correlation for intraoperative open chest imaging of coronary artery atherosclerotic lesions in human beings. J Am Cardiol 1984; 3:1169-1177.

12. Gussenhoven EJ, van Herwerden LA, Roelandt J, Ligtvoet KM, Bos E, Witsenburg M. Intraoperative two-dimensional echocardiography in congenital heart disease. JACC 1987; 9:565-72.

13. Sahn DJ. Intraoperative applications of two-dimensional and contrast two-dimensional echocardiography for evaluation of congenital, acquired and coronary heart disease in open chested humans during cardiac surgery. In: Rijsterborgh H, ed. Echocardiology. The Hague: Martinus Nijhoff 1981: 8-23.

14. Reid CL, Kawanishi DT, McKay CR, Elkayam U, Rahimtoola SH, Chandraratna PAN, Accuracy of evaluation of the presence and severity of aortic and mitral regurgitation by contrast two-dimensional echocardiography. Am J Cardiol 1983; 52:519-524.

15. Goldman ME, Mindich BP, Techholz LE, Burgess N, Staville K, Fuster V. Intraoperative contrast echocardiography to evaluate mitral valve operations. JACC 1984; 4,5: 1035-1040.

16. Herwerden LA, Gussenhoven EJ, Roelandt J, Bos E, Ligtvoet CM, Haalebos MM, Mochtar B, Lecher F, Witsenburg M. Intraoperative epicardial two-dimensional echocardiography. Eur Heart J 1986; 7:386-95.

17. Goldman ME, Guarino T, Fotiades J, Rothschild A, Andrea L, Jethabhai MH, Minddich BP. Impact of in the operative Echocardiography: The first 1000 patients. JACC 1989 13,2:23A.

18. Takomoto S, Kyo S, Adachi H, Matsumura M, Yokote Y, Omoto R. Intraoperative color flow mapping by real-time two-dimensional Doppler echocardiography for evaluation of valvular and congenital heart disease and vascular disease. J Thorac Cardiovasc Surg 1985; 90:802-812.

19. Hagler DJ, Tajik AJ, Seward JB, Schaff HV, Danielson GK, Puga FJ. Intraoperative two-dimensional Doppler echocardiography. J Thorac Cardiovasc Surg 1988; 95:516-22.

20. Sutherland GR, van Daele MERM, Quaegebeur JM. Intraoperative ultrasound monitoring of banding of the pulmonary trunk: a new technique? Int. J Cardiol 1989; 22:395-398.

21. Schlüter M, Langenstein BA, Polster J, et al.. Transesophageal cross-sectional echocardiography with a phased array transducer system: technique and initial clinical results. Br Heart J 1982; 48:67-72.

22. de Bruijn NP, Clemens FM, Kisslo JA. Intraoperative transesophageal color flow mapping: initial experience. Anesth Analg 1987; 66:386-90.

23. Sutherland GR. The role of transesesophageal echocardiography in adolescents and adults with congenital heart disease. In: Erbel, Taijk (ed): Transesophageal Echocardiography (in print).

24. Seward JB, Khandheria BK, Oh JK, Abel MD, Hughes WD, Nichols BA, Freeman WK, Taijk AJ. Transesophageal Echocardiography: Technique, anatomic correlations, implementation, and clinicalapplications. Mayo Clin Proc 1988; 63:649-680.

25. Rice MJ, Seward JB, Edwards WD, Hagler DJ, Danielson GK, Puga FJ, Taijk AJ. Straddling Atrioventricular valve: two-dimensional echocardiographic diagnosis, classification and surgical implications. Am J Cardiol 1985; 55:505-513.

26. Vincent RN, Lang P, Chipman CW, Castaneda AR. Assessment of hemodynamic status in the intensive care unit immediately after closure of ventricular septal defects. Am J Cardiol 1985; 55:526-529.

27. Yeager SB, Freed MD, Keane JF, Norwood WI, Castaneda AR. Primary closure of ventricular septal defects in the first year of life: results in 128 infants. JACC 1984.

28. Lang P, Chipman CW, Siden H, Williams RG, Norwood WI, Castaneda AR. Early assessment of hemodynamic status after repair of Tetralogy of Fallot: Comparison of 24 hour (Intensive Care Unit) and 1 year postoperative data in 98 patients. Am J Cardiol 1982; 50:795-799.

29. Andradle JL, Serino W, deLeval M, Somerville J. Two-dimensional echocardiographic assessment of surgically closed ventricular septal defect. Am J Cardiol 1983; 52:325-29.

30. Ludomirsky A, Huhta JC, Vick W, Murphy DJ, Danford DA, Morrow R. Color Doppler detection of multiple ventricular septal defect. Circulation 1986; 74:1317-22.

31. Oritz E, Robinson PJ, Deanfield JE, Franklin R, Macartney FJ, Wyse RKH. Localisation of ventricular septal defects by simultaneous display of superimposed color Doppler and cross-sectional echocardiographicimages. Br Heart J 1985; 54:53-60.

32. Valdez-Cruz LM, Pieroni DR, Roland JM, Shematek JP. Recognition of Residual postoperative shunts by contrast echocardiographic techniques. Circulation 1977; 55:148-152.

33. Stevenson JG, Kawabori I, Stamm SJ, et al. Pulsed Doppler echocardiographic evaluation of ventricular septal defect patches. Circulation 1984; 70:suppl.I 38-46.

34. Sutherland GR, Smyllie J, Roelandt J, van Daele M, Quaegebeur J. Color flow imaging as intraoperative angiography in ventricular septal defect-advantages and pitfalls. JACC 1989;13,2:75A.

35. Shimazaki Y, Blackstone EH, Kirklin W. The natural history of isolated congenital pulmonary valve incompetence: surgical implications. Thorac Vardiovasc Surg 1984; 32:257-9.

36. Hagler DJ, Taijk AJ, Seward JB, Mair DD, Ritter DG. Double outlet right ventricle: Wide-angle two-dimensional echocardiographic observations. Ciculation 1981; 63:419-428.

37. Macartney FJ, Rigby ML, Anderson RH, Stark J, Silverman NH. Double outlet right ventricle Cross-sectional echocardiographic findings, their anatomical explanation, and surgical relevance. Br Heart J 1984; 52:164-77.

38. Piccoli G, Pacifico AD, Kirklin JW, Blackstone EH, Kirklin JK, Bargeron LM jr. Changing results and concepts in the surgical treatment of double outlet right ventricle: analysis of 137 operations in 126 patients. Am J Cardial 1983; 52:549-54.

39. Musumeci F, Shumway S, Lincoln C, Anderson RH. Surgical treatment for double outlet right ventricle at the Brompton Hospital 1973 to 1986. J Thorac Cardiovasc Surg 1988; 96:278-87.

40. Fontan F, Choussat A, Deville C, Doutremepuich C, Coupillaud J, Vosa C. Aortic homografts in the surgical treatment of complex cardiac malformations. J Thorac Cardiovasc Surg 1984; 87:649-657.

41. Mavroudis C, Rees A, Solinger R, Elbl F. The prognostic value of intraoperative pressure gradients in patients with congenital aortic stenosis. Ann Thor Surg 1984; 38:237-41.

42. Fontan F, Baudet E. Surgical repair of tricuspid atresia. Thorax 1971; 26:240-8.

43. Annecchino FP, Brunelli F, Borhi A, Abbruzzese P, Merlo M, Parenzan L. Fontan repair for tricuspid atresia - experience with 50 consecutive patients. Ann Thorac Surg 1988; 45:430-436.

44. Stellin G, Mazzucco A, Bortolotti U, de Torso S, Faggian G, Fracasso A, Livi U, Milano A, Rizolli G, Galluci V. Tricuspid atresia versus other complex lesions. J Thorac Cardiavasc Surg 1988; 96:204-11.

45. de Vivie ER, Rupprath G. Long-term results after Fontan procedure and its modifications. J Thorac Cardiavasc Surg 1986; 91:690-7.

46. Senning A. Surgical correction of transposition of the great arteries. Surgery 1959; 45:966-80.

47. Mustard WT, Keith JD, Trusler GA, Fowler R, Kidd L. The surgical management of transposition of the great vessels. J Thorac Cardiovasc Surg 1964; 48:953-58.

48. Rastelli GC, Wallace RB, Ongley PA. Complete repair of transposition of the great arteries with pulmonary stenosis. A review and report of a case corrected by using a new surgical technique. Circulation 1969; 39:83-95.

49. Stark J, Rastelli, Anderson RH, Shinebourne EA (eds). Pediatric Cardiology 1977. Churchill Livingstone, Edinburgh 1978; p 540-547.

50. Jatene AD, Fontes VF, Paulista PP et al. Anatomic correction of transposition of the great vessels. J Thorac Cardiovasc Surg 1976; 72:364-70.

51. Quaegebeur JM, Rohmer J, Ottenkamp J, Buis T, Kirklin JW, Blackstone EH, Brom AG. The arterial switch operation - an eight year experience. J Thorac Cardiovasc Surg 1986; 92:361-384.

52. Gibbs JL, Qureshi SA, Grieve L, et.al. Doppler echocardiography after anatomical correction of transposition of the great arteries. Br Heart J 1986; 56:67-72.

CHAPTER XVII

TRANSESOPHAGEAL ECHOCARDIOGRAPHY IN CONGENITAL HEART DISEASE

George R. Sutherland

Oliver F.W. Stümper

Introduction

Since the introduction of transesophageal echocardiography in 1980 as a semi-invasive tool for cardiac imaging [1-2] it has subsequently gained widespread acceptance over the past seven years in the adult cardiac outpatient clinic [3-5] for the investigation of atrial mass lesions [6-7], in the evaluation of mitral prosthetic valve function [8-9], in the assessment of endocarditis and its complications [10-15], and in the evaluation of thoracic pathology [16-19]. The recent increased interest in this technique has been largely due to further developments in the equipment that have provided a combination of high resolution cross-sectional imaging, spectral Doppler and color Doppler facilities for use via a single probe. The major advantage of the transesophageal approach is that it provides excellent insight into cardiac morphology and function especially in cases where a precordial ultrasound examination is difficult or impossible due to lung disease, chest deformity or mechanical ventilation.

Transesophageal imaging is now increasingly being used as a major diagnostic tool in the adult cardiology outpatient clinic. However, experience with this technique in patients with congenital heart lesions remains still limited [20-22] and its precise role in this group of patients is as yet undefined. As the transthoracic ultrasound approach yields complete morphologic and hemodynamic information in virtually all unoperated infants and young children with congenital heart disease, there would appear to be little need for the transesophageal approach in this patient group. However, in these patients major difficulties in obtaining complete diagnostic information from the transthoracic approach are encountered following cardiac surgery via a midline thoracotomy, as acquired fibrous adhesions restrict the precordial ultrasound window. Furthermore, ultrasound imaging in all children becomes more difficult with age due to increasing chest and cardiac size and the natural reduction in the transthoracic ultrasound window. In addition, complex congenital heart disease is frequently associated with either cardiac malpositions, where the heart is completely or partially obscured by the sternum and rib cage, or significant spinal or thoracic cage abnormalities which make ultrasound examination difficult.

Technique

Both the size of the currently available esophageal transducers and the semi-invasive nature of the procedure preclude its use in non-sedated or non-anaesthetised conscious children. Even when general anaesthesia is used to allow probe insertion and placement, the size of the probe, which in most cases exceeds 12 mm maximal diameter, will normally not allow children of less than 8 years to be investigated with safety [23-24].

In adolescents and adults a study can be performed in the outpatient clinic following local anaesthesia of the hypopharynx, to prevent the gag reflex, and, where appropriate, mild sedation of the patient with a short acting benzodiazepine. The patients should have fasted for at least four hours prior to the procedure. The role of antibiotic prophylaxis when performing such studies in patients with complex heart disease is unclear and remains contentious: we do not prescribe this ourselves. The conscious patient is studied lying in the left lateral decubitus position. The probe is introduced into the hypopharynx, with the distal end being partially flexed, and then, after allowing the distal end to straighten and asking the patient to swallow, the probe is advanced to the lower end of the oesophagus. The probe is advanced blindly as no imaging fibres are retained in the current generation of instruments. The technique used is exactly the same as that used during the blind insertion of a gastroscope. Normally no difficulties are encountered with probe insertion, but care should be taken in patients with a history of either cervical spine abnormalities or with suspected esophageal abnormalities.

Monitoring during the study is normally confined to a single lead continuous electrocardiographic recording. This is used to detect any episodes of arrythmias which may be provoked by manipulation of the probe. In our experience, arrhythmias are very rarely induced and where they do occur are transient and of supraventricular origin. Reported complications encountered with transesophageal investigations are exceptional [25-26]. The only major complications in adult patients were reported when transesophageal monitoring was used during neurosurgical procedures [27]. However, informed written consent should be obtained from every patient prior to the procedure.

Scanning Equipment

The transesophageal probes currently available are either phased linear or Phased annular arrays which are mounted on the end of a flexible conventional endoscope. The technique of manipulation of the probe tip using the steering and locking mechanisms is comparable to the technique used in gastroenterology. Most commonly 5-7.5 MHz transducers are used in the construction of esophageal probes, though prototype annular array probes to 10 MHz are bring tested. Nowadays, virtually all of the available equipment allows high resolution cross-sectional imaging and both color and pulsed Doppler investigations, for the simultaneous assessment of morphologic and hemodynamic parameters. More recently a mechanical annular array probe has been developed that also integrates continuous wave Doppler, pulsed Doppler, and color flow mapping in combination with 5.0 to 7.5 MHz cross-sectional imaging. All currently available transesophageal probes, using a modified gastroscope as their carrier, have maximal transducer diameters ranging from about 12 to 16 mm, with the shaft diameter of the endoscope being normally more than 10 mm [28]. Due to the relatively large dimensions of the probe transesophageal echocardiography in the unanaesthetized patient currently remains feasible in adolescents and adults only. Further attempts to miniaturize the transesophageal probes in order to allow assessment of children with congenital heart disease meet with several difficulties: 1. the production of smaller individual ultrasound crystals, and assembling these crystals onto a functioning transducer seem to have reached a critical point in minimal size, 2. the shaft of the endoscope has to contain all the electrical wires plus the steering wires to allow full manipulation of the transducer tip. To overcome these problems both phased annular and linear array prototype probes, based on a pediatric bronchoscope, have been constructed which have a maximal tip diameter of only 8 mm. These probes allow the safe and effective investigation of even small children. However the need for such studies is listed as the precowlied ultrasound approach in this patient population provides complete diagnostic information in the majority of patients.

Advantages and Limitations

Our recent experience in evaluating a range of complex congenital abnormalities by transesophageal echocardiography [29] has revealed many clear advantages of the transesophageal over the precordial approach in adolescents and adults with congenital heart disease, and particular in those who underwent prior corrective cardiac surgery for complex lesions.

These advantages included: 1. improved image quality when compared to precordial ultrasound evaluation in almost every patient, 2. the identification of atrial appendage anatomy, 3. clear demonstration of both normal and abnormal patterns of systemic and pulmonary venous drainage, 4. better definition of atrial septal defect morphology, 5. improved insight in atrioventricular valve and junction abnormalities, both in patients where prosthetic material precludes the evaluation of atrioventricular valve function from the precordial approach and in the complex abnormalities of chordal insertion in criss-cross hearts, 6. a new insight into atrial baffle function following the Senning or Mustard procedure, 7. better evaluation of the morphology and function in patients with a Fontan-type circulation, 8. improved definition of complex subaortic obstruction, and 9. the definition of ascending aortic morphology in Marfan's syndrome.

The major inherent limitations of the esophageal approach in the evaluation of congenital heart disease are: 1. the poor demonstration of cardiac structures that lie some distance from the esophagus (e.g. the anterior and apical part of the trabecular interventricular septum and the right ventricular outflow), 2. poor alignment to the direction of intracardiac blood flow (except for mitral valve and pulmonary vein flow) when performing pulsed wave Doppler studies, and 3. poor patient tolerance of the procedure in the adolescent and young adult age groups. Furthermore, the variety of scan planes obtainable from within the oesophagus are considerably reduced when compared to those available from the transthoracic approach. The esophageal examination with the current generation of single plane probes remains in essence a series of short axis scans.

Assessment of Congenital Heart Disease

All transesophageal investigations should follow a predetermined standardized protocol which will allow a complete assessment of both the morphology and hemodynamic features of any lesion studied. We would suggest the following scheme of investigation: 1. a complete atrial scan including the definition of atrial appendage anatomy, 2. demonstration of the pattern of systematic and pulmonary venous drainage (including a pulsed Doppler registration of pulmonary venous return), 3. documentation of the integrity of the atrial septum, 4. definition of the mode and morphology of atrioventricular connection, 5. assessment of atrioventricular valve structure and function, 6. examination of the integrity of the portion of the interventricular septum which is visible, 7. demonstration of the morphology of the ventricular outflows and semilunar valves, and 8. demonstration of the morphology of the ascending and descending thoracic aorta and proximal pulmonary arteries. A complete study will normally require a routine sequence of transducer manipulations to visualize all possible scan planes from within the oesophagus and the fundus of the stomach [30-31].

The information which can thus be obtained in congenital heart disease by transesophageal echocardiography from each of the different cardiac levels is now described.

Cardiac Position

Precordial imaging in patients with an abnormally positioned heart (e.g. dextro- or mesocardia) is often difficult and incomplete due to the large areas of the heart that are obscured by the sternum or lung tissue. Contrastingly, an abnormal cardiac position does not create any major problems for a transesophageal study although the transducer has to be manipulated in a different way in order to obtain complete information in patients with meso- or dextrocardia. These changes in transducer manipulation are relatively easy to learn and a full imaging study can routinely be carried out in every patient.

Atrial Appendage Anatomy - Atria

One of the major advantages of transesophageal echocardiography is that this technique allows superb insight into the morphology of both atrial appendages, despite either an abnormal cardiac position or any degree of cardiac rotation. Atrial appendage anatomy is reliably identified as cross-sectional imaging from the oesophagus can delineate the precise morphologic features of either atrial appendage. The left atrial appendage is demonstrated as a long, crescentic and crenellated structure (Fig.17-1a). These appearances can consistently be differentiated from those of the short blunt right atrial appendage (Fig.17-1b). Normally the atrial appendage anatomy cannot be defined by the transthoracic approach. Due to the difficulties encountered with direct visualization of appendage anatomy from the precordium situs identification by ultrasound is normally attempted by analyzing the morphology and relationships of the great vessels in the upper abdomen. This method is reliable in approximately 85% of cases of abnormal situs but may give false results, especially in patients with atrial isomerism [32]. Transesophageal echocardiography should appear to be a better technique in cases where ambiguity persists, as it can allow direct indentification of atrial appendage morphology in every patient.

Furthermore, the esophageal approach should be superior to the transthoracic approach in indentifying juxtaposed atrial appendages and for the detailed diagnosis of partitioned atrial chambers (cor triatriatum)[22]. In patients with cor triatriatum and supravalvular mitral stenosis transesophageal echocardiography can provide valuable additional information as the exact site of insertions and extent of these obstructive "membranes" can be clearly demonstrated. Any coexisting atrial septal defect or the abnormal drainage of any pulmonary vein can be visualized. Pulsed wave Doppler sampling can allow assessment of blood flow characteristics across these lesions.

Post-operative evaluation of patients who underwent a Senning or Mustard procedure for correction of complete transposition of the great arteries in the past, is largely facilitated by transesophageal investigations. The complex anatomy of the baffle, both atria, both atrioventricular valves and systemic and pulmonary venous return are easily accessible from the esophagus. Hemodynamically relevant lesions such as baffle leaks or obstructions to systemic or pulmonary venous return are clearly demonstrated by a combination of color flow imaging and pulsed wave Doppler.

Systemic Venous Drainage

Scanning from the oesophagus in a series of short axis cuts derived by positioning the probe at differing levels within the thorax, clearly demonstrates the course and drainage of the superior vena cava. The inferior vena cava can only be visualized at its orifice as it enters the floor of the right atrium. Persisting venous valves (which may be the cause of turbulent flow within the right atrium) are clearly demonstrated with high resolution cross-sectional imaging from the oesophagus.

Abnormalities of systemic venous return, such as a second left-sided superior vena cava entering the heart either directly to the superior aspect of the left atrium, or by drainage via the coronary sinus can be demonstrated. Color flow mapping, as an adjunct to the imaging diagnosis, is of great value in these situations as it helps to identify the abnormal site of venous flow drainage and to exclude any related interatrial flow caused by drainage via the coronary sinus.

Transesophageal echocardiography imaging allied to pulsed wave Doppler can provide invaluable information concerning both the morphology and function of a Glenn anastomosis in patients with absent right atrioventricular connections. Color flow mapping clearly demonstrates the direct communication between the upper (dilated) portion of the superior vena cava and the distal portion of the transsected right pulmonary artery. Pulsed Doppler measurements can be used to determine flow characteristics across the anastomosis and within the right pulmonary artery.

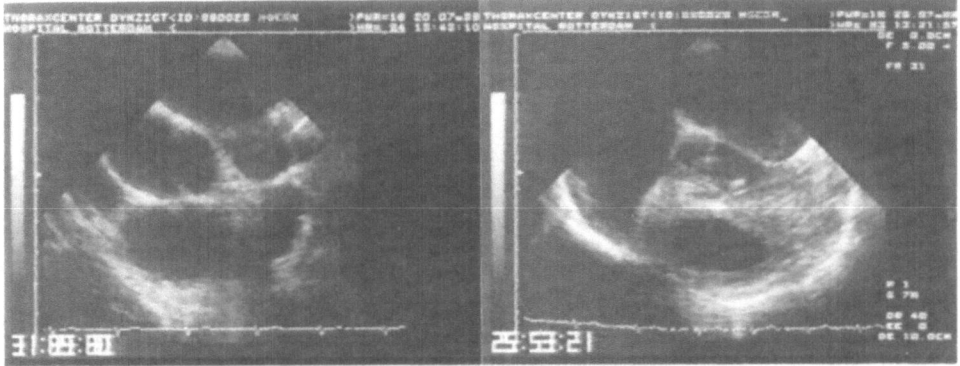

Figure 17-1a: Transesophageal view of a left atrial appendage (LAA). Note the narrow junction with the atrial cavity and the long crenellated cavity of the appendage. Ao = ascending aorta, RVOT = right ventricular outflow tract. b: The atrial appendage (RAA) in the same patient is clearly identified by its junction with the atrial cavity and the blunt and short appendage cavity. (LVOT = left ventricular outflow tract.

Pulmonary Venous Drainage

The identification of individual pulmonary veins and the site of their venous return to the heart is facilitated by using the transesophageal approach. Left and right upper pulmonary veins draining to the left atrium are readily demonstrated by cross-sectional imaging, but the lower pulmonary veins, especially the right are difficult to image. Color flow mapping can improve the ability to demonstrate the exact localization of the orifices of each pulmonary vein. The left upper pulmonary vein and the left atrial appendage are clearly imaged and can consistently be distinguished from each other in every single patient.

As well as demonstrating normal pulmonary venous drainage, transesophageal echocardiography can provide valuable additional information concerning the presence of supradiaphragmatic partial anomalous venous drainage. This ability is of particular importance in older children and adolescents in whom the precordial approach often fails to demonstrate the exact localization of pulmonary venous drainage and coexistence of transatrial flow. Thus the combination of transesophageal cross-sectional imaging, color flow mapping and pulsed wave Doppler investigations can yield maximal information in the investigation of such lesions.

Transesophageal echocardiography is also the diagnostic tool of choice for diagnosing atrial mass lesions, such as atrial myxomas, and is invaluable in the assessment of secondary cardiac involvement by invasive mediastinal tumors, such as malignant lymphomas.

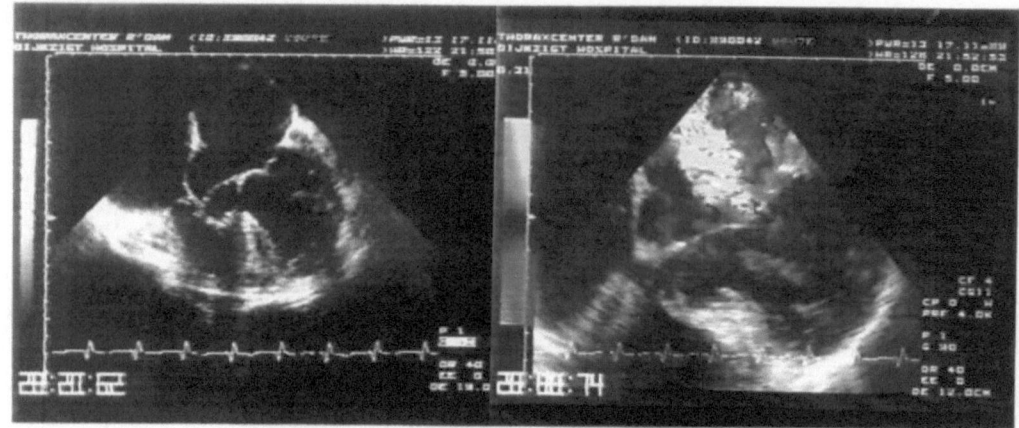

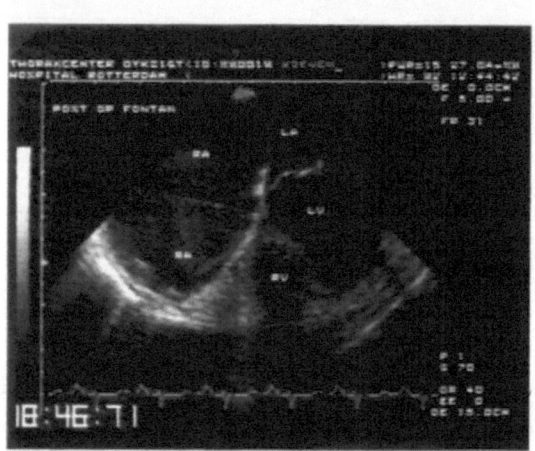

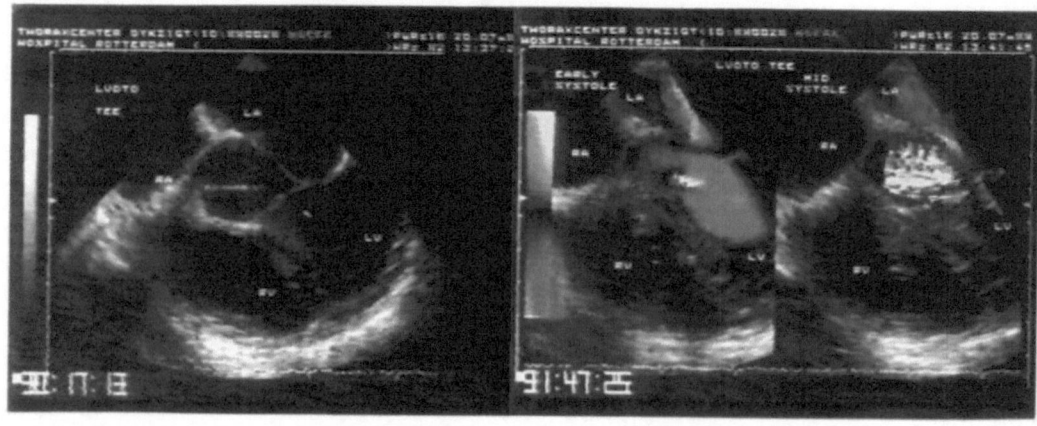

Figure 17-2a : Transesophageal study in an adult patient after repair of an atrioventricular septal defect. The patch used for closure of the atrial defect is bulging towards the right. The mitral valve is assessed in fine detail when scanning a series of four-chamber views. Note the chordal attachments of the superior bridging leaflet into the crest of the ventricular septum (arrow) b: The subsequent color flow mapping study revealed a moderate to severe mitral regurgitation orginating from the mid portion of the line of coaptation. The integrity of the interventricular septum is not reliably documented due to the large distance from the esophagus and the use of prosthetic material in the repair which produces flow masking.

Figure 17-3 : Follow-up study in a patient with a Fontan-type circulation. The right atrium (RA) is massively enlarged and spontaneous contrast was noted during real-time imaging. However no clear evidence for clot formation in the right atrium was detected. The prominent Eustachian valve is seen as thin structure (arrow) dividing the right atrium - no turbulent flow was documentated on the subsequent clor flow mapping study. (LA = left atrium, LV = left ventricle, RV = right ventricle).

Figure 17-4a: Left ventricular outflow tract obstruction. The fibromuscular membrane (arrow) with both its attachments into the interventricular septum and the anterior leaflet of the mitral valve is clearly documented. In this patient any involvement of the subvalvar apparatus of the mitral valve was definitely excluded. (LA = left atrium, LV = left ventricle, RA = right atrium, RV = right ventricle). b: The color flow mapping study shows on an early systolic frame (left) the start of the turbulence at the level of the membrane; the mid systolic frame (right) demonstrates turbulent flow patterns in the entire left ventricular outflow tract. Note that the obstructing gradient cannot be assessed because of an almost ninety degree angle between the Doppler beam and the blood flow.

The Atrial Septum

The major advantage of transesophageal echocardiography in the assessment of the integrity of the atrial septum is that the ultrasound beam strikes the septum almost perpendicularly. Therefore this approach is far less prone to produce false-positive results. Such false-positive results concerning the existence of atrial septal defects are all too frequently encountered when performing precordial studies, and are caused by areas of echo drop-out within the cross-sectional image. The most reliable transthoracic approach for the assessment of the integrity of the atrial septum is the subcostal window, however this is frequently obscured in older children and adults or in the presence of obesity.

From the oesophagus the integrity of the entire atrial septum can be easily assessed with little manipulation of the transducer. High resolution cross-sectional imaging allows differentiation between shunting via a foramen ovale flap valve, a patent foramen ovale or a septum secundum defect.

The exact site of any atrial septal defect, as well as the spatial relationships to the venae cavae, pulmonary veins, coronary sinus and the central fibrous body, are readily demonstrated by transesophageal investigations. Especially in older patients with congenital heart disease associated abnormalities such as partial anomalous pulmonary venous drainage (see previous section), accessory tissue tags of the atrial septum or atrial septum aneurysm formation, and the septum primum and atrioventricular valve abnormalities associated with atrioventricular septal defects, are better visualized from the oesophagus.

In the presence of sinus venosus defects it is possible to demonstrate the exact relationship of the orifice of the superior vena cava to the superior margin of the oval fossa and the right pulmonary veins. In coronary sinus defects the transesophageal approach is superior to transthoracic studies in demonstrating a left persisting superior vena cava as well as demonstrating the exact site and degree of unroofing of the coronary sinus. The precise interpretation of the complex morphology encountered over the range of atrial septal defects, and the associated hemodynamics is largely facilitated by combined color flow mapping and cross-sectional imaging (e.g. single defects vs multiple - especially where there is a fenestrated atrial septum).

Atrioventricular Valves and Connections

The precordial approach to any abnormality encountered on this level is complete and diagnostic in most unoperated patients. Difficulties in accurate ultrasound assessment of atrioventricular valve function are most often encountered after either previous intracardiac repair or following valve replacement. Sequential post-operative assessment of patients who have residual lesions of either atrioventricular valves, and in whom the transthoracic studies fail to produce the information required for patient management, is possible using the transesophageal approach. This technique can provide excellent insight into the morphology and, by means of Doppler investigations, the function of both atrioventricular valves. Most commonly these studies impart a remarkable degree of morphologic detail in the cross-sectional images, and allow better assessment of the degree of atrioventricular valve incompetence (Fig.17-2a/b). These latter points are of crucial importance in assessing patients with 1.Ebstein's malformation of the tricuspid valve, 2. absent vs imperforate atrioventricular connections, 3. double inlet ventricles and 4. criss-cross hearts. Following either atrioventricular valve replacement or valve repair using prosthetic material transesophageal echocardiography is often the only means of obtaining complete information on prosthetic or native valve malfunction.

Furthermore, transesophageal echocardiography is a superb technique for the semi-invasive assessment of patients who have undergone a Fontan-type procedure (with or without a Glenn shunt) in the past (Fig 17-3). This approach can allow direct visualization of the Glenn anastomosis, the right atrial morphology, the blood flow characteristics within the atrium, clot formation, the direct atrio-pulmonary communication and the central pulmonary arteries. In all of these patients, high quality pulsed Doppler tracings of the velocity profiles within each of these structures and anastomoses can be recorded for subsequent detailed analysis. This is routinely not possible from the precordial approach. However, major difficulties are encountered in cases where either a conduit-type connection between the right atrium and the anterior right ventricular outlet chamber or an anterior valved conduit from the right atrial appendage to the main pulmonary artery was created. In these patients transesophageal echocardiography fails to demonstrate the conduit and the valve it contains in most cases. This is due to a combination of its anterior position and the image and flow masking properties inherent in the prosthetic material used in the repair.

The Interventricular Septum

The assessment of an isolated ventricular septal defect by precordial echocardiography is remarkably accurate when using a combination of cross-sectional imaging, continuous wave Doppler and color flow mapping. The only problem area normally encountered in this precordial assessment is in distinguishing a single defect from multiple defects. Thus, the transesophageal approach with its poor ability to visualize the anterior, apical and outlet portions of the interventricular septum has little further to offer in the diagnosis of ventricular septal defects. In fact, only defects in the perimembranous area can be consistently imaged. This is of some value as the majority of moderate or large ventricular septal defects wholly or partially involve this region and thus can be imaged from the oesophagus. However, significant problems do exist with false-positive areas of echo "drop out" when using the transesophageal approach. Furthermore, the cross-sectional image of any ventricular structure obtained from the oesophagus constantly moves in and out of the scan plane. Conclusively transesophageal imaging is not a good technique for the evaluation of congenital ventricular septal defects, when compared to good quality precordial ultrasound studies. This should be borne in mind when the indication for a transesophageal study is formulated.

Ventricular Outflow Tracts

Transesophageal imaging provides excellent imaging of the left ventricular outflow tract, and is a superb technique for demonstrating the range of left heart sub valve obstruction encountered in congenital heart disease (Fig 17-4 A and B). It readily provides much more detailed information on the complex morphology of discrete fibromuscular subaortic obstruction ("subaortic membrane") and its associated abnormalities than the precordial approach [33]. Our recent experience with this technique in assessing fibromuscular subaortic obstruction in adolescents demonstrated that the spectrum of these abnormalities in this group of patients is far more complex than those encountered in young children. This would suggest that the pathology of fibromuscular obstruction may be a progressive lesion. Transesophageal cross-sectional imaging often demonstrates multiple insertions of these "membranes" into 1. the interventricular septum, 2. the region of the aortic valve "annulus", 3. the anterior leaflet of the mitral valve, and 4. the tendinuous chordae of the mitral valve. Additionally, transesophageal echocardiography may also provide substantially more information in tunnel subaortic stenosis and hypertrophic obstructive myopathies when compared to precordial imaging. However, poor alignment to flow normally precludes the use of Doppler measurements for precise quantification of the obstruction gradient. Only the morphology and the color flow map abnormalities can be assessed.

Although transesophageal echocardiography would appear to be the diagnostic tool of choice in adolescents and adults with discrete or "tunnel-like" left ventricular outflow tract obstruction, this technique is incapable of providing any information on the right ventricular outflow tract. This is due to the large distance between the esophagus and this structure.

Arterial Valves and Great Vessels

The aortic valve can be excellently visualized by transesophageal imaging. However, as the sectioning plane from the oesophagus is more or less oblique, Doppler evaluation of blood flow across this valve is limited. The pulmonary valve can be imaged in the majority of cases by an experienced operator as can both the main and proximal portions of the individual pulmonary arteries.

Transesophageal imaging can demonstrate the proximal left and right coronary arteries and the proximal two thirds of the ascending aorta. This technique provides clear advantages over the precordial aproach in: 1. definition of proximal coronary anatomy (which may be relevant in patients with Tetralogy of Fallot who have variable coronary anatomy), 2. identification of supravalvular aortic stenosis, 3. exclusion of acute ascending aortic dilatation or localized areas of dissection in Marfan's syndrome, 4. assessment of vascular rings and 5. assessment of descending aortic coarctation.

Due to interposition of the bronchus between the oesophagus and the aorta, the distal third of the ascending aorta and the proximal part of the aortic arch may not be well visualized. The distal aortic arch and the descending thoracic aorta can easily be imaged. However, in the majority of cases with descending aortic pathology, the transesophageal approach does not contribute any significant additional information, after good quality precordial or suprasternal studies have been performed. In those cases where suprasternal imaging is non-contributory, evaluation of a descending aortic coarctation via the esophageal approach, may provide useful information especially where this is a localized ring-like lesion. However, in complicated cases of descending thoracic aorta pathology, such as long or tortuous coarctations or where there are multiple aortic collaterals supplying lung vessels in complex pulmonary atresia, angiography and/or magnetic resonance imaging, in our opinion, remain the techniques of choice when attempting to make an accurate and complete diagnosis.

Where To Use It

Currently the use of transesophageal echocardiography in congenital heart disease is predominantly restricted to the adolescent and adult outpatient clinic. Referral for such an investigation should be based on the following factors: 1. Is transesophageal echocardiography likely to provide the additional information required for patient management? 2. Should the patient be studied with or without sedation or under anaesthesia? Clearly such outpatient studies are only appropriate where clinical examination and precordial ultrasound studies have failed to achieve a diagnosis and where definitive information can only be obtained from an esophageal study. Appropriate study areas would thus appear to be 1. the atria, 2. atrioventricular valves, 3. left ventricular outflow tract and 4. ascending aorta pathology.

With increasing experience and further technical improvements there will be further applications for this new technique in the near future: 1. intraoperative assessment and monitoring of children with congenital heart disease undergoing corrective surgery (in combination with epicardial studies), 2. monitoring in the intensive care unit in the post-operative period and 3. monitoring of the immediate morphologic and hemodynamic results of interventional catheterization procedures. The use of transesophageal echocardiography in these fields is potentially superior to the transthoracic or epicardial approach as this technique does not interfere with the surgical or catheter procedure, thus eliminating the theoretical risk of infections. Furthermore it provides much better image quality during the post operative period than does the transthoracic approach. The latter is frequently precluded due to entrapped air in the pericardium, mechanical ventilation or the presence of suction tubes.

However, extension of the current applicability of transesophageal echocardiography to infants and small children with congenital heart disease will only be achieved when smaller probes that allow higher resolution imaging become available. The development of multiplane probes, with or without rotational tips, could improve assessment of complex forms of congenital heart disease from the oesophagus.

Summary

Transesophageal echocardiography is a relatively new semi-invasive technique which opens up a new window to the heart. As outlined above, it may contribute information of great additional value for the management of patients with congenital heart disease. Due to the semi-invasive nature of the procedure and the currently existing technical limitations, indication for this procedure should be strict especially in young patients. Transesophageal studies should only be performed in patients where the transthoracic ultrasound approach cannot provide all the information required for patient management, and where the transesophageal technique is likely to yield this extra information. Technical developments in this new field of cardiac ultrasound are proceeding at a great pace so that current limitations to the investigation of small children are likely to be overcome in the near future. This will subsequently increase the potential role of transesophageal echocardiography in congenital heart disease.

References

1. Hisagana K, Hisagana A, Nagata K, Yoshida S. Transesophageal cross-sectional echocardiography. Am Heart J 1980; 100:605-9.

2. Schlueter M, Langenstein BA, Polster J, et al. Transesophageal cross-sectional echocardiography with a phased array transducer system: technique and initial clinical results. Br. Heart J 1982; 48:62-72.

3. Gussenhoven EJ, Taams MA, Roelandt JRTC, et al. Transesophageal two-dimensional echocardiography: Its role in solving clinical problems. J Am Coll Cardiol 1986; 8:975-79.

4. Schlueter M, Hanrath P. Transesophageal echocardiography: Potential advantages and initial clinical results. Practical Cardiology 1983; 9:149-80.

5. Erbel R, Mohr-Kahaly S, Rohmann S, et al. Diagnostische Wertigkeit der transosophagealen Doppler-Echokardiographie. Herz 1987; 12(3):177-86.

6. Aschenberg W, Schlueter M, Kremer P, et al. Transesophageal two-dimensional echocardiography for the detection of left atrial appendage thrombus. J Am Coll Cardiol 1986;7, 1:163-66

7. Thier W, Schlueter M, Krebber H, et al. Cysts in left atrial myxomas indentified by transesophageal cross-sectional echocardiography. Br. Heart J 1983; 51:1793-5.

8. Taams M, Gussenhoven E, Cahalan M, et al. Transesophageal Doppler color flow imaging in the detection of native and Bjork-Shiley mitral valve regurgitation. JACC 1989;13, 1:95-99.

9. Nellesen V, Schnittger I, Appelton CP, et al. Transesophageal two-dimensional echocardiography and color Doppler flow velocity mapping in the evaluation of cardiac valve prostheses. Circulation 1988; 78:848-55.

10. Drexler M, Erbel R, Rohmann S, et al. Diagnostic value of two-dimensional transesophageal versus transthoracic echocardiography in patients with infective endocarditis. Eur Heart J 1987;8 (supp 1): 303-06.

11. Erbel R, Rohman S, Drexler M, et al. Improved diagnostic value of echocardiography in patients with infective endocarditis by transesophageal approach, a prospective study. Eur Heart J 9; 1:43-53, 1988.

12. Gussenhoven EJ, van Herwerden LA, Roelandt J, et al. Detailed analysis of aortic valve endocarditis: Comparison of precordial and epicardial two-dimensional echocardiography with surgical findings. JCU 1986; 14:209-11.

13. Geibel A, Hofmann T, Behroz A, et al. Echocardiographic diagnosis of infective endocarditis additional information by transesophageal echocardiography? (abstract) Circulation 1987; 76.IV:38.

14. Daniel WG, Schroeder E, Nonnast-Daniel B, Lichtlen PR. Conventional and transesophageal echocardiography in the diagnosis of infective endocarditis. Eur Heart J 1987; 8 Suppl J: 287-292.

15. Polak PE, Gussenhoven WJ, Roelandt JR. Transesophageal cross-sectional echocardiographic recognition of an aortic valve ring abcess and a subannular mycotic aneurysm. Eur Heart J 1987; 8:664-666.

16. Borner N, Erbel R, Braun B, et al. Diagnosis of aortic dissection by transesophageal echocardiography. Am J Cardiol 54: 1157-58, 1984.

17. Erbel R, Mohr-Kahaly S, Rennoliet H, et al. Diagnosis of aortic dissection: the value of transesophageal echocardiography. Thorac Cardiovasc Surg 35; 2:126-33, 1987.

18. Engberding-Render F, Grosse-Heitmeyer W, Most E, et al. Indentification of dissection or aneurysm of the descending thoracic aorta by conventional and transesophageal two-dimensional echocardiography. Am J Cardiol 1988; 59:717-19.

19. Taams MA, Gussenhoven WJ, Schippers LA, et al. The value of transesophageal echocardiography for diagnosis of thoracic aorta pathology. Eur Heart J 1988; 9:1308-16.

20. Hanrath P, Schlueter M, Langenstein BA, et al. Detection of ostium secundum atrial septal defects by transesophageal cross-sectional echocardiograophy. Br Heart J 1983; 48:350-8.

21. Morimoto K, Matsuzaki M, Tohma Y, et al. Diagnosis and quantitative evaluation of atrial septal defect by transesophageal 2D color Doppler echocardiography (abstract). Circulation 1987; 77.IV:39.

22. Schlueter M, Langenstein BA, Thier W, et al. Transesophageal two-dimensional echocardiography in the diagnosis of cor triatriatum in the adult. JACC 1983; 2:1011-15.

23. Cyran SE, Kimball TR, Meyer RA, et al. Efficacy of intraoperative Transesophageal echocardiography in children with congenital heart disease. Am J Cardiol 1989; 63:594-598.

24. Ament M, Christie D. Upper gastrointestinal fiberoptic in pediatric patients. Gastroenterology 1977; 72:1244-48.

25. Geibel A, Kasper W, Behroz A, et al. Risk of transesophageal echocardiography in awake patients with cardiac disease. Am J Cardial 1988; 62:337-9.

26. Khandheria B, Seward J, Oh J, et al. Safety of transesophageal echocardiography in awake patients: Experience with 400 procedures. (abstract) JACC 1989; 13,2:225A.

27. Cucchiara RF, Nugent M, Seward JB, et al. Air embolism in upright neurosurgical patients: Detection and localization by two-dimensional transesophageal echocardiography. Anaesthesiology 1984; 60:353-5.

28. Roelandt JRTC, Sutherland GR, Geuskens R, Taams MA, Fraser AG. Transesophageal echocardiography: New developments and clinical indications. (submitted)

29. Sutherland GR, Geuskens R, Taams M, Gussenhoven E, Hess J, Roelandt J. The role of transesophageal echocardiography in adolescents and adults with congenital heart disease. (submitted)

30. Schlueter H, Hinrichs A, Thier W, et al. Transesophageal two-dimensional echocardiography comparison of ultrasonic and anatomic sections. Am J Cardiol 53:1173-1178, 1984.

31. Seward JB, Khanderia BK, Oh JK, et al. Transesophageal echocardiography: Technique anatomic correlations, implementation, and clinical applications. Mayo Clin Proc 1988; 63:649-680.

32. Huhta JC, Smallhorn JF, Macartney FJ. Two-dimensional echocardiographic diagnosis of situs. Br Heart J 1982; 48:97-108.

33. Poppele G, Krueger W, Langenstein B, Hanrath P. Membranose subvalvulare Aortenstenose. Nachweis mittels transthorakaler und transesophagealer 2-D Doppler echokardiographie. Dtsch Med Wochenschr 1988 113(31-32): 1224-8.

Developments in Cardiovascular Medicine

43. S. Sideman and R. Beyar (eds.): [3-D] *Simulation and Imaging of the Cardiac System.* State of the Heart. Proceedings of the International Henry Goldberg Workshop, held in Haifa, Israel (1984). 1985   ISBN 0–89838–687–X
44. E. van der Wall and K.I. Lie (eds.): *Recent Views on Hypertrophic Cardiomyopathy.* Proceedings of a Symposium, held in Groningen, The Netherlands (1984). 1985
                ISBN 0–89838–694–2
45. R.E. Beamish, P.K. Singal and N.S. Dhalla (eds.), *Stress and Heart Disease.* Proceedings of a International Symposium, held in Winnipeg, Canada, 1984 (Vol. 1). 1985   ISBN 0–89838–709–4
46. R.E. Beamish, V. Panagia and N.S. Dhalla (eds.): *Pathogenesis of Stress-induced Heart Disease.* Proceedings of a International Symposium, held in Winnipeg, Canada, 1984 (Vol. 2). 1985   ISBN 0–89838–710–8
47. J. Morganroth and E.N. Moore (eds.): *Cardiac Arrhythmias.* New Therapeutic Drugs and Devices. Proceedings of the 5th Symposium on New Drugs and Devices, held in Philadelphia, Pa., U.S.A. (1984). 1985   ISBN 0–89838–716–7
48. P. Mathes (ed.): *Secondary Prevention in Coronary Artery Disease and Myocardial Infarction.* 1985   ISBN 0–89838–736–1
49. H.L. Stone and W.B. Weglicki (eds.): *Pathobiology of Cardiovascular Injury.* Proceedings of the 6th Annual Meeting of the American Section of the I.S.H.R., held in Oklahoma City, Okla., U.S.A. (1984). 1985   ISBN 0–89838–743–4
50. J. Meyer, R. Erbel and H.J. Rupprecht (eds.): *Improvement of Myocardial Perfusion.* Thrombolysis, Angioplasty, Bypass Surgery. Proceedings of a Symposium, held in Mainz, F.R.G. (1984). 1985   ISBN 0–89838–748–5
51. J.H.C. Reiber, P.W. Serruys and C.J. Slager (eds.): *Quantitative Coronary and Left Ventricular Cineangiography.* Methodology and Clinical Applications. 1986
                ISBN 0–89838–760–4
52. R.H. Fagard and I.E. Bekaert (eds.): *Sports Cardiology.* Exercise in Health and Cardiovascular Disease. Proceedings from an International Conference, held in Knokke, Belgium (1985). 1986   ISBN 0–89838–782–5
53. J.H.C. Reiber and P.W. Serruys (eds.): *State of the Art in Quantitative Cornary Arteriography.* 1986   ISBN 0–89838–804–X
54. J. Roelandt (ed.): *Color Doppler Flow Imaging and Other Advances in Doppler Echocardiography.* 1986   ISBN 0–89838–806–6
55. E.E. van der Wall (ed.): *Noninvasive Imaging of Cardiac Metabolism.* Single Photon Scintigraphy, Positron Emission Tomography and Nuclear Magnetic Resonance. 1987
                ISBN 0–89838–812–0
56. J. Liebman, R. Plonsey and Y. Rudy (eds.): *Pediatric and Fundamental Electrocardiography.* 1987   ISBN 0–89838–815–5
57. H.H. Hilger, V. Hombach and W.J. Rashkind (eds.), *Invasive Cardiovascular Therapy.* Proceedings of an International Symposium, held in Cologne, F.R.G. (1985). 1987   ISBN 0–89838–818–X
58. P.W. Serruys and G.T. Meester (eds.): *Coronary Angioplasty.* A Controlled Model for Ischemia. 1986   ISBN 0–89838–819–8
59. J.E. Tooke and L.H. Smaje (eds.): *Clinical Investigation of the Microcirculation.* Proceedings of an International Meeting, held in London, U.K. (1985). 1987
                ISBN 0–89838–833–3

Developments in Cardiovascular Medicine

Developments in Cardiovascular Medicine

78. M.M. Scheinman (ed.): *Catheter Ablation of Cardiac Arrhythmias*. Basic Bioelectrical Effects and Clinical Indications. 1988 ISBN 0–89838–967–4
79. J.A.E. Spaan, A.V.G. Bruschke and A.C. Gittenberger-De Groot (eds.): *Coronary Circulation*. From Basic Mechanisms to Clinical Implications. 1987
 ISBN 0–89838–978–X
80. C. Visser, G. Kan and R.S. Meltzer (eds.): *Echocardiography in Coronary Artery Disease*. 1988 ISBN 0–89838–979–8
81. A. Bayés de Luna, A. Betriu and G. Permanyer (eds.): *Therapeutics in Cardiology*. 1988 ISBN 0–89838–981–X
82. D.M. Mirvis (ed.): *Body Surface Electrocardiographic Mapping*. 1988
 ISBN 0–89838–983–6
83. M.A. Konstam and J.M. Isner (eds.): *The Right Ventricle*. 1988 ISBN 0–89838–987–9
84. C.T. Kappagoda and P.V. Greenwood (eds.): *Long-term Management of Patients after Myocardial Infarction*. 1988 ISBN 0–89838–352–8
85. W.H. Gaasch and H.J. Levine (eds.): *Chronic Aortic Regurgitation*. 1988
 ISBN 0–89838–364–1
86. P.K. Singal (ed.): *Oxygen Radicals in the Pathophysiology of Heart Disease*. 1988
 ISBN 0–89838–375–7
87. J.H.C. Reiber and P.W. Serruys (eds.): *New Developments in Quantitative Coronary Arteriography*. 1988 ISBN 0–89838–377–3
88. J. Morganroth and E.N. Moore (eds.): *Silent Myocardial Ischemia*. Proceedings of the 8th Annual Symposium on New Drugs and Devices (1987). 1988
 ISBN 0–89838–380–3
89. H.E.D.J. ter Keurs and M.I.M. Noble (eds.): *Starling's Law of the Heart Revisted*. 1988 ISBN 0–89838–382–X
90. N. Sperelakis (ed.): *Physiology and Pathophysiology of the Heart*. (Rev. ed.) 1988
 ISBN 0–89838–388–9
91. J.W. de Jong (ed.): *Myocardial Energy Metabolism*. 1988 ISBN 0–89838–394–3
92. V. Hombach, H.H. Hilger and H.L. Kennedy (eds.): *Electrocardiography and Cardiac Drug Therapy*. Proceedings of an International Symposium, held in Cologne, F.R.G. (1987). 1988 ISBN 0–89838–395–1
93. H. Iwata, J.B. Lombardini and T. Segawa (eds.): *Taurine and the Heart*. 1988
 ISBN 0–89838–396–X
94. M.R. Rosen and Y. Palti (eds.): *Lethal Arrhythmias Resulting from Myocardial Ischemia and Infarction*. Proceedings of the 2nd Rappaport Symposium, held in Haifa, Israel (1988). 1988 ISBN 0–89838–401–X
95. M. Iwase and I. Sotobata: *Clinical Echocardiography*. With a Foreword by M.P. Spencer. 1989 ISBN 0–7923–0004–1
96. I. Cikes (ed.): *Echocardiography in Cardiac Interventions*. 1989
 ISBN 0–7923–0088–2
97. E. Rapaport (ed.): *Early Interventions in Acute Myocardial Infarction*. 1989
 ISBN 0–7923–0175–7
98. M.E. Safar and F. Fouad-Tarazi (eds.): *The Heart in Hypertension*. A Tribute to Robert C. Tarazi (1925–1986). 1989 ISBN 0–7923–0197–8
99. S. Meerbaum and R. Meltzer (eds.): *Myocardial Contrast Two-dimensional Echocardiography*. 1989 ISBN 0–7923–0205–2

Developments in Cardiovascular Medicine

100. J. Morganroth and E.N. Moore (eds.): *Risk/Benefit Analysis for the Use and Approval of Thrombolytic, Antiarrhythmic, and Hypolipidemic Agents.* Proceedings of the 9th Annual Symposium on New Drugs and Devices (1988). 1989   ISBN 0-7923-0294-X
101. P.W. Serruys, R. Simon and K.J. Beatt (eds.): *PTCA - An Investigational Tool and a Non-operative Treatment of Acute Ischemia.* 1990   ISBN 0-7923-0346-6
102. I.S. Anand, P.I. Wahi and N.S. Dhalla (eds.): *Pathophysiology and Pharmacology of Heart Disease.* 1989   ISBN 0-7923-0367-9
103. G.S. Abela (ed.): *Lasers in Cardiovascular Medicine and Surgery.* Fundamentals and Technique. 1990   ISBN 0-7923-0440-3
104. H.M. Piper (ed.): *Pathophysiology of Severe Ischemic Myocardial Injury.* 1990   ISBN 0-7923-0459-4
105. S.M. Teague (ed.): *Stress Doppler Echocardiography.* 1990   ISBN 0-7923-0499-3
106. P.R. Saxena, D.I. Wallis, W. Wouters and P. Bevan (eds.): *Cardiovascular Pharmacology of 5-Hydroxytryptamine.* Prospective Therapeutic Applications. 1990   ISBN 0-7923-0502-7
107. A.P. Shepherd and P.A. Öberg (eds.): *Laser-Doppler Blood Flowmetry.* 1990   ISBN 0-7923-0508-6
108. J. Soler-Soler, G. Permanyer-Miralda and J. Sagristà-Sauleda (eds.): *Pericardial Disease.* New Insights and Old Dilemmas. Preface by Ralph Shabetai. 1990   ISBN 0-7923-0510-8
109. J.P.M. Hamer: *Practical Echocardiography in the Adult.* With Doppler and Color-Doppler Flow Imaging. 1990   ISBN 0-7923-0670-8
110. A. Bayés de Luna, P. Brugada, J. Cosin Aguilar and F. Navarro Lopez (eds.): *Sudden Cardiac Death.* 1990   ISBN 0-7923-0716-X
111. E. Andries and R. Stroobandt (eds.): *Hemodynamics in Daily Practice.* 1990   ISBN 0-7923-0725-9
112. J. Morganroth and E.N. Moore (eds.): *Use and Approval of Antihypertensive Agents and Surrogate Endpoints for the Approval of Drugs affecting Antiarrhythmic Heart Failure and Hypolipidemia.* Proceedings of the 10th Annual Symposium on New Drugs and Devices (1989). 1990   ISBN 0-7923-0756-9
113. S. Iliceto, P. Rizzon and J.R.T.C. Roelandt (eds.): *Ultrasound in Coronary Artery Disease.* Present Role and Future Perspectives. 1990   ISBN 0-7923-0784-4
114. J.V. Chapman and G.R. Sutherland (eds.): *The Noninvasive Evaluation of Hemodynamics in Congenital Heart Disease.* Doppler Ultrasound Applications in the Adult and Pediatric Patient with Congenital Heart Disease. 1990   ISBN 0-7923-0836-0
115. G.T. Meester and F. Pinciroli (eds.): *Databases for Cardiology.* 1991 (forthcoming)   ISBN 0-7923-0886-7
116. B. Korecky and N.S. Dhalla (eds.): *Subcellular Basis of Contractile Failure.* 1990   ISBN 0-7923-0890-5
117. J.H.C. Reiber and P.W. Serruys (eds.): *Quantitative Coronary Arteriography.* 1991 (forthcoming)   ISBN 0-7923-0913-8
118. E. van der Wall and A. de Roos (eds.): *Magnetic Resonance Imaging in Coronary Artery Disease.* 1991 (forthcoming)   ISBN 0-7923-0940-5

Developments in Cardiovascular Medicine

119. V. Hombach, M. Kochs and A.J. Camm (eds.): *Interventional Techniques in Cardiovascular Medicine*. 1991 (forthcoming)   ISBN 0-7923-0956-1
120. R. Vos: *Drugs Looking for Diseases*. Innovative Drug Research and the Development of the Beta Blockers and the Calcium Antagonists. 1990 (forthcoming)
                                        ISBN 0-7923-0968-5

Previous volumes are still available

KLUWER ACADEMIC PUBLISHERS – DORDRECHT / BOSTON / LONDON